THE
BILL
SCHROEDER
STORY

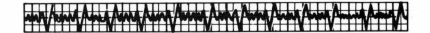

THE
BILL
SCHROEDER
STORY

The Schroeder Family
with Martha Barnette

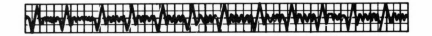

William Morrow and Company, Inc.   New York

Library of Congress Cataloging-in-Publication Data

Barnette, Martha.
  The Bill Schroeder story.
  1. Schroeder, Bill—Health. 2. Heart—Surgery—
Patients—United States—Biography. 3. Heart, Artificial
—Complications and sequelae. 4. Heart—Surgery—
Patients—Family relationships. I. Title.
RD598.35.A78S33 1987   362.1'97412'00924 [B] 87-5607
ISBN 0-688-06893-6

Printed in the United States of America

First Edition

1 2 3 4 5 6 7 8 9 10

BOOK DESIGN BY CONRAD CARLOCK

We would like to dedicate this book to all those who have suffered or walked alongside the agonizing complications of heart disease—but especially to an individual whose love for life, his family, and God gave him courage to help mankind.

May this book show the Bill Schroeder we all knew and loved. May God be with him.

ACKNOWLEDGMENTS

This book is meant to show how a family, focused in the public eye, traveled alongside their father and husband through an extraordinary medical experiment. There are hundreds of people involved with *The Bill Schroeder Story*. We would like to thank every one of them for their contributions; they will always have a special place in our hearts.

In particular, we would like to thank all of Bill's relations, who helped fill in background information, especially his brothers, Jerry and Paul; and Margaret's brothers, Frank, John, and Riley Huff; and her sister, Nora Fleck. We wish to thank Bill's fellow workers at the Crane Naval Weapons Support Center and his classmates from the Jasper High School class of 1950.

For giving insight into Bill's failing health that led to the artificial heart, we wish to thank J. P. Salb, M.D.; Phillip R. Dawkins, M.D.; and the Jasper Memorial Hospital staff.

A great deal of thanks goes to Humana Inc., and especially to Humana Hospital-Audubon for arranging interviews and making information available. In particular, we would like to thank the hospital administrator, Bruce MacLeod; the second-floor C.V.U. and C.C.U. nursing staff, especially John Lammers, Sandy Chandler, Laura Wood, and Bill Binggeli; the security team, especially Captain Tom Biondolillo; the public-relations staff, particularly George Atkins, Donna Hazle, Bob Irvine, and Linda Broadus; the Total Artificial Heart (TAH) technicians, Larry Hastings, Brent Mays, Melissa Williams, and Lawrence Barker; the home health-care nurses, Cheryl Ailiff, Trish Haaker, and Elizabeth Bryant; also all the therapists, the respiratory personnel, the technicians, aides, and hospital employees.

We would like to thank the Humana Heart Institute team, especially Kevan Shaheen, Gary Rhine, and Polly Brown. To all the doctors, particularly Allan M. Lansing, M.D., Ph.D.; Gary

7

Acknowledgments

Fox, M.D.; Albert B. Hoskins, M.D.; Sam Yared, M.D.; Julio Melo, M.D.; Ronald Barbie, M.D.; A. Attum, M.D.; C. Dannaher, M.D.; M. Grimaldi, M.D.; Z. Masri, M.D.; D. Scullin, M.D.; C. Dobbs, M.D.; W. Epstein, M.D., D.M.D.; J. Meffert, M.D., D.M.D.; Robert Jarvik, M.D.; and Lawrence Mudd, M.D.; we extend our gratitude.

We want to thank Bill Strode for his wonderful pictures, which captured the joys as well as the frustrations. We thank Sheryl Snyder and Bill Hollander of Wyatt, Tarrant, and Combs for legal counsel. We would also like to thank the Barney Clark, Murray Haydon, and Jack Burcham families for their support and friendship.

For all the book arrangements we want to thank our agent, Gail Ross, and Adrian Zackheim and Mary Ellen Curley of William Morrow and Company.

Of course, a very special thanks to William C. DeVries, M.D., who made this story possible. We thank him for devoting his time and skills to give us twenty-one special months with Bill, and we will always consider him a part of our family.

For the many hours spent alone and for their patience, understanding, and support, we must thank our families and fiancés: Bob, Vicki, and Bobby Bohnert; Patti, Melanie, and Abbie Schroeder; Terri, Tracey, and Lukas Schroeder; Julie Schroeder; Glenn Humbert; and Lori Schmidt.

Finally, a special appreciation to Mel Schroeder and Martha Barnette. Without their determination, encouragement, and support of this project, *The Bill Schroeder Story* would never have been told.

Jasper, Indiana
April 1987

And from Martha Barnette

I am grateful to the Schroeder family for trusting me with their story. They have been wonderful to work with, freely turning over diaries and documents, graciously enduring long hours of interviews, and making suggestions that vastly improved the manuscript.

Thanks also to Humana Inc., which granted every interview that I requested, and especially to Dr. DeVries for several hours of candid discussions.

I would not have undertaken this project without the support of my mentors, Sandy Hayden and Deborah Weiner. They helped me through each step, from dreaming the dream to proofing the final draft.

Not only has medical-technical writer Gail McGowan Mellor been generous with her own copious research, but her influence on my thinking and writing has been profound, and I am grateful.

Several people contributed to this effort in uniquely creative ways: Ellen Armour, Oriana Castillo, Ellen Ewing, Nancy Flowers, M.D., Robin Garr, Cannan Graves, Patti Hagewood, Leonard Latkovski, Julia McGrew, Pat Owen, Judy Rosenfield, Marty Spiegel, Jorge D. Tarafa, Nanci Thomas, Mona West, and Lisa Yankowy. Thanks also to Dawn Ripley for transcribing assistance.

And to my parents, Henlee and Helen Barnette, and my brothers, Jim, Wayne, and John—who were the first to teach me what "family" is all about.

Louisville, Kentucky
April 1987

Then Oz said to the tin woodsman, "I think you're wrong to want a heart. It makes most people unhappy. If you only knew it, you're in luck not to have a heart."

"That's a matter of opinion," the woodsman replied.

—DR. WILLIAM C. DEVRIES, quoting *The Wizard of Oz* at a lecture on medical ethics, March 18, 1985

All I wanted to do was, number one, to get myself healthy. Number two, I wanted to be able to help other people. And if I can succeed in any of those two, I'll feel like my mission's been accomplished.

—BILL SCHROEDER, the world's second man with a permanent artificial heart, on nationwide television, December 9, 1984

PROLOGUE

His strength was seeping away with every hour. Margaret sat on the side of the bed, stroking his arm, just wishing she could give him a little bit of her own life. Her husband wasn't saying anything, but she knew that even now, especially now, Bill Schroeder hated to be kept waiting. He'd been in this hospital almost two weeks, had let them run all kinds of tests—and the doctors still hadn't said for sure that he could get that artificial heart.

The doctors back home had said that without a new heart, Bill would die in less than a month. His diabetes and age ruled out the possibility of a human heart transplant. He was down to the last resort. If the doctors here really were going to choose him for the artificial heart, it would have to be soon. If not . . .

The door opened, and Dr. William DeVries walked in, trailed by several members of his medical team. The tall, sandy-haired surgeon was smiling as they formed a half-circle around Bill's bed.

"Well, Bill," DeVries said, "we've decided to go for it. You're now officially a candidate for the artificial heart."

"Fine with me," Bill said quickly. "When do we do it?"

First, DeVries explained, they'd have to read over and discuss a seven-page consent form, to make sure that Bill understood everything. DeVries would read it to him now and Bill would sign it. They'd go over the whole thing again, twenty-four hours later, then Bill would sign it again to show that he knew what he was doing. Margaret reached for Bill's hand. The lanky surgeon sat down beside them and began reading aloud.

". . . I recognize that the ventricles—the larger two of the heart's four pumping chambers—from my own natural heart will be removed . . ."

13

Margaret couldn't believe it. It was like a dream. *They really are going to give him the artificial heart.*

". . . risks include: (a) emboli or blood clots which may lead to stroke, kidney loss, liver, bowel or lung dysfunction, or damage to other organs or body functions . . ."

She squeezed Bill's hand. *We made it. We really made it! Bill's going to get himself that artificial heart.*

". . . During his life with the Total Artificial Heart, Dr. Clark experienced kidney and lung problems, a pneumothorax, which is air in the lung cavity, valve breakage, seizures, bleeding complications, and depression. He remained hospitalized during the entire hundred-and-twelve-day period . . ."

Bill didn't say a word. He just watched DeVries and nodded every once in a while. After hanging on this long, he certainly wasn't going to quit now.

". . . No representations or guarantees have been made to me either that the procedure will be successful, or the length of time or the level at which the Total Artificial Heart will function . . ."

At least now we have a chance. I'm going to bring him home with me and we can be a family again.

". . . I understand that the materials which are made public, as described in this paragraph, will protect my modesty and be within generally accepted bounds of good taste . . ."

Oh, come on, Dr. DeVries. You know we trust you. You just get Bill better.

". . . I acknowledge by my signature to this special consent form that I have read and understand the foregoing, including the risks involved . . ."

Margaret thought he would never finish reading. *Of course* she wanted the doctors to save her husband. Bill was only fifty-two, with everything to live for—their grandbaby due in the spring, their third son's wedding four months away, just the chance to come back home and live out whatever time he had left with his family. DeVries could read that thing backwards and sideways if he wanted to, as long as he gave Bill that artificial heart.

"Do you have any more questions?" DeVries asked. "Anything at all?"

"No," Bill answered. "I understand everything." He reached for the pen.

14

It was like an answer to prayer, the thought of Bill getting well again. He had really shown those doctors that he was their man: a positive attitude, a strong will to survive, cherished goals to live for, and a close family to support him until he got back on his feet.

Margaret couldn't wait to tell the kids.

CHAPTER ONE

At parties, he was the hefty guy introducing himself to everybody, the one gathering people around to hear his latest jokes. At the office, he was the worker who always arrived first, and often stayed long after everyone else went home. At wedding receptions, he was the bear of a man sashaying around while he modeled the bridesmaids' hats, who kept dragging everybody back onto the dance floor until the band finished playing for the night. At yard sales, he was the guy who drove halfway across Dubois County before sunrise in order to get the best bargains. At baseball games, he was the parent who yelled throughout the game—coaching from the bleachers, rattling a cowbell, and tooting a bullhorn—even during lulls in the action.

You could pick out Bill Schroeder anywhere.

He was born and raised in Jasper, a small southern Indiana town surrounded by acres and acres of cornfields, pastures, and forests. Even as a teenager, Bill's energetic, fun-loving personality impressed his classmates: A SENSE OF HUMOR AND WIT TO ENLIVEN THE BLUEST OF DAYS they put under his picture in the 1950 Jasper High School yearbook. The year he graduated he also fell in love with a shy, skinny girl named Margaret Huff, who worked with his mother at Sakel's, the town's only drive-in restaurant.

Margaret had just moved to Jasper from the hilly countryside a few miles away. The first time she brought Bill to her folks' farmhouse for supper, her father sat at the table studying this city boy in icy silence. Bill glanced around, wondering how to make everyone feel comfortable. Finally, he picked up his plate and loudly slurped all the juice off the beans. Margaret's family couldn't help laughing, and Bill quickly won her father's approval.

From then on, it was always the two of them—Bill, the center

17

of attention, master of ceremonies, and Margaret, standing to one side, watching proudly, only half-embarrassed by his jokes. Shortly after they became engaged, Margaret developed rheumatic fever and had to move back to the farmhouse. On weekends, Bill would drive out from Jasper, spread a quilt on the ground, then scoop her up in his arms and carry her into the sunshine, where they'd spend quiet afternoons dreaming about going off to see the world. They got that chance when Bill enlisted in the air force and returned from basic training to marry her.

His people weren't happy with the engagement at first because Margaret wasn't Catholic—in a town where most of the five thousand residents had strong German Catholic roots. The Jasper phone book was packed with names like Heichelbech, Schwing- hamer, and Gelhausen, with twice as many Schmidts as Smiths. Bill himself had served as an altar boy at St. Joseph's, the ma- jestic Bavarian-style church overlooking the town square, and even considered following in the footsteps of his two uncles who had become priests. But folks in Jasper had a saying: "You can always tell a German. You just can't tell him *anything*." Bill was German through and through, and he married Margaret on Sep- tember 2, 1952.

For their honeymoon, they drove to Bill's new assignment as a cook at Fort Bragg, North Aarolina, vowing that they'd never come back and say they couldn't make it on their own. That pat- tern would continue throughout their lives: Margaret and Bill, side by side, loving the adventure of traveling to someplace un- known. Over the next fourteen years, they would have six chil- dren, and Bill's assignments would take him to South Carolina, a frozen outpost in Newfoundland, Saudi Arabia, Texas, and finally Michigan. Margaret and their growing family went along with him, except for his tour in the Middle East, during which she and the kids lived with her parents at the farmhouse. Being back home only served to remind Margaret of how glad she'd been to leave behind that rugged life—backbreaking work, no indoor plumbing, and home remedies for all but the worst illnesses.

By the time the family moved to Michigan, Bill had worked up to sergeant and taken on the stressful job of air-traffic control- ler. He was once sent on a secret mission—on a radar ship dur- ing the Cuban missile crisis. His Michigan assignment stretched into five years. Now he and Margaret were in their early thirties. Their oldest daughter, Monica, and three sons, Mel, Stan, and

Terry, were in grade school. Another daughter, Cheryl, was still a toddler, and their last child, Rod, had just been born. Hand-me-down clothes passed right down the line. To help provide for his growing family, Bill worked extra jobs on weekends, such as pumping gas or painting houses. Somehow he also found time to be active in the Knights of Columbus organization, and attained the title of Grand Knight at his local post.

Family fun in Michigan was always homemade. They'd dress the children in pajamas, fill a grocery bag with popcorn and a jug with Kool-Aid, pile them into the car, and park in the front row at drive-in movies. As a special treat, they might play minia-ture golf. The kids always looked forward to "Devil's Night," an annual event around Halloween when pranksters egged houses or rang doorbells. The kids enjoyed it, of course, but Bill had a blast. He'd crouch in the shrubbery with a high-pressure hose, just itching for some young punks to try something. Or late at night he'd put a thumbtack on the doorbell button of their house, camouflage the sharp end with black tape, then tiptoe indoors and listen for the next victim who tried to ring the bell.

For the first time, Bill's young family had lived somewhere long enough to feel settled. But that sense of security was soon to be disrupted. Margaret suffered from rheumatoid arthritis, which swelled her hands and stiffened her fingers so badly that she couldn't even change a diaper. Back in Jasper, Bill's mother, who was still in her early sixties, died suddenly of a heart attack. Not long afterward, Bill's father lost a leg to complications from dia-betes, and was now having a difficult time caring for himself in the small white frame house where Bill grew up. In addition, Bill found out that his next assignment would be in the Philippines.

He felt backed into a corner. He'd spent fourteen years building a military career, lacking only six more years to retire-ment and a good pension. But he couldn't leave Margaret behind to look after six kids while her arthritis was getting worse. Be-sides, his father needed someone at home to help out around the house. Bill thought it over and made up his mind. He would bring his family back to Jasper.

So in 1966 they crowded in with Bill's father, Alois, in the house on the corner of Mill and Sixteenth streets. Bill found work in the same wood factory he had left to join the service, but rest-lessly scanned the classifieds for something better. He got a fed-eral job at the U.S. Naval Weapons Support Center, about forty miles away in Crane, Indiana, where the navy stockpiled ammunition. He started out on the assembly line, and by taking night classes for several years, he worked up to a top position as a quality-assurance supervisor.

It was a demanding job, and eventually his schedule required him to work ten-hour shifts, four days a week. The workday started at 6:00 A.M., but sometimes he was at his desk as early as 4:30. He'd brush off his co-workers' warnings to slow down, insisting he did better work in the early-morning quiet.

Bill quickly earned a reputation at Crane as a natural leader and comedian. He was constantly adding to a manila folder that already bulged with off-color jokes and cartoons, and he always carried a new one in his pocket to pass around. He also told jokes on his CB radio during the long commute, going by the handle "Silly Billy."

He found his niche in the federal employees' union, where he became the toughest negotiator. Bill was now a hulking, intimidating figure, with more than two hundred pounds on his six-foot frame. His domineering, demanding personality served him well at the bargaining table. Poised across from management, with more moderate union members to his right and left, Bill led the charge into arguments, demanding far more than could ever be conceded. When management resisted, Bill pounded the table with his fist, jumped to his feet, and yelled at his opponents nose-to-nose. Then his fellow negotiators eased in and used milder tactics to get what they really wanted. That strategy won Bill nearly all his cases, and earned him the nickname "Bull" Schroeder. He liked to think of himself as an advocate for the rights of the little guy, and no matter how small the case, he was always hell-bent on winning.

Union work had to be done during his off time, so after a long day at Crane, Bill often disappeared into the office he set up in the basement at home. He read the newspaper daily to track down legislation that affected his workers, and if an article raised questions, Bill never hesitated to call his representatives in Washington to find out the answers himself. He also represented his union at meetings throughout the country.

Bill's leisure time revolved around his family, but even then he was constantly in motion, as if the only way he could relax was to work some more. The children all had early-morning paper routes, and on Sundays, when the paper was thicker, Bill and Margaret and the kids would all pile in the car and drive the routes together, then attend early mass at St. Joe's. As they grew older, Bill taught them all to camp and fish and hunt. He and the boys spent months building a cinder-block cabin on a lake.

Bill was an avid sports fan, and always intensely competitive. He managed his kids' Little League teams, and sometimes worked as an umpire. If irate parents griped about his calls more than once, Bill would throw his hands over his head and bellow: "TIME OUT!" Then he'd shove back his face mask, march up to the fence, point at the offender, and yell: "If you think you can do any damn better, then you get your ass out here! We're looking for volunteers all the time!"

Bill also loved to dish it out from the sidelines. He got so disgusted with the officiating at one Jasper High basketball game that he wadded a popcorn box and beaned the bald-headed ref, then turned around with everybody else to see who'd thrown it. Even in card games around the kitchen table, Bill hated to lose— and usually made sure he didn't, badgering everyone into staying in the game until his luck turned and complaining to his partner about a stupid play.

When his son Terry ran cross-country, Bill, stopwatch in hand, would wait alongside the path on the last hilly half-mile, then run beside Terry for a few yards at full speed, yelling at him to pick up the pace. When Terry pitched for the Jasper High Wildcats, Bill attended every game. When Stan played defensive linebacker for the Wildcats, his teammates learned to expect that at half time ol' "Wild Bill" would hurry down from the bleachers to do some coaching of his own, slapping shoulder pads and strolling down along the bench to give unsolicited advice.

In many ways, Bill was just an overgrown kid himself. Whenever it snowed he was the first one out on the slopes, doing a belly flop onto an inner tube then piling the kids on his back for the ride of their lives. On Margaret's birthday he'd lead them in a chase through the house to corner her so they could all give her a spanking—but Margaret never managed to do the same to Bill on his birthday because he was too big and feisty for them to hold down.

Bill loved to poke around at auctions and yard sales, always proudly hauling home things that nobody else wanted, like the car that fell apart right after he bought it, or a necklace for Margaret made from hundreds of safety pins. He was always ordering new gadgets from catalogs, such as shoes to massage Margaret's feet, "Like 1,000 Fingers"; if Bill saw a new product on TV with "o-matic" in its name, he was sure to be ordering one before midnight.

When Margaret inherited her forty-acre share of the family farm, Bill decided to make it their special place, where they'd retire to live the simple life: hard work, sweat, sun, fresh air. What he probably liked the most about the wooded lot was that there was always so much to be done on the place: a big garden to tend, brush and weeds to clear, grass to mow, and, eventually, the perfect spot to build a house. Bill liked nothing better than to take off his shirt and work all day on some project. He built a barbecue with concrete blocks, put in a pond and stocked it with catfish. He took the kids hunting in the woods. In the fall he would gather walnuts, spread them behind the car, drive back and forth to crush them, then freeze them for making cakes, pies, and snacks. In the spring he took Margaret and her sister Nora to hunt mushrooms there, always striding twenty paces ahead of them, bragging that he'd bring back the biggest batch.

He hauled a mobile home to the farm so the family could stay on the weekends. In the evenings he would string up Japanese lanterns and treat family and friends to his homemade barbecue. Afterward, he and Margaret would sit in a swing he set up near the pond, watch the moon rise over the hills, and try to spy deer in the woods.

For every special occasion—birthdays, holidays, christenings, graduations, and weddings—Bill loved to throw a big party, don a three-piece suit, and act as emcee. He'd spend weeks planning and kept a meticulously updated, permanent file of names and addresses of people to invite. He loved to cook and would always whip up something special, like a fancy dessert or his mom's special dressing. On Thanksgiving, Christmas, and New Year's, of course, the Mill Street house was crowded with big, boisterous family gatherings.

Bill was a traditional kind of guy who didn't show physical affection with his sons or tell them, "I love you." He figured he didn't have to tell them; they'd know by the things he did for them. If they ever needed his help, all they had to do was ask.

The kids rarely saw tears in his eyes. It happened once after the youngest had started school, and Margaret took a part-time job in a five-and-dime store. One afternoon, while setting up a store display, she grew faint and fell from a ladder, and was taken to Jasper Memorial Hospital. Doctors discovered that she'd suffered a mild heart attack. As Bill broke the news to their kids, he wept. After a number of scary and uncomfortable tests, the doctors concluded that Margaret's heart problems could be controlled with medication. Bill had always been very protective of Margaret; now he was even more careful to keep her from overexerting her delicate heart—even cutting down the backyard clothesline so she wouldn't be tempted to hang up laundry in nice weather.

A few years later, when his own father died, the family saw him cry again. Bill and Margaret had helped take care of Alois at the Mill Street house until the end. As the diabetes got worse, Alois's other leg had to be amputated, but he still managed to get around in a wheelchair or by using wooden legs and crutches. Although Margaret had prepared him special meals recommended by the doctors, Alois was always just as stubborn as his son, and he would hobble out of the house after supper and drive his specially equipped car to Dairy Queen for dessert.

Meanwhile, Bill was neglecting his own health. In 1979 he had a routine checkup by the family doctor, J. P. Salb. Dr. Salb was a tall, soft-spoken, bespectacled physician who'd seen the Schroeder kids through the usual childhood illnesses and injuries, and had followed Margaret's arthritis and heart ailment. He was a little older than Bill, and was accustomed to the respect and responsibility that come with being a small-town doctor. Bill liked to kid him just the same, sometimes teasing that J.P.'s latest trip to a medical seminar sounded a whole lot more like a vacation to him. Both Salb and Bill were big Jasper Wildcats fans, and if they ran into each other at a game, they'd sit together.

Dr. Salb found that Bill, like his father, had developed diabetes. It could probably be controlled with a low-salt, low-sugar diet, the doctor said. Bill ought to follow the diet anyway, since he was about fifty pounds overweight. Bill had also smoked for years; by now he was up to two packs a day. Salb suggested that he cut out the cigarettes and slow down his workaholic lifestyle. The doctor also understood his patient well enough to know that Bill wouldn't heed such advice if he didn't want to. As far as Bill Schroeder was concerned, there were two ways to do things: the wrong way, and Bill's way.

23

Besides, he felt fine as long as his diabetes was under control. He was a powerful man, entering the prime of life, a good provider who'd worked his way to the top in a responsible job. He'd won the respect of his fellow union members. He had a devoted wife, six decent kids nearly raised, and five grand-children. He'd worked hard to earn the good life, done everything he was supposed to to make the American Dream come true—and now he was on the verge of reaping his rewards.

He soon obtained one of them—getting elected president of the American Federation of Government Employees' Sixth District, which encompassed Indiana, Kentucky, and Ohio. Because he was so good at getting what he wanted, Bill sometimes rubbed co-workers the wrong way. Nevertheless, his election meant that they respected his abilities. After he served this term, Bill figured that he'd go for a national office in the union.

Around this time, Bill developed a more persistent smoker's hack. He noticed he had some trouble breathing when he exerted himself at the farm. Like everyone else, he'd read all the statistics about smoking, and even though he'd tried to quit before, it was now more pressing to stop. He did it in typical fashion: He just threw away his cigarettes and toughed it out, cold turkey. The first few weeks he was grouchy and nervous, popping mints every time he craved nicotine. But for Bill it was just an-other battle of will, another fight he refused to lose.

On a follow-up visit, Dr. Salb again urged Bill to ease up at work and consider early retirement. "You know you have a family history of heart disease and diabetes," Salb told him. "There are all kinds of things you love to do in your off time. Why not just start enjoying yourself now?"

That was ridiculous, Bill said. He still had to bring in money to support his family, and besides, he loved his work. The only major physical exertion at his job was climbing a flight of stairs every day. Again, there was no arguing with him. So Bill kept up his high-stress desk job and the long commute—and con-tinued to work like all-get-out around the house or at the farm on weekends.

In the fall of 1982, after a weekend at the forty acres, Bill and Margaret were returning to Jasper in their pickup truck. The weather was unusually warm, and Bill was happily tired and sweaty from a hard morning's work. As usual, he was kidding Margaret about something or other as he drove along. Suddenly his eyelids drooped and his head fell back. He let go of the steering wheel and slumped against her.

"Bill! What are you—?"

He didn't move.

"BILL!" Margaret grabbed the wheel and kicked his foot off the accelerator. Bill lay against her, a dead weight, as she eased the truck off the road. "Bill!" Margaret yelled. "If you're doing this for meanness, you and I are in trouble!"

Then she saw that his lips were pale and his bare chest and face were wringing wet with sweat.

"Bill! What's the matter?"

He slowly opened his eyes and frowned. "I'm okay," he said.

"Well, you're not driving back to Jasper, that's for sure," she said as she got out and came around to the driver's side. By the time they reached the outskirts of town, Bill was feeling better. Margaret headed straight for Jasper Memorial, but when they neared Mill Street, Bill muttered, "Turn here."

"But Bill, we've got to get you to the emergency room!" she said.

"TURN HERE," Bill insisted.

"But Bill—"

"I said, 'Turn,' dammit. Don't I look fine now?"

"But honey, we've got to get you checked out at the hospital. You just fell over—just passed out!"

Bill looked straight ahead. "I know it's my diabetes. I'll take care of it when we get home."

"But Bill, it might be something really wrong."

"I ain't going up to no crazy hospital and pay good money to sit around all afternoon."

Margaret looked at him for a long moment.

"And the kids," Bill added. "Don't you go worrying them with this either, you hear?"

Margaret bit her lip. There was no arguing with him. She turned up Mill Street.

CHAPTER TWO

January 8, 1983. That day Bill had gone to Dr. Salb's for a physical. He'd been having stomach pains and often felt tired, but the exam turned up nothing out of the ordinary. Afterward, he and Margaret decided to take off for the afternoon along with Cheryl. They drove to a shopping mall in Evansville, about fifty miles away. While Cheryl was making a purchase, Margaret and Bill tried out one of those machines that measure blood pressure and pulse for a quarter. Margaret's read: AVERAGE. Bill's read: POOR—SEE YOUR DOCTOR. They both got a good laugh out of that. After all, Margaret was the one with the bad heart.

On the drive back, Bill's stomach pains grew worse. He went through a whole roll of antacid mints, trying to ease the burning under his breastbone. Still, he insisted on driving back himself, telling Margaret and Cheryl that it was probably the burger and fries they'd had at a fast-food restaurant on the way. "Stuff's poison," Bill grumbled. But the pain persisted through the evening.

Late that night, Bill and Margaret watched some TV with Cheryl and Terry in the living room. Rod went upstairs to bed. From time to time, Bill still winced and put his hand to his chest. Margaret kept asking him, "Honey, are you *sure* you don't want to go to the emergency room?" Bill just shook his head, *No*. Finally, he and Margaret went to get ready for bed. A few minutes later, Margaret called from the bedroom with a voice that sounded strange:

"Cheryl!"

Cheryl went in and found her father slumped across the bed, moaning. Her mother was standing over him helplessly. Cheryl called for Terry. Bill's face was pale and clammy, and he was grabbing at his chest with one hand.

"Okay," Terry said. "Let's get him to the hospital." Bill

frowned, and tried to talk about the terrible pain in his chest. He couldn't feel anything in his left arm. The pain became so intense that he began to pass out, wake up for a few seconds, then pass out again.

"Come on, Dad," Terry ordered. "We're going." When Terry tried to help him stand, Bill collapsed against him. Terry and Cheryl draped Bill's arms over their shoulders and dragged him outside. There was no time to get Rod. Getting Bill into the car was like trying to lift a 220-pound sack of grain. Cheryl drove, speeding through the dark streets, running red lights like crazy.

At the hospital, they dragged Bill out of the car, put him in a wheelchair, and rushed him into the brightly lit emergency room. Margaret wouldn't leave his side. As Terry and Cheryl tried to handle the paperwork, hospital workers started all kinds of tests on Bill, taking his blood pressure, monitoring his heart, trying to get him to answer questions. Bill had now broken out in a cold sweat and was trembling all over. A nurse telephoned for doctors, but they were slow in coming, so she took matters into her own hands. She wheeled Bill toward an elevator bound for the intensive-care unit, with Margaret and the kids hurrying alongside. Once inside the elevator, the nurse told Margaret it looked like a heart attack.

That couldn't be, Margaret thought. Not Bill. She and the kids followed as far as they could go until Bill was whisked into the ICU. The door closed behind him, and Terry and Cheryl held their mom as she finally let herself break into tears.

In the meantime, Dr. Salb got a call at home—something about a Schroeder having a coronary. As he sped toward Memorial, he thought, *I wonder how bad she is?* Once inside the hospital, Salb rounded a corner on the way to the ICU, saw Margaret standing there, and stopped short.

"Margaret!" he said. "You mean it's *Bill*?" She'd been just as surprised as he was. Before the nurse mentioned it, the possibility that Bill was having a heart attack had never occurred to Margaret. Not someone as strong and active as Bill. While Salb went to check on him, Margaret, Terry, and Cheryl found a waiting room. Terry called his brothers and Moni. By that time, it was past midnight, and for the Schroeder kids, the phone ringing in the dark hinted at the bad news before they even answered.

After what seemed like a long time, Dr. Salb came back to talk to Margaret. Before he could say anything, she quickly searched his eyes for answers, and prayed that his words wouldn't confirm what she saw.

"Margaret," Salb said gently, "I'm afraid it *was* a heart attack. A bad one. We don't know if he'll make it or not." Margaret began to cry again softly. "It's going to be touch-and-go for a while," Salb said.

"Can we see him?" Terry asked.

"Only for a minute," Salb answered. "Right now we have to make sure he stays quiet. The first forty-eight hours will be the most crucial. We'll need to get him stable. Then we can assess how much muscle damage this thing did to his heart. The best I can tell you is just to keep waiting and hoping. Try to get some rest if you can, because it's going to be a while."

One by one, the other kids arrived, red-eyed from crying on the way over. They each slipped in to see him, just long enough to say that they loved him. They returned to the waiting room, numb, thinking of all the other things they wished they'd told their father—things that now they might never get a chance to say.

Toward morning, the nurses began allowing Margaret and one other family member visit for ten minutes every hour. Bill looked terrible. His skin was cold and pasty, his hair looked wet and slicked back, and he was lying so still that he looked dead. Between visits, Margaret stood at the glass door of the ICU, just looking at Bill and blaming herself. Why had she let him drive back from Evansville? Why hadn't she made him lie down that afternoon? Bill had kept saying it was indigestion. If she'd known it was his heart, she could have reached into her purse and given him some of the nitroglycerin she carried for her own heart. She felt terrible about not thinking of it earlier. Why didn't she insist on taking him to the hospital after he'd passed out at the wheel that time? The knowledge that no one could ever have convinced him to go—Bill could just be so bull-headed sometimes—was small comfort now.

Margaret kept a vigil at Bill's side for as long as the nurses would let her, holding his hand, kissing his forehead, stroking his cheek, whispering that she loved him. The rest of the family practically camped out in the waiting room for the next two days, taking turns visiting Bill for a minute or two at a time. They would squeeze their father's hand and tell him they loved him. Bill could talk now, but he didn't say much and he tired easily. It was very hard to see this bear of a man, their dad, looking so weak, so scared and disappointed—sometimes even crying help-lessly.

The heart attack—the doctors called it a "myocardial in-farction"—had damaged Bill's heart muscle, but just how badly was still not known. The doctors told Margaret that Bill faced a long, slow recovery, and that he absolutely *must* give up that hectic pace of his. There remained a possibility that Bill would have another heart attack at any moment, so the doctors were also considering a coronary-bypass operation.

About a week later Bill was moved to a regular coronary-care room. Margaret stayed at his side for the next couple of weeks, lingering past visiting hours, crocheting when he fell asleep—sometimes falling asleep herself in a chair by his bed. The kids would try to get her to leave for a while, but they couldn't pull her away from him. Bill had taken care of her for so many years, and she wasn't going to let him down now. Within a few days, the family could see that Bill was feeling better because he began taking charge again and bossing people around from his hospital bed. When the dietary department sent up the wrong order for his dinner, Bill phoned the kitchen to demand that they get it right. After his food arrived cold more than once, he dialed the hospital administrator and the dietitian to set up a meeting so he could give them a piece of his mind. When he thought the nurses were loafing, he disconnected his monitors and waited to see how long it took them to come running.

"Bill!" Margaret chided him, trying not to laugh. "You shouldn't do that to them!"

"Well, hell," Bill muttered, "they're supposed to be look-ing after me, not gabbing up at the nurses' station. They keep you awake all night yakking, then come in and bother you when you're trying to sleep. They're getting paid good money to sit around on their butts."

Some nurses did find Bill gruff at first—until they realized he really wanted them to dish it right back to him. So, when Bill called on the intercom to demand a cold beer, they'd humor him. "It's on its way," they'd answer. Five minutes later, he'd call again. "*Where's* my beer? Can't a guy get decent service around this joint? I'm paying good money to be in this here hospital, you know."

Margaret, only halfway embarrassed, would take the nurses aside and try to explain that Bill didn't even like beer. "It just seems like he gets thirsty for it in the hospital for some reason," she said. But secretly, Bill's rambunctiousness made her happy: He was getting better.

He was discharged on January 20 with a handful of prescriptions: Nitrol ointment and Isordil to ease his chest pain; Lanoxin to improve his heart's pumping power; NPH insulin for his diabetes; and instructions to follow a strict low-salt, low-sugar diet. He weighed more than two hundred pounds, and the doctors told him that the extra weight was straining his heart. A week later, under doctor's orders, he began mild exercise sessions in cardiac rehab.

Bill's physicians also recommended that he have a cardiac catheterization to determine whether the heart's arteries were so badly clogged that a coronary bypass should be considered. The test carried some risks, and might well be unnecessary. But after discussing it with the doctors, Bill decided that percentages were in his favor. Besides, the doctors recommended it, and Bill was always inclined to take the advice of professionals he trusted, so he agreed to the test.

He knew something of what to expect because Margaret had had a catheterization to check her own heart. A cardiologist inserted a long tube, or catheter, through a blood vessel in his groin, then snaked the tube up through the artery and directly into his heart. Then a special dye was injected through the catheter, which, under X rays, revealed the outline of Bill's heart while it was beating. Bill insisted on having the X-ray monitor turned toward him so he could watch the process himself. The test revealed growing blockages in two of his coronary arteries, the large vessels that nourish the heart muscle with blood. Without an open-heart operation to bypass those blockages, Bill risked another severe heart attack, one which could be deadly this time.

Bill asked many questions about the operation. How long would it be before he could go back to work? Would he be able to mow or chop wood? Once the doctors explained that he could probably build up to a fairly normal activity level, Bill was determined to go for it. He decided he'd just get his bad heart fixed and go back to work as soon as possible. The doctors told him that no one could say for sure, but the standard estimate was that a bypass could add as much as ten years to someone's life. The rest of the family also had high hopes for the surgery, because he seemed so optimistic, and was taking charge as usual.

So in March 1983, two months after his heart attack, Bill checked into Jewish Hospital in Louisville, Kentucky, some ninety miles away. His surgeon would be Dr. Allan Lansing. Bill had heard of him; Lansing's surgical group boasted the largest practice in Kentucky and had impeccable credentials. Suave and silver-haired, Lansing inspired confidence with his sure, resonant voice, and his way of taking a person's hand in both of his when they met. Bill liked him instantly.

In a standard coronary bypass, surgeons remove part of a vein from the leg, then attach one end of the vein to the aorta and the other to the coronary artery, thus providing an alternate route for the blood to bypass blockages in the coronary vessels. In Bill's case they would take a vein from his arm, because, years earlier, he'd had varicose veins removed from his leg. Once again, the family gathered for the ordeal: the brief visits to squeeze Bill's hand and tell him they loved him, the waiting rooms, the drawn faces of other families there with their own worries, the hours dragging by. Finally, the doctors came back to say that Bill was doing just fine, and that the family could see him in intensive care. As the Schroeders quietly walked through the intensive-care section, they passed several other patients who looked pale and lifeless. Each of them was connected to a respirator by means of a fat tube that went through the mouth and into the throat. At the end of the row, Bill lay with his eyes wide open, angrily gesturing for someone to remove the tube from his mouth. It was uncomfortable at best, and as his anesthesia began to wear off, it created a terrible gagging sensation. Afterward, Bill complained loudly and long that he never wanted to go through that again.

As they say around Jasper, Bill came through like a dose of salts. He wasn't intimidated by a big-city hospital, and once again he flirted with the nurses, joked with the doctors, and griped about the food. Ever the consumer advocate, Bill kept records of all treatments, medicines, and supplies he received to make sure that he wasn't charged for anything he didn't get. When the bill for his bypass arrived later, Bill noted that even though he'd only been given oxygen for two days, the hospital had charged him for oxygen over the course of his entire stay. He caught the error and saved the insurance company a few hundred dollars.

Bill was determined to recuperate quickly. As his discharge date neared, he grew increasingly impatient. He couldn't wait to get back to work. He was discharged from Jewish Hospital after nine days, which was about average for such an operation. Like other heart patients, Bill had lingering chest pain for a few weeks, mainly because of having to cough up mucus from his lungs. His breastbone still felt raw where Dr. Lansing had fastened it back together with fine wire, and the coughing tugged on it. He learned to ease the pain by hugging a pillow to his chest when he coughed.

Despite doctors' orders to slow down, Bill's heart attack only made him more determined to overcome the problem by himself. Instead of frightening him into slowing down, his bad heart seemed to drive him to prove something. He figured that the bypass had given him a new lease on life—ten extra years at least. Besides, he was worried about how to pay this last hospital bill, keep his job, and provide for his family. They were holding his job for him at Crane, and he was anxious to get back as soon as possible and start bringing home a real paycheck. He was convinced that if he just kept exercising, took all his medications, and watched his diet, he could beat this disease. As always, when Bill was convinced that he was right, nobody could argue with him.

Back in Jasper, Bill attended cardiac rehab sessions religiously, arriving early for workouts. He'd pedal the exercise bike even past the point at which it became hard for him to breathe. The nurses would notice his face turning pale with a hint of pain, and they'd have to persuade him to stop. "Oh, I'm fine," he'd insist. "It's Margaret I've got to worry about." He was always talking about Margaret, about her fragile heart, about her arthritis flare-ups. She was the one who needed taking care of, he told them. He could look after himself just fine.

Bill returned to work in just a few weeks—much sooner than anyone at Crane had expected. Bill was overjoyed to be back on the job, to have a place he had to go to each day, and to have responsibilities to other people. His family and co-workers urged him to take it easy, but now he was working even harder to catch up on what he'd missed. He set his sights on running for a national office in the union.

A couple of months after the bypass, Bill started having stomach pains again. He figured they were just heartburn, since they usually seemed to come around mealtime. He was given a GI exam of his digestive tract, but nothing wrong showed up. Bill also noticed that increasingly when he worked outdoors he had to stop and catch his breath. Must be all those years of smoking cigarettes, he figured.

One night in June, Bill suddenly awoke with his heart racing. He felt an overwhelming sense that someone was trying to suffocate him. In a panic he jumped out of bed and stood in front of the open window, trying to get some fresh air. The spell lasted only a few minutes, but during the next few days, it happened again and again. And for some reason, he gained several pounds within one week; he now tipped the scales at 236.

Reluctantly, Bill checked back into Memorial on July 1, 1983. Doctors ran more tests and the diagnosis was grim: severe congestive heart failure. That meant that the damage from his heart attack had been so extensive that the heart muscle was growing too weak to pump sufficient blood to meet his body's demands. It beat faster and faster but pumped less per beat. As a result, his kidneys released a substance that caused fluid retention, and excess water seeped into his tissues, especially into the chest cavity. Bill's lungs were filled with fluid, like soggy sponges. In what would become an all-too-familiar routine, doctors drained the excess fluid with diuretics, so that he lost about twelve pounds at a time, most of it water. His heart's waning ability to pump enough blood left him constantly weak and tired.

At Dr. Salb's suggestion, a conscientious young internist from Jasper, Dr. Phillip R. Dawkins, began following Bill for his heart problems. And when Bill was discharged a few days later, Dr. Dawkins sent him home with the following regimen: go on a low-sugar, low-salt diet; take 40 units of NPH insulin daily and monitor his blood sugars at home. Also he had to take one 0.25-mg Lanoxin tablet daily, to make his heart beat more efficiently; one 100-mg Aldactone tablet daily, to help rid his body of excess water; one 40-mg Lasix pill daily for the same reason; one Bactrim-DS tablet daily to guard against bladder infection; one tablespoon of Mylanta II after meals and at bedtime for indigestion; one 300-mg Tagamet tablet daily for stomach pains; one 0.5-mg Halcion tablet at bedtime, as needed, to sleep.

Dawkins emphasized that Bill had to start eating a healthy low-calorie diet. That was no problem because Bill liked to cook, just as he had in the air force. Coming up with tasty, healthful meals would be a welcome challenge. Dawkins also warned him to take it easy. But nobody could persuade him to do that. It drove Bill crazy to have to sit around the house and rest.

That summer Terry came by the house one day after work and found his dad pushing the garden tiller in the backyard.

"Hey, Dad! You don't need to be doing that."

"Well, hell," Bill groused, "if I don't do it, it won't get done. I don't see you out here doing this."

"Here, Dad," Terry said, reaching for the tiller. "Give it to me. You take it easy."

They argued and Terry grabbed the tiller. Bill knew he was too weak to pull it away from his athletic son, so he grudgingly let Terry take it. Terry took up where his dad left off, but Bill continued to watch over him like a factory foreman.

"Hey!" Bill yelled. "You're not doing it right!"

Terry kept on.

"Hey! You missed a spot there!" Bill yelled. "Here. Here, let me do it."

"I'm doing just fine, Dad. Don't worry."

"No, look," Bill said, both hands gripping an imaginary handle. "Look, you hold it like this."

Finally, Terry stopped and straightened up. "Dad, I know how to do this. See? You're the one who showed me how, remember? You just go inside. Get some rest." Terry turned back to his work.

"Well, hell, if you're going to do something, you ought to do it right," Bill said. "Use your head, dammit! That's what it's there for! Use your head!" Bill disappeared into the house.

Terry kept on tilling. A few minutes later, around the side of the house, he heard the hum of the weed-eater.

"Aw, DAD!"

Scenes like that were repeated again and again. After a few weeks, Bill managed to get permission from his doctors to return to Crane. But he found he couldn't do as much as he had before. There seemed to be more stairs on the flight up to his office. From time to time, he had dizzy spells, a side effect of the Lasix. And when the water pills took out too much potassium from his body, he'd get leg cramps.

Bill's lungs continued to fill with fluid, which necessitated regular trips to the hospital. He told the family that he felt as if he was trying to breathe under water. And in a sense, he was trying to do just that: Every time they drained his chest at the hospital, quarts of fluid would be removed. He'd feel better for a few weeks, then slide right back down to where he was before.

The long, humid southern Indiana summer just made it that much harder to breathe outside, forcing him to spend more and more time cooped up indoors. He often found it easier to breathe if he sat with his head between his knees. It was as if the fluid were spreading out more shallowly along his lungs instead of just pooling at the bottom. Bill would be doing something around the house and then have to sit down, shaking his head in disbelief. "I can't get my damn breath. I just can't get my damn breath!" He seemed surprised that his own body could be letting him down. Bloating became such a problem that Bill could eat very little for a week but still gain three pounds.

Bill thought he had won his battle with heart disease by having the bypass, but now it was turning into a long siege. He began seeing Dr. Dawkins about twice a month. Bill liked to think of his treatment as a task they had to work on together, like partners, trying to discover the right balance of drugs to control his problems. It was like the trial-and-error process of finding out what's wrong with a car. Adjust one thing, and if the problem is still there, adjust something else. The only way was to experiment with different combinations of "beta blockers," calcium-channel blockers, nitroglycerin, potassium, Capoten. Dawkins set aside fifteen minutes for each appointment, but usually it took just a couple of minutes to figure out what to try next. The rest of the time they'd visit like old pals, talking about Jasper High sports, quail hunting, or the latest cartoon Bill was carrying in his coat pocket.

It became harder and harder for Bill to carry on his work at Crane. That fall he even passed out at his desk, and his supervisors ordered him home for the rest of the day. Stubborn as always, Bill insisted on driving the forty-mile trip back by himself.

In early winter, Bill began having severe chest pains that felt like a softball knotting up tightly under his ribs. He couldn't stand the idea of going into the hospital again, but he had no choice. The doctors again ordered bed rest and switched around his medications. During that hospital stay, Bill decided to organize a Schroeder family reunion. Nine of his eleven aunts and uncles were still living, and, as the eldest nephew, Bill felt a responsibility to bring everybody together for one big family gathering. He called a local community center and reserved it for a weekend that coming summer. He wrote out and mailed scores of invitations. Again, he was glad to have some kind of project to work on while confined to bed.

During the next few weeks, he'd feel a little better and try to return to work. Then he'd overdo it and get worn down again. On March 2, 1984, he was hospitalized for acute and chronic congestive heart failure. A few hours after admission, when Bill was napping in his hospital room, he awoke with that suffocating feeling he'd had before. He called a nurse, and was rushed to intensive care. Once again, he was stabilized, and after a couple of days, he was sent home with a sackful of medications: insulin, Lanoxin, Procardia, Nitrol ointment, Bactrim, Restoril, Valium, Bumex tablets, and Slow-K potassium. By now he'd grown so weak that at times he had to use a cane to walk.

Bill finally had to admit that he wasn't getting better. It tore him up to do it, but he had to retire from Crane and file for disability. He had worked so hard, accomplished so much, and was now so close to reaping all the rewards he was due. But he didn't talk much about it with fellow workers, and when they gave him a big going-away party, he tried to keep up a cheerful front.

Retirement was frustrating for Bill; it made him feel so useless. He hated not having to get up in the morning and go somewhere. He no longer had a hectic schedule to shape his day, or co-workers seeking his help in pleading their cases against management, or meetings to call, or complaints to file.

He couldn't even do things around his own house anymore. It was spring. Hell, he ought to be out fishing or tilling the garden at the forty acres. The family planted another garden that year in the backyard at the Mill Street house. Bill would go out there early in the morning carrying a hoe and a bucket. He'd hoe one row, turn the bucket upside down, and sit down to rest. He'd hoe another, rest, then hoe another. He strapped a dandelion digger to a broom handle and took a chair out in the front yard to dig dandelions; he'd pull up all the weeds within his reach, then move his chair to another part of the yard. On good days, he'd overdo it and suffer the consequences. On bad days, he'd get frustrated because he could do so little. He felt he had to do something, anything—he kept saying he never wanted to reach the point where all he could do was watch soap operas on TV.

It became so hard for Bill to breathe lying down that now he had trouble sleeping. He'd prop pillows under his back to ease the congestion in his lungs, or go into the living room and try to catch a few hours' sleep sitting up in his easy chair. Like many people with severe congestive heart failure, Bill often felt uncomfortably hot, so he'd just sit on the edge of the bed with his face right in front of the air conditioner. Or sometimes in the middle of the night, he'd leave the house and drive around the empty Jasper streets with the air conditioning turned as high as it would go.

The more he had to stay home, the more Bill looked forward to spending time with his kids. By now they were all just about grown—Moni, Mel, and Stan all had kids of their own. Rod had just graduated from high school and gotten a job in a wood factory, just as Bill had. Sometimes Rod would drive him up to Crane for the day to see how things were going with the union. Or Bill would call Cheryl or Terry at work, ask what they were doing that afternoon, and hint that maybe they'd like to go out to eat or to a yard sale or something. When any of the kids came by to take him fishing, Bill would be waiting on the front porch, all decked out in his fishing gear, a tackle box at his feet. Margaret would pull them aside and whisper that Bill was so eager he'd been sitting there, ready to go, for almost an hour.

The house had always been a stopping-off place for all of them. They never needed an invitation or to call ahead. It wouldn't be the same if they didn't drop by every once in a while for a home-cooked meal, to borrow a five or a ten until payday, or watch a ball game over a couple of beers. Especially now that Bill was home all the time, he was increasingly determined to be in charge of the cooking. Usually, each day around lunchtime, at least a couple of the kids dropped by the house. In fact, if they didn't show up for a couple of days, they would hear about it from Dad: "Well, damn, I fixed you a great lunch and you didn't even come by!" Now the kids and Bill were just beginning to enjoy each other as adults. They'd talk about the Jasper Wildcats, or argue politics, with Bill always holding the Democratic party line. That spring they got into a lively argument over whether Geraldine Ferraro would make a good vice-president. Bill pounded the kitchen table, saying, "She's the best damn candidate for the job! If a woman's got the damn qualifications, then she should be in the White House!"

From time to time, Bill would keep the grandkids. He'd put Mel's little girls, Melanie and Abbie, on his lap and tell them stories, or have them teach him some sign language, which they learned from their mother's deaf brother-in-law. They showed him how to make the sign for "I love you" by holding up his thumb, forefinger, and pinky. It became his secret shorthand signal to them.

In May Bill began having more chest pains and problems with low blood pressure. Again, Dr. Dawkins adjusted Bill's medications, adding regular doses of Capoten to regulate his blood pressure, and told him to attach a fresh Nitro-Dur patch to his

38

chest every day, so that the nitroglycerin, absorbed through his skin would ease the pain in his chest. Dr. Dawkins made a regular practice of writing letters to his patients after each office visit to review their progress. And in a June letter, the doctor noted that Bill was feeling the best he had since his heart attack, and that Bill had reported that he was able to get out and fish and even hoe in the garden occasionally. The physical exam showed that his weight was 211 pounds, and that his lungs were clear. Maybe they were gaining on this disease after all.

Bill's big project during those summer weeks was the family reunion, and he pulled it off in true Schroeder style. In July about two hundred relatives converged on the community center in Celestine. Bill, of course, was master of ceremonies. He made sure his aunts and uncles had seats of honor at a long table at the front of the hall, then kept everybody laughing by going right down the row, telling stories on each of them. He told one on a couple of uncles who carried big automatic shotguns whenever they went quail hunting. "Oh, yeah," Bill said, "they'd be sure to hit quail with those things, all right! Of course, they had a hard time finding any pieces afterward!" Bill enjoyed himself tremendously, and looked better than he had in a long time. He always seemed energized by being around lots of people. The reunion was such a hit with the family that they agreed to have another one in two years.

That August, during Strassenfest, Jasper's annual street fair, Bill and Margaret went a few blocks over to the courthouse square to watch some of the activities: the barstool races, the band playing in the beer garden, and the annual parade. But Bill couldn't do nearly what he'd been able to in previous years. Instead of walking around, striking up conversations and introducing himself to everybody, he had to find a cool, shady spot to sit and watch all the activity go past him.

By this time, Terry had become engaged to his girl friend Julie, a secretary from Jasper. They were planning a wedding for the coming March, but even now, Bill was kidding his future daughter-in-law, nagging that she'd better hurry up and pick out a wedding dress. Even though he was teasing, it was clear that he couldn't wait to see another one of his kids get married.

In late August, Bill's main physical complaint was that he felt dizzy whenever he stood up. His blood pressure was low: 65/50 while sitting down. Dr. Dawkins suspected that the Capoten was causing Bill's lightheadedness, so he cut the dosage.

But it was becoming clear that no juggling of medications was going to get Bill as healthy as he was before his first heart attack. He was growing weaker and having to work harder for each breath. The bypass alone wasn't going to be enough.

In early September, Dawkins noted in a letter to Bill that despite the reduction of the Capoten, his dizziness had returned. "You discontinued the Capoten on your own and are feeling better," Dawkins wrote. "However, you are still quite weak." Bill had also developed leg cramps, so the doctor added one Quinamm tablet at bedtime to ease them.

Dawkins wasn't sure, but now he feared that Bill might even be suffering a series of small heart attacks, or infarctions.

With each infarction, more of the heart muscle turned to scar tissue. Meanwhile, the fatty buildup in Bill's coronary arteries was slowly starving his heart of blood, thereby causing cardiomyopathy, literally, "heart muscle disease." Bill was living on a fraction of his heart—a fraction that would only get smaller. His last hope would be to replace that heart. In the summer of 1984, Dr. Dawkins decided to look into the possibility of getting Bill a human heart transplant.

Heart transplants were becoming increasingly common, thanks to recent advances with drugs used to battle the body's natural tendency to reject foreign tissue. But transplant recipients had to meet certain eligibility guidelines. The criteria varied at medical centers across the nation, but they usually required patients to be fifty years old or younger and to be generally free from other chronic diseases. Dr. Dawkins feared that Bill would be disqualified on the grounds that he was fifty-two and diabetic. So he checked with Dr. Lansing's group, which had moved across town from Jewish Hospital, which was a not-for-profit institution, to Humana Hospital-Audubon, run by Humana, a for-profit hospital chain based in Louisville. But at the time, the team was still setting up its transplant program. Dawkins called Jewish Hospital, but got the same reply. He also contacted a transplant surgeon in Indianapolis, whom Dawkins knew to be diabetic himself. However, diabetics were considered too risky, and again the answer was no. Dawkins told Bill that the best they could hope for was to keep adjusting medications.

That August the newspapers were full of the startling news that a controversial, world-famous heart surgeon was joining Lansing's group in Louisville. Dr. William DeVries was the University of Utah Medical Center surgeon who had implanted an artificial heart called the Jarvik-7 in Seattle dentist Barney Clark two years earlier. DeVries told reporters that he had become frustrated by delays in the university's ethical review process and by the lack of funds for his research. Clark's surgery and postoperative care during the 112 days he lived with the device cost about $250,000, and DeVries complained that he had to spend almost all his time raising money for more operations instead of treating patients. Dr. Lansing, who had traveled several times to Utah to study artificial heart surgery with DeVries, had persuaded Humana to fund DeVries's research for up to one hundred artificial heart implants, provided that the first few went well. DeVries wouldn't receive a salary from Humana, but would be a partner in Lansing's practice and thus have access to Audubon's facilities and staffing services. It was an offer the forty-year-old surgeon felt he couldn't refuse.

An artificial heart, Dawkins thought. If they couldn't maintain Bill Schroeder on medications, then that would be his only hope. It was a long shot. It was experimental. No one knew much about it. Dawkins wasn't sure whether Bill's age and diabetes would disqualify him for an artificial heart in the same way they had for a human heart transplant. It could be that Bill's previous coronary-bypass surgery had left too much scar tissue inside his chest. Or Bill might not even want to try it. Dawkins did some checking and learned that the artificial heart program guidelines required prospective patients to be ineligible for a human heart transplant and that their heart disease be so advanced that they were in "Class IV," meaning they had fewer than fifty days to live. Bill hadn't reached that stage yet, but he might soon. If worse came to worst, Dawkins felt he owed it to Bill to investigate this last option.

In October Bill's teeth became badly infected, probably as a result of the diabetes. The infection became so severe that his dentist said he would have to remove all of Bill's uppers. Even though he tired very easily now, Bill insisted on going to the dentist by himself. When the phone rang about an hour after he'd gone, Margaret felt an odd sense of dread. Yes, it was someone from Jasper Memorial—Bill had collapsed in the dentist's office and was back in intensive care.

"Oh, my God. I'll be right there." Like anybody else whose loved one suffers a long illness, Margaret made the next moves automatically: gathering supplies from home, calling the family members to relay the sad news, making sure Rod and

Cheryl could manage without her for several days, tucking away her worries and fears.

When she reached the hospital, the doctors told Margaret that Bill had suffered another major heart attack. *Oh, God, no*, Margaret thought. He was already so weak. How in the world could he stand any more? Margaret resumed her now-familiar spot at Bill's bedside, holding his hand, rubbing his arm. Bill looked worse than ever, lying there so miserable and defeated. He couldn't go on this way. *He'll never live through another one of those attacks*, she thought. Bill seemed to be thinking the same thing. The next day, when Dr. Dawkins and Dr. Salb walked into his room and closed the door, their faces confirmed those fears.

"Well, Bill," Salb began, "the news isn't good. I know I don't have to tell you that every month you're getting weaker. You've just about run out of heart."

"I understand," Bill said softly.

"We could just let you go, and see how you continue to do on medication," Salb said. "But it's only going to get worse. You might live for several more weeks that way, but that's about all. I'm afraid we're down to the last option."

Margaret's hand tightened around Bill's.

"The only other thing we have to offer—and it is the *very* last resort—is that artificial heart they're trying down in Louisville," Dawkins said. "Now, I really don't know all that much about it. I don't even know if you'd be a candidate for one, what with your diabetes and your age and all. I just don't know. And even if you *are* eligible, you might not want to try it. There's only been one other patient in the world who's had one."

"Yeah, I know," Bill said. "Barney Clark."

"Right," Dawkins said. "It's highly experimental. I don't know what it can offer you. You could get one and see what happens. Or you can go on like you are now, and you'll live for a few more weeks at the most."

Bill nodded. He'd known he was getting worse, but that didn't make it any easier to hear the doctors say it out loud and speak with such finality. "Well, I don't know anything about an artificial heart either," Bill said. "But I'd like to go and take a look at it. Can you call and get me an appointment?"

"Sure, I can do that for you," Dawkins said.

"And I'd like for you and Dr. Salb to be there, if that's possible."

The doctors promised him they would.

"Thanks, guys," Bill said.

Later that morning as Bill dozed, Margaret began calling the kids, one by one, to tell them that the doctors had said Bill was really going to die soon. Telling them was as hard as hearing it herself—probably worse. She hated to think of them being so worried and scared, knowing that their dad was steadily fading away from them.

She reached Mel first, at Kimball International, a Jasper-based manufacturer of furniture and pianos, where he worked as an electronics engineer. Mel hurried to the hospital on his lunch break, and ran into Margaret in the lobby as she was leaving to get some more clothes and supplies. They hugged each other tightly, trying to hold back the tears, to be strong for the other one. They choked up when they tried to talk, but there wasn't much to say anyway.

Upstairs, as he stood in the doorway to Bill's room, Mel saw his dad sitting on the edge of the bed, dangling his feet, staring into space. It was so hard to believe that this same man was really his dad—the dad who'd always been so powerful, who always got his own way, who had an answer for everything. Now, sitting there in his pajamas, shoulders sagging, his father looked so damn scared.

Finally, Bill noticed his son. Mel swallowed, managed a weak "Hi, Dad," walked over, and sat next to him on the bed. Bill looked at his son for a long moment, glad to see him, then looked away.

Bill tried hard to draw a deep breath. "Well, I got the bad news today," he said. Just like that, like he'd lost his job or something. Mel put his arm around his father's shoulders. "Yeah," Mel said. "I know." Both men stared ahead at the floor. Mel could feel Bill crying softly and shaking his head. "I don't know what I'm going to do," he kept saying.

Mel rubbed his back. "I sure wish there was something I could do, Dad." Bill put his hand on Mel's knee. It had seemed that there was always something Bill could do about any problem. He'd always faced difficulties with such optimism and resolve, and always found the answers, through pure determination if nothing else. But there was no argument now. Neither father nor son felt a need to be strong in front of the other. So, side by side, they wept quietly.

As they sat there, it seemed to Mel that the bad news must already have traveled all over the hospital wing. Before that day, nurses and doctors would pop their heads in the door every couple of minutes to tease Bill or take some ribbing from him. Now the whole hallway seemed strangely quiet, as if everyone was walking past the room without saying a word.

After a few minutes, there was a knock at the door. "Can I come in?"

Bill and Mel each made a quick movement to wipe the last of their tears. When Bill recognized his cousin Kenneth, he straightened, smiled, and waved him in. "Sure, come on, sit down." Bill said. Somehow, as Kenneth asked the usual hi-how-are-you questions, Bill began to brighten and look a little more like his old self.

"Yep, they gave me the bad news today. The old ticker's about had it," Bill said, patting his chest. "Looks like I'm going to go down to Louisville and check out the artificial heart. Yeah, they've been doing research on it for a long time now, you know, and I'm going to get me an appointment to go down there. I guess that's what's next."

Mel couldn't believe it. His father was talking as if it would be a simple procedure, as if he'd suddenly become some kind of expert on artificial organs. "They've only done one before," Bill was saying, "but I feel I've got a little better chance than Barney Clark. See, they say he had a lot of other things wrong with him besides. But except for my diabetes—and my heart, of course—I'm in pretty good shape otherwise . . ."

The rest of that day and the next, the other kids came to the hospital, one by one. It was hard to know what to say to him now. Any other problem he would have just worked into the ground. This was different.

Stan visited Bill along with his wife, Terri. Stan was the son who'd always had the most run-ins with his dad, the one who'd been grounded most often, usually over the typical mischief teenage boys can get into. But he redeemed himself in Bill's eyes by playing football for the Jasper Wildcats. And after he got out of the army, found a municipal job in Jasper, and settled down with Terri, he seemed to straighten out. He and Terri, a beautician, had eloped, and of course, since Bill couldn't stand the idea of his son not having a wedding reception, he organized one for them along with Terri's parents.

Now as he stood beside his dad's hospital bed, Stan didn't know what to say, except that he loved him and appreciated all the times he had stuck by him, even when Bill disapproved of his actions. Stan was relieved to be able to mention one other thing.

"Well, Dad, at least there's *some* good news."

Bill looked at him wearily. "What?"

"Terri's pregnant!" Stan said. "Due in May!"

Bill's eyes lit up briefly. "Better be a boy," he said.

Stan had known Dad would say that. Bill had five other grandchildren—Mel's little girls, Abbie and Melanie, Stan's six-year-old daughter, Tracey, and Moni's children, Vicki and Bobby—and certainly didn't love them any less. But his whole family knew that Bill was a traditional German who desperately wanted a *Schroeder* grandson to carry on his name.

Bill began talking about what he'd do with a Schroeder grandson: take him fishing up at the forty acres, teach him to play Wiffle ball in the backyard, sneak him out to Dairy Queen for sundaes. But somehow his words sounded hollow. Spring was awfully far away.

That day, when Terry finished his job driving a delivery truck for a meat-packing company, he and his fiancée, Julie, visited Bill. Lean and athletic, Terry was a carbon copy of his father otherwise—the loudest and most stubborn of the family, the one who was always clipping jokes and cartoons for Bill's collection.

Now he tried to cheer up his dad by reminding him that the wedding was only four months away, and he was sure Bill would be there to see it. When Julie mentioned that she still hadn't picked out a dress, Bill tried to tease her, but again it looked like he was trying to keep up a brave front. How Bill wanted to be at that wedding! But they all knew he might never get the chance.

Cheryl came in with her boyfriend, Glenn. Cheryl had a good secretarial job at Kimball International, and Glenn worked for the company in maintenance.

Since Cheryl still lived at home, she and Glenn often joined her parents in such activities as gardening, playing cards, and going to yard sales. Even though Cheryl had seen the steady decline of her father's health day by day, she still couldn't believe it as he tearfully told her that he didn't have long to live.

She searched for the right words. "You don't know that for sure, Dad. You never know what could happen."

Bill mentioned that he was going to look into the possibility of an artificial heart, and Cheryl seized on that hope, trying to encourage him.

"See, Dad? We won't give up hope yet. You'll just have to take it easy for a while." She figured it must be some kind of device like a pacemaker—and she knew that plenty of people were walking around with those.

When Rod, the youngest, visited Bill the next day, they both knew that he wouldn't stay very long. Rod was the most nervous and high-strung of all of them. He was the one who was different—while the others had inherited their parents' straight, dark hair and deep brown eyes, Rod had fair, curly hair and blue eyes. He was fresh out of high school, still lived at home with Cheryl and his parents, and worked at the wood factory. When Rod and his girl friend, Lori, stopped by to see him, Bill was soon urging them to go on home, understanding that hospitals always made Rod jittery.

Moni, the oldest, was the only one who'd left the area. She was now a three-hour drive away in Sparta, Illinois, where she and her husband, Bob Bohnert, who was also from Jasper, lived. Bob worked for a coal-mining company and Moni worked part-time in a nursing home. They had a teenage daughter, Vicki, and a younger son, Bobby. Her folks had never liked the idea of her moving so far away, but the Bohnerts made regular trips home to Jasper and hadn't missed a Thanksgiving or Christmas there yet.

As soon as she heard the news, Moni returned to Jasper. She couldn't believe how weak her father had become, and had to try to hide her surprise. Like the other kids, she told him she knew that he'd hang in there. Dad would never be a quitter, and even though they didn't know anything about this artificial heart he kept mentioning, they were all encouraged to see that he wasn't about to give up.

Bill had to wait three weeks for an appointment with Dr. DeVries. Humana Hospital-Audubon was still in the process of obtaining federal authorization to have an artificial heart program. The Food and Drug Administration, which oversaw research on experimental medical devices, had already approved DeVries to perform seven implants, after which the agency would reassess his work and decide whether to allow him to do any more. But Audubon's facilities also needed FDA approval, which was expected to come in early November. Dr. Salb and Dr. Dawkins had to be in Louisville on November 8 for a doctors' symposium anyway, so they arranged for Bill to meet DeVries then.

Bill was certainly sick enough to stay at Jasper Memorial. However, there was nothing more to be done for him, so he insisted on going home. The next three weeks were his worst yet. As the days and nights dragged on, Bill had to fight harder and harder for every breath. His family could only imagine how frightening that must be, like trying to breathe through a straw that was almost stopped up.

Now Bill was lucky to get two hours' sleep a night. As soon as he lay down, fluid would fill his lungs. Coughing fits shook his whole body. His face would turn bright red, as if it were going to burst. He would go into the living room and sit up all night. Margaret would pull up a chair in front of him, put his head on a pillow in her lap, rub his back, and just wish she could do more for him. Bill would whimper and cough and listen to her as she talked to him, trying to keep his spirits up, reminding him that pretty soon they would go down to Louisville for the meeting about the artificial heart. From her room, Cheryl could hear her father coughing and moaning. She'd lie awake listening for his next breath, afraid that each one would be his last.

If Bill tried to walk, he could manage only a few steps at a time, from chair to chair, or chair to wall to doorframe. Just moving from the bedroom to the bathroom wore him out. Anytime he tried to walk, everyone would tense up, ready to catch him or help him back into his chair. Bill was still a proud man who hated to be a burden to anybody. He'd work his way around the house by himself, and wouldn't ask for or accept anybody's help unless he stumbled and fell.

Sometimes it seemed that the possibility of that artificial heart was the only thing keeping Bill alive. The rest of the family secretly doubted that he would ever make it to the Louisville meeting with DeVries, or if he did somehow, that anything would really come of it. They let him hang on to that hope mainly to buy him a few more days' time. Something as strange as having an artificial heart was the kind of thing that happened to other people. Not to your own dad.

When the kids stopped by the house, they'd find their parents exhausted. Often one or two would come over after work to let Margaret catch some sleep after a long night up with Bill. One afternoon, as he struggled to carry on a conversation with Margaret and some of the kids, Bill kept shifting in his vinyl La-Z-Boy chair, sometimes bending over to catch his breath. Finally, he grumbled something and slowly made his way to the bedroom.

Margaret followed, knowing what she would find: Bill lying on his side, all doubled up, trying to breathe, and there'd be nothing for her to do but rub his back. The kids stayed behind, sensing that Bill had left the room so that they wouldn't see him cry.

That day Bill's body wouldn't even allow him the relief of a few tears. Whenever he began to cry, he ended up gasping for air between sobs. Margaret called for the kids to come. He was lying there curled up, his face all red while he struggled to breathe. Margaret gave them a look that said, "*Do* something!" They stood over him and discussed whether to take him to the hospital, but he put a stop to such talk. There wasn't anything that could be done for him at the hospital, he insisted. He was at home where he wanted to be. After he lay still for a few minutes, Bill regained a more regular rhythm of shallow breaths. Then he sat up for a while and dozed, exhausted, while the family talked to each other in low voices.

That kind of scene happened again and again. Now the kids tiptoed quietly in the house, which had been a noisy, bustling, dropping-in place. As Bill's strength seeped away, he became more and more grouchy. He was very moody now, and it was hard to tell what might set him off. If the kids talked too loudly, he might blow up in anger. Or he might not. If he opened the refrigerator and discovered that they were out of milk, somebody would catch hell for it. At times, he seemed to be waiting for somebody, anybody, to start an argument. Other times, if something happened that seemed sure to set him off, he wouldn't say a word, as if he'd just given up caring about anything. When the grandkids visited, they would stare in confusion at the grandpa who used to pick them up and swing them in the air and race them to the car on the way to buy ice cream.

CHAPTER THREE

Thursday, November 8, 1984. The day of Bill's appointment had finally come. Mel, who lived on a small farm several miles from Jasper, agreed to meet his folks in a factory parking lot in nearby Ferdinand and drive the remaining seventy miles or so to Louisville. He arrived early in his pickup truck, but his parents were already waiting for him. He could see that his father had had a terrible night; he knew that meant that Mom must have been up all night, too.

Mel parked his truck and took over the wheel of the vinyl-topped Ford LTD, which the family had nicknamed "The Boat." Bill rode in the front seat, his eyes closed, concentrating on his breathing. Margaret kept up a steady flow of talk from the backseat, mostly to keep Mel awake and assure Bill she was there. From time to time Bill coughed loudly, and Margaret would reach up to massage his shoulders.

They found their way to Audubon, a huge new hospital just east of downtown Louisville. Bill needed help getting out of the car, and had to pause and rest every few steps as he and Margaret walked toward the entrance. Bill, wearing a sport shirt and slacks, insisted on carrying his briefcase, the one he used to carry around on his union business. Now it contained his medical records, a legal pad, and a tape recorder. The three of them took seats in the lobby and waited for the doctors from Jasper. After what seemed like a long time, an admitting clerk asked if they needed help. Bill told him they were to meet their doctors from Jasper and a cardiologist named Dr. Dageforde, who was going to give him an "echo" scan. Bill had gone through this test before, in which ultrasound was used to observe blood flow through arteries in his neck. There was some confusion about whether Bill had to register as a patient. Finally, the clerk had Dr. Dageforde paged and had Bill fill out some forms. Margaret and Mel just watched, unsure of what they were getting into.

Soon a young man in a white coat strode up. "Mr. Schroeder? I'm Dr. Dageforde." Bill slowly stood up to shake hands. He was breathing a little easier now because it was cool inside the hospital. Dageforde told Mel and Margaret to wait in the lobby for the doctors while he took Bill for the scan. As he and Bill started down the hall, Dageforde walked ahead briskly, asking what medications he was taking. They'd gone about twenty paces when Bill leaned against the wall and bent over, gasping for breath. "Whoa!" Bill said, holding up a hand. "Can't keep up with you there."

Dageforde turned and looked behind him. "Oh, I'm sorry—here, let me get you a wheelchair!" Meanwhile, Mel and Margaret were signing papers the clerk had handed them, although Margaret felt uneasy. "I didn't know we were going to have to do all *this*," she said. Bill was just going for an interview with the doctors—what was all this paperwork about? Dr. Dawkins, Dr. Salb, and another Jasper physician, Dr. K. A. Volz, finally showed up, and soon Dageforde returned to take the doctors on a tour of the hospital. Mel and Margaret waited for Bill, and within a few minutes, a nurse wheeled him back. He was tired and sore from the test.

Margaret and Mel wheeled Bill to the second-floor wing that housed the offices of Humana Heart Institute International, the hospital's center for cardiovascular disease. They were escorted to a small, windowless conference room, where they rejoined Dageforde and the doctors from Jasper. They took seats around a long table and made small talk while waiting for Dr. DeVries. Bill opened his briefcase and took out the tape recorder and the legal pad. He'd written some questions on the pad in his precise, all-capitals printing, and had left several lines underneath each one for the answers. He planned to tape the meeting so all the kids would know what had been discussed.

A tall, thin man in a white coat approached the open door. He was flipping through a chart and talking over his shoulder to a nurse at the same time. He was frowning as he looked over the chart one last time and handed it back to the nurse.

Then he looked up and smiled. He had a friendly, boyish face, and was so tall that his sandy hair almost grazed the top of the doorframe. "Hi, I'm Bill DeVries," he said, holding out a huge, freckled hand to the Schroeders.

My God! This was the surgeon who implanted the artificial

heart in Barney Clark, the guy who was all over TV and on national magazine covers. Here he was, smiling and shaking everyone's hand, just like a regular person, looking right into their eyes and calling them by name. After introductions all around, Dr. DeVries settled into a chair.

Even though Bill was weak and tired—and even though he was sitting across from a world-famous heart surgeon—he was determined to be in charge. This was going to be like any other meeting he'd ever conducted with big shots. He'd prepared carefully, and was going to get them to answer all his questions before he left. He asked the doctors if he could tape their discussion so he could play it at home for the family.

That was fine, DeVries told him.

Bill switched on the tape recorder. For a moment, no one spoke. Finally, DeVries said, "Hard to know where to start, isn't it?"

"Well," Bill began, "let me start out and tell you what I know of it. And if I'm getting off track, stop me and put me back on the right track."

DeVries held up a hand. "Okay, let me just tell you where we are right now as far as the whole process first. That may save some of your questions."

Bill nodded, and DeVries began explaining: Artificial hearts had been used in humans three times before. Dr. Denton Cooley of Houston had twice used an artificial heart to keep patients alive for several hours until they received human heart transplants, once in 1969 and again in 1981. Both patients died of complications within three days. The model Cooley used wasn't exactly like the one DeVries had used in his first recipient, Barney Clark, two years before.

DeVries said that while he was in Utah he had to get his artificial heart program approved by the Food and Drug Administration. After moving to Louisville, he had to go through even more paperwork to get approval to do the implants at Audubon. By coincidence, he said, just hours ago, the FDA gave the go-ahead to do artificial hearts at the hospital here. "So right now, this hospital is certified and ready to go. Essentially we're now officially looking for patients. It so happens you're the first one that's come in, because we haven't made any announcement yet. But all of the regulations and things like that are approved," DeVries said.

"Well," Bill said, "I want to speak on what I think I know so far. And I just gained this knowledge yesterday, on television, from Channel Eleven." The night before, on *Hour Magazine*, he said, a Seattle doctor had described an electric artificial heart he was developing that would be powered by a battery belt.

DeVries explained that the device shown on TV was still in its early stages and wouldn't be ready for testing for a few years. He said that scientists had been working with artificial hearts since around 1965, and the government had contributed about $200 million in research. Work was being done at several centers, such as Penn State, the University of Utah, Houston, and Stanford.

The door opened, and in walked Dr. Lansing, the silver-haired surgeon who'd done Bill's bypass at Jewish Hospital and recruited DeVries to Louisville. "Dr. Lansing!" Bill said, like he was presiding at a meeting and welcoming a latecomer. Bill waved him over, and introduced the doctors and family members.

DeVries continued: "The electric heart is being developed, but right now it has not reached a point for practical use. I implanted about fifteen or sixteen electric hearts, and the longest we've ever had a survivor has been about fourteen days. The Pennsylvania State group had an animal that lived about a month. So that is in the future—probably *will* be the heart of the future."

At present, he said, the most effective heart in use—the one used in Cooley's patients and in Barney Clark—was the "air-driven" heart.

"The artificial heart that we're talking about is one that's implanted in place of your own heart. The diseased heart is actually removed. The machine is put in right in the same place.

"It has basically two moving parts, one for the heart's right side and one for the left side." DeVries made a small *o* with his thumb and forefinger, then held it against the left side of his white coat, just above belt level. "Two tubes about this big around come out through the abdomen, air is pumped in and out through those tubes." The puffs of air make the heart move so that it pumps blood, he said. "The blood doesn't come outside of the body—it stays inside where it's supposed to be. The air goes in and out through the tubes, and a machine outside the body pumps the air in."

Bill looked puzzled. They'd hook him to a machine that pumped air? Then that wasn't the heart he'd heard about after all. He couldn't picture it.

"How big is the machine?" he asked.

"The main machine is about the size of a shopping cart. It's on wheels," DeVries said. "Weighs about two hundred thirty pounds." It was called a "Utahdrive."

Mel looked at his father, stunned. *A 230-pound shopping cart?*

DeVries explained that the tubes connecting Bill to the machine were about eight feet long. "So you're connected to that machine. You can move around with it, you can push it around, and your mobility is about the same as in a wheelchair." He added that the FDA had also approved testing of a new, much smaller pump, about the size of a large handbag. "It can go on your shoulder like a camera case. You could move around pretty freely on that." The FDA had also given approval to try out the small pump for a few hours at a time.

"Hopefully, we can wean you off the big machine and use the small one all the time. That's something you can carry around and have essentially normal mobility. You wouldn't be able to swim," DeVries said with a smile. "But you could maybe play golf or bowl, or something like that."

Margaret still couldn't get over the idea of all these big-time doctors sitting here talking to her and Bill and Melvin—not just ones from Jasper, but some of the best in the world. She had some questions, but felt tongue-tied around such important people.

"So," Bill asked, "the machine that you're talking about now—if I decided to go through with this—would be the shopping-cart–sized one?"

"Yeah, you'd have to be put on that machine and then stabilized. And then sometime in the period right after surgery, we would put you on the small machine and test how well you do on it." If everything went well, they'd switch him back and forth between the larger and the smaller machine, building up more time on the portable one. The plan would be to taper off from the big machine, but that goal was one of the "side branches" of the project, DeVries said.

"So," Bill said thoughtfully, "you'd be more or less confined or restricted at first."

"Yeah, you would be at first," the doctor said. "I mean, you'd be attached to a machine. You have to assume that you're going to be attached to a machine for the rest of your life—of one type or another. Now three or four years later—as electric hearts come out—if a new heart were developed, which would make your life better, you might be able to go on to one of those. But we wouldn't have any way of knowing about that right now." Bill would have to weigh his current quality of life against that afforded by the device, and then choose between the two. But it was still very hard to imagine what life with that machine would be like.

Now Bill asked about something he'd heard on the TV program. "I'm right in saying that the capacity, the output of the heart, would be about eighty percent?"

Actually, DeVries said, the Jarvik-7 heart was able to put out as much as fifteen liters of blood a minute—twice as much as Bill would need for normal activity.

"That's fine," Bill said quickly. He told them how he'd had to stop and rest just walking down the hospital corridor, and that often he had to sit with his head between his knees to catch his breath.

"Let me also just go through a little bit about the process of what we do," DeVries said. "If you were to decide that you were real interested in this and wanted to pursue it, then what we would end up doing, basically, is try to educate you. We'd show you the device, give you a lot of literature to read, and answer all the questions you have. You'd have time to think it over. Then we would get your own physicians involved, so they understand, and can give you advice." One of Barney Clark's doctors had initially advised against the operation, but changed his mind after looking over the program. That kind of give-and-take and questioning was important, DeVries said, and Bill should rely on his doctors to advise him in the same manner.

"If you felt that you wanted to go ahead with it, then we'd have you evaluated by the committee here. It would involve a couple of cardiologists who had never seen you before, so they could form their own opinion of whether or not you medically were fit. Also, a social worker, a psychiatrist, a nurse—basically just to see that all the requirements were met. Then we would accept you as a patient, and work out the medical details, and your details of the way you want to go ahead and set the date."

Dr. Salb spoke up. "How long a period of time are we talking about there?"

"That could be a day, or a matter of months, or six weeks," DeVries replied. "It just depends on how things go. If someone were deteriorating rapidly, we would have to move fast."

But it was also important for Bill to be sure about his decision. "We don't want to talk anybody into anything, you know. We just want to be sure you—"

Bill interrupted. He wanted them to know that he had the right attitude. "No, I'm optimistic about it. I'm the kind of person that has an open mind, and I believe in changes. And I believe in challenges, too, unless the odds are just not there. There ain't no way to tell how long I could live. I could have another heart attack tomorrow—there's no way of knowing.

"If I knew I would have no more than six months to live, I'd want the mechanical heart. But if you decide there's another year left with my own heart, taking quantity versus quality, I'd definitely say, 'Forget about the mechanical heart.'"

"Sure, that makes perfect sense to me," DeVries said. "I feel the same way you do about it. I wouldn't want to offer you anything that I wouldn't do myself. I think the question really is, When do you feel it's the right time? I think in making that decision, you've got to rely on the people in this room who know you, and know your medical condition."

"Well," Bill said, "the drawback now that I see is being sort of confined and restricted."

"Yeah," DeVries said.

"That would be a drawback, that's for sure. What about the financial expenses?"

No problem there, DeVries answered. Humana was underwriting the cost of the experiments. "You wouldn't have a hospital bill or a doctor bill or anything cost-related. As far as when you went home with the thing, we are working out ways that that could be worked on." Obviously, he said, Humana would like to get as much as possible out of any third-party payor, and a social worker would help work out such insurance matters. Humana would pick up the rest of the tab. "The real good news is that it's not going to cost you. We look at it this way: You're taking part in a very creative type of research that's going to help other people. And we're going to get really exciting answers to help other people like you. In addition, we hope you're going to get a good quality of life out of it, and it will help you live. That's the trade-off."

Dr. Dawkins asked DeVries whether Bill's diabetes would disqualify him.

Initially, DeVries said, they'd planned to screen out dia-

55

betics, but later decided that if the disease could be controlled with insulin, it would probably pose no problem.

Salb asked, "When he leaves here, are you optimistic that he'll leave here with the smaller unit?"

"We would hope so," DeVries answered. "If I were to say to you, 'You're going to be in the hospital the rest of your life,' that may not be something you want to do. May not be what I want to do, either." Once Bill was well enough to be discharged, he'd move into a nearby apartment just purchased by Humana—a "halfway house" where artificial heart patients could spend a few weeks or months adjusting to being outside the hospital.

DeVries said he didn't know how long Bill would have to stay in the hospital. "It may take a month, may take two months. I don't know." By that point, Bill would be using the shopping-cart–sized "drive system," with intermittent periods on the smaller machine.

"In other words, if he wanted to go for a walk, he would go on the small system: go out, walk around, come back in the house. Reading, watching TV, or whatever he wanted to do at home, he'd go on the big system. Now, as to the weaning process, we really don't know how that's going to come. Hopefully, we'd get the small system going, but I would say you should assume you'd be going home on the big system."

Mel was still curious about exactly how the equipment worked. After all, his training was in electronics.

DeVries said that the small drive system was powered by nickel-cadmium batteries like those in video cameras. The Utah-drive, the big machine, ran on electricity from a wall outlet. The Utahdrive also had to be plugged into wall outlets for air compressors, which supplied puffs of air that powered the heart. But if they had to move the machine away from a room with a compressed-air source, the machine could run temporarily on air tanks.

"The big one sounds awkward and cumbersome, and looks awkward and cumbersome," DeVries acknowledged. "But right now it's the one we have the most experience on, and it's the most reliable, if you're just choosing to move around the room or around the house. But ultimately we'd really like to see someone use the little drive system all the time."

"Say the electricity went off or something like that," Bill said. "I want to make certain—"

"It charges automatically and stores electricity in it with battery cells," DeVries said. If the power ever went off, the machine's alarms would sound. The Utahdrive's battery cells would keep it running for another several hours on its own.

Margaret tried to imagine what it would be like to be responsible for all this space-age machinery, to watch over it back at the house in Jasper. Finally, she spoke up. "May I ask something? If, like you said, he would be able to come home, perhaps—if something goes wrong then, are you saying he has to come back here?"

"Yeah, we'd have to come out and help then," DeVries said. They could probably monitor a lot of the machine's activity through telephone-to-computer hookups. Months earlier, he and Dr. Lansing had implanted artificial hearts in calves in Utah which they still monitored via computer lines every day. "But this is all conceptualized," DeVries acknowledged. "We haven't done any of this, except with the animals. But it would be the type of thing that we would try to work out."

Computers? Phone lines? Margaret wanted to make sure she understood what they expected her to do. "You're talking about me. At home."

"Yeah," DeVries said. "Yeah, I would like to have him where you're living now, and carry on your life there. Ideally that's what we would like to have. It may take a while to get there, but that would be our goal."

Bill was jotting down answers under his questions. Then he asked whether DeVries would mind if Dawkins observed the surgery.

DeVries had no problem with that, and said that in fact it would be good to have someone whom Bill trusted explain everything to him from a somewhat different perspective.

Mel couldn't believe it. Mom and Dad were already talking about having the surgery and bringing him home, but they still didn't really know how these devices were supposed to work. "I'm sure there's been some tests or something to see how long that thing can keep someone alive," Mel said.

Yes, DeVries told him, they had data from two kinds of longevity tests. They'd tested artificial hearts in a laboratory, having them pump water until they wore out, which sometimes took as long as six years. They'd also tested the hearts in calves and sheep. That was rougher on the Jarvik, and the animals usually lived only four or five months, although one was now approaching a year with the device.

Lansing added that there were other problems with animals: "One, they outgrow the machine. They're young animals and they get to be bigger than the heart can handle. Secondly, it's very difficult to prevent infection occurring in animals, because they're very hard to keep clean. Humans can look after themselves. The third thing is that these are mechanical devices, and probably in humans some type of blood-thinner would be used to protect you against any kind of clots forming anyplace. And that is very difficult to maintain in the animals.

"So, the animals outgrow it, there's a problem of infection, and that of clots forming—none of which should occur in a good human situation," Lansing said. "That's why there's no reason to do more and more animal experiments—because you've learned all you can. The experimental condition itself limits what you can learn. Because of the tremendous amount we can learn, we feel that it's appropriate to offer this now to humans. But until we know how you or somebody else does, we really don't know for sure how well it's going to work."

"That was one of my other questions," Bill said. "The possibility of blood clots." He knew that many people whose heart valves were replaced with mechanical ones had to take blood-thinners to prevent clots.

"What would be the compatibility of medications with the mechanical heart?" Bill asked.

"So far, we haven't had any difficulty at all," DeVries answered. "As Dr. Lansing said, you'd have to be on blood-thinners. But a lot of people we operate on are under those conditions. It means taking a pill a day." DeVries foresaw no problem with taking insulin, but added, "I think you have to realize that that would be one of the risks you would be taking." He doubted any other drugs now prescribed for Bill would pose problems. With an artificial heart, improved circulation would probably cancel the need for many of those medications, although he might have to take others, such as the blood-thinner Coumadin.

Bill wondered what would happen if he needed some other surgery. "I anticipate sometime I'm going to have to have varicose veins removed from my leg."

"Yeah, we would be involved in that, because, first of all, I'm sure the surgeons wouldn't want to take you as a patient unless we were right there to make sure we knew what was going on," DeVries said. "We'd have to allow your blood to clot again for a short while. What we would do is stop the Coumadin and put you on some IV medicines until the time of the surgery. And then we would do the surgery, then start back up again. It's like people with heart valves—when they have teeth pulled or varicose veins or major surgery, they have to adjust their medications."

Bill mentioned that his upper teeth had to be pulled because they were infected. DeVries told him that would have to be done before the surgery to minimize the risk of further infection.

Mel looked at his dad in disbelief. He sounded as if he were already making plans for the operation.

Bill asked, "If I want to take a shower, what do I do? Disconnect myself?"

"No," DeVries answered, grinning. "You just take a shower."

"With it all on?" Bill asked.

"Yeah, you'd look exactly as you look now. The only difference is you'd have two tubes coming out here," DeVries said, again pointing to his side. "The tubes come out and they're connected. They have a little special fuzzy cloth called 'velour.' Your skin actually grows into that fuzzy tube, and thus prevents infection from going in from the outside."

Velour? Fuzzy tube? It was still very hard to imagine.

"If you want to shower, you just take a shower," DeVries was saying. "And you'd be very careful to keep the connections clean and maybe put some ointment on them." Barney Clark couldn't take a shower until about a month after his implant, but he'd also been treated with a number of drugs that impaired his body's ability to heal.

"His death was not attributed to the mechanical heart?" Bill asked.

"No, his death was not related to the artificial heart," DeVries said. "His death was probably related to the fact that he got the flu and vomited one night. Some of the vomit went into his lungs, and he got infected. We treated him with an antibiotic and it actually cleaned out his lungs very well." One of the side effects of the antibiotic was that it killed some necessary bacteria in his bowel. Clark's death was actually a complication of the antibiotic.

They discussed the fact that Clark had suffered many more

medical problems than Bill had. Clark had also been a longtime smoker, DeVries noted.

Bill jotted some more notes, then joked that Dr. Salb had told him to quit smoking. "But he never told me about *these* after-effects. Now I'm in this position." Everyone chuckled.

Bill turned serious again. "I don't have any more questions," he said. "The way it sounds is that you've improved somewhat on the mechanical heart since Dr. Clark's days."

"Yes, we have," DeVries said. "The biggest improvement has been the possibility of having a small drive system. I think that's really important. Dr. Lansing and I have real strong feelings, too, about some of the other improvements to make. But the only way you make improvements is by taking those steps and learning. That's why it's exciting if you can be a part of something like this."

"And I understand, too," Bill said, "that further on down the road that probably it'll get better—"

DeVries interrupted. "If something came along that we thought would improve your quality of life—and again you've got to realize that the only place in the entire world this can be done is right here—"

"Right," Bill said.

"—and we're trying to keep up on the very edge of it. If something comes along that we think would be better, we'll sit down and discuss it with you—all the risks and complications and possibilities, and you would ask us questions just like we're doing here," DeVries promised.

Bill put down his pen. "I don't have any further questions other than that."

Mel did. How long, ideally, could the heart be expected to pump inside a human being?

"Well," DeVries said, "I was looking for something like two years, three years, with Barney Clark. That's what I felt. If anybody asked me—if the press asked me—I would never say that. But that's my own personal feeling about it. I think that people are stronger than animals, cleaner than animals, and we know more about people than we know about animals." So, humans ought to outlive the experimental animals, DeVries said, turning to Lansing. "What do you think?"

"In some of the animals, we've already virtually removed the mechanical heart and replaced it with another pumping system," Lansing said. "So it can be changed—"

"It *can* be changed," Bill repeated.

"As an improved model came about—or, if it wasn't doing exactly what it should—part of it can be changed, or all of it can be changed. The parts are sort of interchangeable," Lansing said. "And you would be opened up again; it would mean another operation." Replacing parts would be a difficult challenge, he said, but if necessary the original implant could certainly be replaced or repaired.

Bill nodded. "The procedure of the operation is similar to a bypass?"

"The incision would be through the breastbone," said DeVries, tracing an imaginary line down his chest, "and everything else would be exactly the same except it wouldn't involve an incision in the legs. The actual operation would be here. Your heart is removed, and the device would be put in exactly where your heart is right now."

Bill coughed and struggled to breathe for a moment. Margaret spoke up. "I just have one more question: Like, when he would leave the hospital and come home, or go to this other place or something, he won't just be 'sent home,' and he won't just be forgotten about. I mean, we will be in contact?"

Lansing smiled. "You'll probably be asking to be left alone a little bit!"

"Oh." Margaret laughed hesitantly.

"It's exactly the opposite," DeVries said. "You may be having too many people around—"

"You know, it's kind of scary," Margaret said.

"—and that's something else you may need to talk a little bit about," DeVries said. "The thing that surprised Dr. Clark and his wife the most about the procedure wasn't necessarily that he was still alive after it. It wasn't that he was able to walk around, that he had a little more activity. What they were most surprised with was all of the public hoopla that went on around them. That's something you've got to think about. It's impossible to describe what happens when this goes on. Everybody recognized his name all around the world, little kids were writing him letters all the time, and his wife, Una Loy, was photographed wherever she went. That can be okay. It can also be a real hassle. And it may end up that you can't walk down the aisle at the supermarket anymore without people coming up and asking you about how things are going.

"So that's something you kind of have to adapt to. You end

up being a celebrity overnight. It may be fun for about twenty minutes, but then it fades. It gets boring real fast. So you're not going to get put off in a corner where nobody will recognize you," he said, grinning. "I'll guarantee you that."

"Well," Margaret said, "I wasn't interested in other people so much. I just don't want the *doctors* to forget me."

"No, I think you'll find that it's a very tight team around here," DeVries assured her. "And it involves a tremendous amount of people who dedicate a lot of their lives to make sure it goes well. I think you'll find that they are really highly competent professional people who are not going to let anything go undone."

"That's good to know," Margaret said.

"So there's support from every direction," DeVries said. Margaret nodded.

Then Dr. Salb asked DeVries, "You mentioned possibly two months or maybe more in the hospital and then in the apartment. About how long in the apartment before possibly, ideally, would you like to see—?"

DeVries estimated that even if everything went perfectly, Bill would be in the hospital at least a month, maybe two months if complications occurred. Then he might live in the halfway house as few as three months or as long as a year. "I don't know. We're just guessing. I've never even been through that before," DeVries said. Barney Clark had never left the hospital and spent most of his 112 days in intensive care.

Salb pressed to know what the ideal scenario would be. "I just don't know the answer to that," DeVries said. But, he added, once scientific innovations are begun, improvements follow quickly. "I think we've seen it with the space races you know. I mean, Sputnik goes up and all of a sudden, everything started coming in." The same might happen with the heart's drive system. "The thing is mushrooming so fast, we might have drive systems that would enable you to go home in a couple of months very easily, and not even have to use the big drive system. The Utahdrive may end up in the trash heap."

Salb asked, "While they're living at the halfway house will there be any chance of excursions from there?"

"We hope so," DeVries said. "Especially if the drive system's working well. That battery pack lasts about four hours and if you felt comfortable with it, you could carry an extra one with you."

"How about, like, going to a ball game?" Bill asked.

"I would hope to do something like that," DeVries replied. "I really would."

"He would have availability to community activities?" Salb asked.

"I can't promise that," DeVries said, "but I would hope that—let me get the portable drive just to show you what it looks like. It's right in my office here."

After DeVries left the room, Bill began coughing again. He fought for a deep breath, shook his head, and exhaled wearily.

Margaret rubbed his back. No one spoke. "Big sigh, isn't it?" she said.

Salb turned to Lansing. "We're talking about, you know, quality of life and quantity of life. That's what Bill and Margaret are concerned about."

Lansing nodded. "This is not something you make a decision about rapidly. You lower the possibilities, think about it, then you watch how you're getting along. You keep this in your back pocket as a possibility . . ."

DeVries came back carrying what looked like an oversized camera case.

"That's the shoulder pack," Bill said.

"And it just goes on your shoulder like this," DeVries said. He pointed to a pair of holes on the side. "And see? This is where the two tubes come in." It opened like a squat little brief-case to reveal what looked like a circuit board and a long, boxlike battery.

DeVries closed it again and handed the portable to Mel, who hefted it, then passed it to Margaret.

"See that?" DeVries smiled. "Probably a little lighter than your purse, isn't it?"

"You know how much it weighs?" Bill asked.

"About eleven pounds," DeVries said.

"Eleven pounds! Aw, I've caught fish bigger than that," Bill said.

DeVries laughed. "I haven't, I'll tell you that. You're going to have to show me where those fish are."

Margaret was still studying the portable pack. "That wouldn't be that terrible to carry around," she mused. "It'd feel like a big shoulder bag—a little bit heavier."

"Yeah, that's basically the drive system," DeVries said.

"You'll have to think about it. I'll give you some material to read. Read it and ask questions and then come back. I don't think this is the type of decision you can make right away, you know. We wouldn't want that."

But by now it was clear that Bill wouldn't take too much time to decide. "One thing that really I don't want to miss is, we have a son getting married in March," Bill said. "So I'm worried about that."

"How many children do you have?" DeVries asked.

"Six," Bill answered quickly.

DeVries grinned. "I've got seven, so I know what that's like."

"Yeah, I'm sure." Bill raised his eyebrows and returned the doctor's knowing smile.

Salb turned to Margaret. "You have anything?"

She began slowly, "When he is in the hospital, will I be able to—"

"You'll spend a lot of time with him," DeVries assured her. "We found that it was particularly important to have Una Loy Clark there a lot of the time. We felt that it was really important to have someone there with him who cared about him and was helping him through and supporting him. That's really critical. You just can't do something like this by yourself."

Bill decided it was time to lighten things up: "How will this increase my sex life?"

"Just turn up the drive system!" Lansing said, laughing.

"Do I have to use *two* batteries?" Bill asked. "She'd get a charge out of that!"

"I'm going to leave!" Margaret retorted. Everybody laughed.

DeVries asked the other doctors a few standard questions about Bill's lung problems and ulcers, then briefly flipped through the rest of Bill's records. When DeVries reached the last page, Bill spoke up: "Well, the only thing I can say in conclusion is that I appreciate everybody's time, sitting down and talking with me. It's been very interesting—"

"I hope we can help you," DeVries said.

"—and if I decide to do it, I'll feel like I've got the best in the world. And I'll give it a try."

"No corners will be cut, I'll tell you that," DeVries said. "You'll get the best that's available."

"I feel that way, too," Bill said.

"Why don't we get your medical records and get a chart assembled on you here," DeVries said. He would put together some material for the doctors and the Schroeders to read.

"I think," Salb said, "we should get together and talk to Bill and Margaret and the family, so we can resolve a lot of things and get some appropriate questions for next time."

"Good, good," DeVries said. "Don't hesitate to call and talk with us—myself or Dr. Lansing. We're always here."

Salb asked what could be done if Bill had another sudden heart attack.

"We'd have to move fast," DeVries said. The surgeon suggested that if Bill decided to have the operation, he could sign the consent form in advance, and keep it with him in case they had to do an emergency procedure.

"That's the only thing I fear," Dawkins said. "That we're just so close."

"I don't think that's something I can answer. But I think it's one of the questions you ought to be asking them," DeVries said to Bill, nodding at the Jasper doctors. "I hate to put them on the spot, but you've got to get some indication of what your life expectancy is like. I don't know how to answer that question." He shrugged. "They may know or they may not."

There was one other consideration, DeVries said: If another patient was chosen before Bill, the medical team would have to decide whether it had the resources to deal with two artificial heart patients at once. "But," DeVries added, "as far as I'm concerned right now, you look like you'd be a very good candidate."

Bill realized that he was going to be arguing the biggest case of his life. He wanted that heart. If they could do only one patient at a time, he'd have to show the doctors that he was their man.

He asked how far he could let his health deteriorate and still be considered for the heart.

DeVries answered that they'd prefer to operate when Bill's body was still in fairly good condition. If Bill suffered another heart attack, he could be in serious trouble.

"Okay, thank you again for all your time," Bill said, as if wrapping up a meeting with management. "And it was my pleasure meeting you." Bill reached out to shake hands with each of the doctors.

Mel turned to his mother in disbelief. "He's going to do it, isn't he?"

Margaret knew too.

While Mel went to get the car, Margaret wheeled Bill down to the lobby. This time, he didn't need help getting into the car. In fact, he seemed like a different man—better than he had looked in the past three weeks. He was standing taller, breathing easier, even laughing. On the drive home, he talked up the meeting and how much he liked the doctors. At best, he figured, he'd spend a couple of months in the hospital, three to four months in the apartment, and be home in time for summer. He'd take a pill a day to prevent blood clots and throw away his Lasix forever. Start on a machine about the size of a shopping cart, but build up time on the small portable system, so he could come and go as he pleased. Then get new, improved models as all the refinements started coming in. Fishing, ball games, weddings, maybe even bowling. "Hell, he said I could do everything but swim," Bill kept saying. The car crossed over the Ohio River, back into Indiana. At the Georgetown exit, they stopped for something to eat.

When they finished, Bill was surprisingly full of energy. He *had* to tell somebody. "Hey!" he said. "As long as we're this close, let's stop in and see Cousin Truman and Vivian over in English!"

"Bill!" Margaret couldn't believe her ears. "Are you sure you don't want to go back home and rest?"

"Hell, no!"

"But Bill, shouldn't we call them first? We can't just drop in like that!"

"Hell, they're family. You don't need an invitation. We're in the neighborhood, so let's just stop in and visit a while! Come on. Turn here, Melvin."

Mel pulled into the driveway, but no cars were around. It didn't look like anybody was home, so Mel started backing up. "Wait a minute," Bill said. "Somebody may be there."

Mel looked back at his mom. They couldn't believe this. Mel shrugged. "Okay. I'll go knock."

Bill was already opening the door on his side.

"Dad! You stay here, and I'll—"

"No, *you* stay here."

Mel settled back in his seat. He knew there was no arguing if Dad's mind was made up.

Bill walked to the door, knocked, and leaned against the door as he waited. He knocked again.

"C'mon, Dad," Mel said. "Nobody's home."

Bill motioned for them to wait. "Maybe they're out back," he said and started to go around the side of the house.

Mel turned to his mom. "Geez! Can you *believe* him?"

Margaret shook her head. She was worried for Bill, of course. But she also felt a surprising excitement. Suddenly her husband seemed so much like his old self, it was possible to believe that maybe the artificial heart really could make him well again.

Bill didn't waste any time. That evening he called the kids over to the house to hear the tape, and set up a meeting for the following evening with the family, Dr. Salb, and Dr. Dawkins. Even though the doctors had said this wasn't a decision that should be made quickly, Bill felt a sense of urgency. First, he knew that he could have another heart attack anytime, which, if it didn't kill him then and there, could make him ineligible for the artificial heart. Second, he was having to compete for the artificial heart, and someone might come along and take his place. Third, Moni had heard on the news that a potential candidate from Illinois was being screened at Audubon.

The family gathered at seven o'clock that Friday night in a conference room at Memorial Hospital. The mood was somber as they took their seats around a long mahogany table—it was so different from the other times when a bunch of Schroeders gathered together. They were waiting for Stan to show up, and Bill was getting impatient and irritable. "Dammit, you call a meeting and people don't show up on time . . ." Moni couldn't get away from her nurses' aide job in Sparta, Illinois, so Bill had mailed her a copy of the tape. Finally, Stan came in and tiptoed to a seat. Bill, as usual, conducted the meeting, but he seemed quieter than usual. Margaret slipped her hand into his.

"Okay." Bill turned to the doctors. "We're here to discuss the artificial heart. Now, I want it all out on the table. I want you to tell me how long I got. Don't hold nothing back."

"Well," Dr. Salb began gently, and looked around the room. "You all know that Bill hasn't been getting any better.

And at this point, we can't expect him to. He's just about run out of heart. He's in what they call Class Four, which means he's at the very last stage of end-stage heart disease." Salb paused and glanced at Bill. "Of course, it's impossible to say for sure. But our best guess is that he has about forty days to live."

Bill swallowed hard and blinked several times. Margaret and some of the kids quietly wiped away tears. It wasn't a surprise, really. On some level the family had known for a long time that Bill was dying, but it was still so painful to hear. Before, there had always been hope: change his medicines, make him rest, watch his diet, maybe even get a human heart transplant. Now they had run out of possibilities. Now there was nothing left—nothing except an artificial heart that nobody knew much about.

"We really can't tell you all a great deal about what it would be like," Dawkins said thoughtfully. "As you know, only one other man ever had one of these. And he had lots of complications. I don't know if you all have read the consent form, but it lists all kinds of things that could happen, like strokes, infections, or one of the mechanical valves breaking. But specifically I can't tell you what's going to happen. It's all so new that Dr. Salb and I have never had any experience with one."

"Okay," Bill said abruptly. "Anybody got any questions?"

Even though the kids had listened to the tape the night before, none of them knew what to think, much less what to ask. They asked a few faltering questions about what kind of life Dad could expect, how soon he could come home after the operation. Dawkins and Salb could tell them little more than what they themselves had learned only by reading about it. It was discouraging to realize that no one else alive had faced such a decision, so strange to think there was no place to look for answers.

Stan turned to Dr. Salb, who'd seen him through all his boyhood accidents and football injuries. "If you were in Dad's shoes," Stan asked, "would you have it done?"

Salb had to think for a moment. He'd never really considered what he himself would do. All he knew was that this man whose family he'd cared for over the past twenty years was sure to die otherwise.

"Yes," Salb replied thoughtfully. "I think I enjoy life as

much as your dad does. If I knew I was going to die of heart disease, well . . . sure"—he paused—"sure, I'd grab at any straw I could."

Terry shifted in his chair. "What about Mom? Can she handle all this with *her* heart? Won't this be pretty tough on her?" The other kids looked at him impatiently. They were here to talk about Dad, about getting him well. That was what they were concerned with now. Besides, Mom had always backed Dad, no matter what.

The situation seemed simple enough: Dad's heart was giving out, while the rest of his body was in fairly good shape. If he just got a new heart, and it worked, he could keep on living. Who could argue with that?

"Anybody got any more questions?" Bill asked. The kids shook their heads. "Well, if nobody has any more questions"—Bill made a fist and softly rapped the table—"I say, 'Let's go with it.'"

Although it was a relief to know that Bill was taking control of the situation as always, that he was going to hang tough and go for it, everyone was still in shock. "I feel it's going to help me," Bill told the doctors. "And even if it doesn't, it may help the next guy. Somebody somewhere along the line is going to have to do it. And if I'm in line for it, it might as well be me."

The whole family was choked up. Margaret pulled Bill's arm in close against her side and stroked his hand. That was her Bill. He would never give up—he loved his family too much to do that. The doctors sat in silence, and Dawkins wiped his own eyes.

Bill coughed and cleared his throat. "So, how do we get started? You going to call them?" he asked Dawkins.

"Yes, I guess I can," the doctor answered, looking almost as stunned as everybody else.

"When?" Bill asked.

"Well . . . I guess I can go ahead and call them now." The young doctor reached for a phone on the wall behind him and dialed Audubon. *This isn't really happening*, the family kept thinking.

Bill looked around the table. Such a good-looking bunch of kids, after all, their faces so serious now, and so scared.

"DeVries isn't in," Dawkins said. "I'll try again later."

"Okay," Bill said. "I know we all want to thank the doctors for their time. Meeting adjourned." The family went back to the

house for something to eat. As they relaxed into the more familiar atmosphere of gatherings at home, more questions began
trickling out.

"Hey, Dad," Mel asked, "are you *sure* Humana's going to
pay for everything?"

Bill blew up. "Dammit! You heard the doctors! They said
on the tape they'd pay for it. We've got it on tape! All you want is
my money! I'm sitting here dying, and all you care about is
money?" Now Bill was yelling. His face turned bright red, and he
began gasping for breath. "Some son! The doctors say this is my
last chance and he wants to know how much it's going to cost
him!"

Mel held up his hands. "Whoa, Dad! Take it easy." Everybody was afraid Bill was going to have another coronary right
there. Bill started to cough. They tried to calm him down.
"Hey," Mel was saying gently. "Hey, I'm sorry. I just didn't know
if maybe we should try to get something in writing or whatever . . ."

As the eldest son, Mel had felt obliged to step into his
dad's shoes while Bill was sick, to take responsibility for matters
such as family finances. But now he felt terrible asking about
them; he probably didn't have any right to talk about money when
his dad had only one hope left. And he was afraid that if Bill got
upset, he might really have another heart attack right there. "It's
okay, Dad," Mel said. "Just forget it."

A few minutes later, the phone rang. Bill grabbed it.
"Hello. Yes. Yes . . . that's right. Okay . . . okay. Fine.
Yeah, thank you. See you then." Bill hung up and looked around
at his family. "Humana. They said to be there Sunday at ten
A.M."

It was settled. If they had any more questions now, they
didn't ask them. Who were they to question their dying father's
last chance to live?

That night after the family left, Bill had trouble breathing
again. He sat bent over in his chair while Margaret rubbed his
shoulders. She kept up a steady stream of talk to encourage him
and take his mind off the pain.

"Yep, we'll go up there and get you that artificial heart,
honey, and then you'll be all better . . ."

"They've got to try it on somebody," Bill muttered. "Might
as well be me—"

"Oh, I know you'll make it work, Bill."

"Maybe they'll make all kinds of improvements, and I can get a newer one in a year or two. If it doesn't help me, maybe it'll help somebody else down the road. . . . Who knows? Maybe even one of the grandkids someday—"

"Oh, you'll get that heart and come home and then you can do everything like you used to, hon."

"Maybe they'll learn something that can help *you*," Bill said.

CHAPTER FOUR

The next day, Saturday, Bill insisted on attending a wedding reception for a relative. He spent the whole time hunched over a table just inside the door. Often he had to stop in midconversation to cough; that alone was enough to wear him out. His appetite had been dwindling steadily, and now he barely picked at the plate Margaret brought him. It was so different from past gatherings when he'd pile food on his plate and dance until no one could keep up.

He told some uncles and cousins that he was going to Louisville to check out the artificial heart, but no one in Jasper had any idea what that meant. An artificial heart sounded strange, something that could never really happen to anyone they knew. But they were pleased that Bill was as determined as ever to fight to the end. He also told them that Humana insisted that the plans be kept secret, but again this really didn't sink in. What could be so secret about a heart operation?

Just before ten on Sunday morning, November 11, Bill and Margaret arrived at Audubon with Mel and Rod. Bill was so weak now that he had to walk into the hospital supported by his sons. They went to the front desk, where, as he'd been instructed, Bill asked the receptionist to page Dr. Dageforde.

The receptionist was rarely asked to page doctors to meet someone in the lobby. "Can I tell the doctor who's waiting for him?" she asked.

"Never mind who it is," Bill answered, recalling Humana's instructions to keep his surgery secret. "Just tell him to come down here," he said in a hush-hush way, as if he was an undercover agent. Bill seemed so serious and insistent that the receptionist finally summoned the cardiologist.

Margaret began filling out the paperwork for admitting him to the hospital, still unsure just what she was signing. Dageforde

73

and the boys accompanied Bill as he was taken in a wheelchair, first downstairs for a chest X ray, then up to a room in the second-floor cardiovascular unit. Suddenly there were some half a dozen nurses around Bill, all working to get him into a hospital gown and settled in bed, starting intravenous lines in his arms and getting several tests under way at once. He was put on oxygen, administered through a clear thin tube with plastic prongs that fit into his nostrils. He was breathing easier almost immediately. They also gave him insulin because all his other ailments had sent Bill's blood-sugar levels out of control. He had almost no appetite and was growing weaker from lack of nutrition. But despite his deteriorating physical condition, Bill's spirits seemed to perk up at the realization that he had finally made it to the hospital, to the top artificial heart team in the world. Now the real challenge would begin, one he could do something about: proving to those doctors that he was the one they wanted for the artificial heart. He was determined to hold on long enough to get it.

No private room was available yet, so Bill was placed with another heart patient in a room divided by a curtain. They exchanged pleasantries, but Bill didn't mention why he was there. That evening after Mel and Rod drove home, Margaret stayed up with Bill until he fell asleep around midnight. Then she found her way down the hall to a waiting room where several other people already slept. A nurse gave her a blanket and pillow, and she tried to sleep propped between two chairs. This was too uncomfortable, so she stretched out on the floor and dozed until daylight.

Around noon on Monday, Bill was put in a private room near the end of the second-floor hallway. Margaret was pleased to see that the room had a small couch with a foldout bed where she could sleep. Throughout the day and the rest of the week, Bill and Margaret were rarely alone. A never-ending parade of hospital staffers trooped in and out of his room with new tests to run or a new specialist for the couple to meet.

Bill endured dozens of tests to determine whether he was mentally and physically able to stand the stress of the experimental surgery and a recovery that could take any number of turns into the unknown. Apparently, doctors from every specialty wanted to run his or her "base line" tests to determine how the different systems in Bill's body would react to the artificial heart—from his red blood cell count to his sleep patterns. Each time someone showed up to perform a test, Bill questioned who ordered the study and why. He cooperated as soon as he understood what the procedure involved, why it was important and who thought so. He was determined to understand everything that was going on. On a white legal pad, he kept a list of all the doctors who came to see him, again in his precise all-capitals printing. But as the list got longer and longer, his handwriting became more faint and wobbly, and finally he stopped. He was getting weaker by the day.

The test data were collected for the screening committee, which would decide whether Bill was a suitable candidate. The panel, set up to comply with FDA regulations, consisted of two cardiologists, a psychiatrist, a nurse, a social worker, and Dr. DeVries. Bill had lengthy interviews with each, and Margaret also talked with them. For Bill the conversations were less a time to learn about the Jarvik-7 than to convince the heart team that if anybody could make it work, he could. Bill tried to impress on them his strong will to live and healthy attitude about life, how active he'd been before his heart problems, the goals he wanted to live for, and the fact that he had a close and supportive family.

Throughout the week, Bill and Margaret met several more staffers who would play important roles in their lives if Bill was to receive the heart. Polly Brown, a nurse, had coordinated Dr. Lansing's team for years, and now supervised virtually all the activities of the heart institute staff. She quickly impressed Margaret and Bill as someone with a knack for getting things done, who would see to their needs, whether it was as simple as getting an extra pillow or as difficult as tracking down a doctor for a conversation.

Bill and Margaret were also reintroduced to nurses Kevan Shaheen and Shirley Moore, who had cared for Bill at Jewish Hospital at the time of his bypass, and had later moved with Dr. Lansing to Audubon Hospital. Both women worked as "patient coordinators," informing families about what to expect from the moment the heart patients entered the hospital until after their discharge. The Schroeder family would see a lot of Kevan and Shirley if Bill was chosen as an artificial heart candidate.

Several other nurses had been trained for the artificial heart team, including Laura Wood, coordinator of the coronary intensive-care unit, located on the second floor between the heart institute's offices and the regular rooms for heart patients. Sandy

Chandler, a petite nurse with a very outgoing personality, spent much of that week looking after Bill. Several male nurses would also form part of the team. In addition, two artificial heart technicians would oversee the workings of the machinery itself. Larry Hastings, a soft-spoken young man, had accompanied DeVries from Utah, where he had performed the same duties for Barney Clark, and had probably spent as much time as anyone with Clark during his 112 days with the Jarvik heart. Brent Mays, a physician's assistant with Lansing's practice, was also trained as a technician.

Privately, some members of the medical team doubted that Bill was the right patient for the project. Those who remembered his stay at Jewish Hospital knew that he was hardly what they called "medically compliant." If, for example, Bill disagreed with a postoperative diet or exercise regimen, they could forget about convincing him to follow it. Even at Audubon, he complained when staffers administered medications or ran tests differently from the way he'd always seen it done. By now, Bill had spent plenty of time in hospitals, and stubbornly insisted on having things his way. Some staffers worried that after receiving the artificial heart, Bill might refuse to undergo any experimental tests he considered unnecessary.

At this point, then, it was still uncertain whether Bill would be chosen for the operation. DeVries told the Schroeders that Bill's infected teeth would definitely have to be removed before he could be considered—and even then there would be no guarantees. For Bill there was no question. On November 14, he was given general anesthesia, and an oral surgeon removed all his upper teeth. The doctors feared that the gums might not heal well because of his diabetes, poor nutrition, and generally deteriorating health. However, Bill recovered from the surgery right on schedule. The family was encouraged. By now, they figured, he must be a fairly strong contender for the heart.

Then Bill developed severe abdominal pains. The doctors found he had gallstones, which would have to be removed before he could be cleared for the artificial heart. DeVries warned the family that because Bill's body was so fragile, the stress of yet another operation under general anesthesia could be extremely dangerous—perhaps as risky as the artificial heart surgery itself, because in the latter operation, Bill's failing heart would have to function only until the heart-lung bypass machine took over and the Jarvik-7 replaced it forever.

Bill didn't hesitate. He had come this far, and he certainly wasn't going to quit now. Three days after his dental surgery, the Schroeder family gathered at the hospital before the gallbladder operation. They tried to prepare for the worst, but they also sensed that Bill was more determined than ever to hang on. Surely the doctors wouldn't go to all this trouble if they didn't consider Bill a likely candidate.

Dr. Philip Rosenbloom had him in and out of the gallbladder surgery in less than half an hour, and during the next two days, Bill seemed to be doing as well as they could hope. He was constantly receiving intravenous drugs to keep his blood pressure from dipping too low and to improve his heart's output. Now that his infections were clearing up, the doctors felt that the diabetes could probably be controlled by diet instead of with insulin. But his abdominal pains persisted; they were apparently caused by fluid buildup in his liver, a result of his poor ciculation. If Bill was going to get that artificial heart, he would have to have the operation very soon.

Although the family was largely unaware of it, other preparations for the world's second permanent artificial heart implant were going on behind the scenes. For months, nurses, doctors, and technicians from Audubon's artificial heart team had crisscrossed the country in private jets to confer with their counterparts in Utah. Now, like actors preparing for opening night, they rehearsed the roles they would play in the historic surgery. They regularly held dry runs in the operating room, checking and double-checking equipment and procedures. A nurse would climb onto a stretcher to pose as a recipient, and the team would practice every step, including transporting patient and Utahdrive down the hall between the operating room and coronary intensive-care unit.

At the same time, the Humana corporation itself was preparing to step into the international spotlight. When DeVries had announced his move to Louisville four months earlier, Humana's eight-member corporate PR staff set to work on an elaborate plan. They were keenly aware that other hospitals had been criticized for less-than-efficient handling of news about dramatic surgeries: When doctors had transplanted a baboon heart into the body of Baby Fae at Loma Linda University in California, officials came under fire for releasing incorrect information. The University of Utah Medical Center had been caught off guard by the intense media interest in Barney Clark's operation, and had to set up a makeshift press headquarters in the hospital cafeteria. Security at Utah was also a problem: Someone had broken into DeVries's office and stolen two Jarvik-7s, valued at more than fifteen thousand dollars each. Also, one day when DeVries rounded a hospital corridor, a photographer sprang from a laundry bin and began snapping pictures.

Humana faced a tricky decision. If the private company tried to keep the artificial heart experiment a secret, the press was sure to accuse them of a cover-up. The staff and the patient's family would probably be harassed by reporters seeking scoops. Humana officials decided that the best option would be to provide thorough, accurate information in formal briefings that would be open to all media.

Humana was particularly sensitive to publicity concerns because the company was often criticized by those who found something wrong with the idea of corporate medicine for profit— even though the same critics seemed to find nothing wrong with individual doctors practicing medicine for profit. Others worried that a private firm which financed medical research might be tempted to influence scientists' conclusions for its own gains. The fact was, DeVries had been unable to carry on any research at all—couldn't even begin to seek answers to scientific questions— because the money just wasn't available from nonprofit organizations.

Humana was never shy about acknowledging that its commitment to the artificial heart provided a priceless opportunity for free advertising. In a savvy marketing move a couple of years earlier, the company had rechristened all of its hospitals so that the first word in their names would be Humana. Therefore, a worldwide audience would soon hear of Humana Hospital-Audubon and Humana Heart Institute International. However, the company was also taking a risk: If the experiments went poorly, such widespread publicity might backfire.

In the summer of 1984, Humana's director of public affairs, Robert Irvine, was transferred from the corporate office in downtown Louisville to oversee public relations for the heart institute. Donna Hazle, Audubon's public-relations director, was assigned to handle hospital security. George Atkins, a Humana vice-president, would coordinate the overall PR plan. Dr. Lansing was tapped to serve as the program's "chief clinical spokesman." He would provide daily briefings to the press to ensure that accurate medical information was dispensed by an authoritative source. To deter overaggressive news photographers, Humana contracted with Black Star, a photographic distribution firm, for an official photographer, Bill Strode, to chronicle the patient's experience in hundreds of pictures that would be released to the press. Medstar, a film company specializing in medical subjects, would tape several features about the artificial heart program and film the implant operation itself.

While Bill was being screened for the artificial heart, construction workers downstairs were scrambling to convert a hospital classroom into a state-of-the-art briefing area for some 150 members of the media. A room next door was equipped with desks, twenty-five phones, and jacks for one hundred more. The PR staff, meanwhile, was assembling a hefty three-ring briefing book, slick graphics, and videotapes about all aspects of the artificial heart program. They escorted DeVries and Lansing to meetings with the local press, on the condition that the interviews not be published until Audubon received FDA approval for the implants. They sent invitations to the national media for a "technical briefing" with Drs. Jarvik, Lansing, and DeVries on November 19—before the implant was performed—so that many questions could be answered in advance. They arranged to rent blocks of rooms at a local hotel, and promised reporters a shuttle service from their doorstep to the hospital. In fact, the PR staff even considered providing the doctors with home-to-hospital limousines to discourage TV crews from staking out the doctors' parking lot.

Like the medical team, the PR staff were keenly aware that their effort was an experiment in which they would have to expect the unexpected. But when the technical briefing was held on November 19, they were flabbergasted to see more than one hundred reporters from all over the world packed into the new briefing room. Humana officials knew instantly they'd never be able to accommodate the additional 150 or more reporters expected to cover the actual surgery. So they hurriedly rented a huge downtown convention center, equipped it with radio and TV outlets, video screens, phone banks, and bulletin boards to post hourly updates and photos.

The Schroeders didn't pay any attention to the fanfare around them. All they cared about was keeping Bill alive just a few more days.

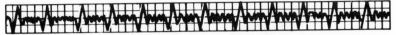

Chapter Five

Friday, November 23. As soon as Bill signed the consent form making him a candidate for the artificial heart, a short, bespectacled man came into his room carrying a couple of cameras. It was Bill Strode, the official Humana photographer. He began taking pictures right away while DeVries continued to talk with Bill and Margaret.

Earlier that week, the surgeon had said that if Bill was indeed chosen, the operation would probably be performed the following Tuesday or Wednesday. But now, he told them, because Bill's condition was deteriorating so rapidly, the surgery was being moved up to Sunday.

Bill nodded. "Sooner the better."

Within minutes, Donna Hazle, Aububon's PR director, brought in a press release announcing Bill's operation. Margaret gave it the once-over. So strange to see something like that written up about her own family. "Looks fine to me," she said.

Bill reached out a weak hand. "Let me see that." His half-closed eyes shot open. "Aw, Margaret! Use your head. They got our damn name spelled wrong! Come on, use your head."

She looked again. *Shroeder*. "Well, they sure did. How about that?" It was just a press release anyway—who really cared? Bill did. Damned if he was going to go through all that and then let them put out his name spelled wrong.

When Mel called during his lunch hour, Margaret told him to spread the word to the kids in Jasper that the operation would be sooner than expected. She'd call Moni, who was planning to leave her home in Illinois for Jasper that evening, and Terry, who had driven with Julie to Atlanta for her sister's wedding. Margaret told Mel that Humana had given strict instructions not to say anything about Bill's surgery until the press release went out that evening. Polly Brown, Lansing's head nurse, had also warned that they should bring valuables from home, especially family photo albums, to the hospital for safekeeping. Someone had broken into Barney Clark's house after his operation and stolen things like that.

Even though the instructions sounded ridiculous, Mel passed them on to Stan, Rod, and Cheryl. The Schroeders figured there would have to be some media coverage of the operation. Maybe a write-up and a picture of Bill in the Jasper *Herald*, like the time he caught an eighteen-pound snapping turtle. Maybe an AP story, or an interview on Channel 7 in Evansville. The staff at Humana had tried to warn them, but the family couldn't imagine that all hell would break loose.

Until it did.

That night, Cheryl and Glenn invited another couple over to the house on Mill Street for a quiet evening of playing cards and watching TV. Glenn was dealing at the kitchen table when the phone rang. Cheryl answered. A voice said:

"Hello, is this the Schroeder residence?"

"Yes."

"Who is this speaking?"

"This is Cheryl."

"Are you Bill Schroeder's daughter?"

"Yes," said Cheryl.

"Well, this is —— at —— TV News in Louisville. What do you think about your father getting an artificial heart?"

"I . . . I . . . don't know what you're talking about," she said.

"Do you mean to tell me that you were not *aware* that your father is getting an artificial heart?"

"Well, I—" Glenn was pointing at the TV. Bill's picture was on the screen.

"Ma'am," the reporter continued, "were you not aware—?"

"Well . . . yes," Cheryl said. "Yes, I was aware."

"And would you tell me how you feel about it? Are you optimistic that—?"

What was she supposed to say? "Uh, I'm sorry. We just really don't have anything to say right now."

"Could you describe what kind of man your father is?"

"I'm really sorry, okay? I've got to go."

As soon as she hung up, the phone rang again. Another reporter. What if she said something wrong? "I'm sorry," Cheryl said. "We don't have any comments to report right now." She had no idea what to say.

She hung up. It rang again. She picked it up, snapped the switchhook to get a dial tone, and called Mel.

"Mel, people are calling here like crazy! They're wanting to know how we feel about Dad!"

"All right, just stay calm," Mel said. "Just tell them you have no comment. And whatever you do, don't let them in the house. Remember what happened to the Clarks."

"Okay, if you say so." As soon as she put down the phone, it rang again. Glenn was trying to explain things to their astonished guests when there was a knock at the front door. "Somebody else get the phone this time," Cheryl said.

A TV reporter and cameraman were on the front porch, and wanted to come in and talk. "I'm sorry," Cheryl said. "My brother told me not to let anybody in the house." She didn't know how she was going to get rid of them.

"Well, how about if we just come in and see what the inside of your house looks like, maybe take some shots of those pictures on your wall?"

She had to laugh. That *was* ridiculous. "No, you don't want to see what the inside of *this* house looks like."

"Hey, don't worry. We can make it look real nice," the cameraman said.

By the time Cheryl got rid of them, Glenn was talking on the phone to a reporter from CBS. People were pounding on the front and back doors. She and Glenn looked at each other. "What IS this?" Cheryl didn't know whether to laugh or be scared. The phone rang again. They took it off the hook.

Up at the Jasper High basketball game, it was halftime. Stan and Rod were hanging around in the parking lot. A couple of police cars screeched up to where the town's mayor was chatting with friends.

An officer got out of one car. "Mayor, it's chaos up on Mill Street! We need to bring over some reinforcements from here."

"What's wrong?"

"Something about a Schroeder getting an artificial heart. Nobody can get through up there." The mayor recognized one of the Schroeder boys. "What's going on?"

"Well," said Stan, "I think Dad's going to get him an artificial heart."

Moni had already left for Jasper before Margaret tried to call her. Moni and her daughter, Vicki, had taken the car, while Bob and little Bobby rode in the truck. Moni wasn't really listening when the news came on the radio: ". . . doctors at . . . operation . . . William Schroeder . . ." Her back stiffened and she turned up the volume. ". . . because his condition is rapidly deteriorating. The fifty-two-year-old Jasper native has six children and five grandchildren."

"What? WHAT?" That was all. She punched the buttons, looking for another newscast. There was no place to stop and phone. She stepped on the gas.

When they reached Jasper, Moni and Bob stopped at a filling station. Moni went in to pay, and heard two men asking the clerk for directions to 1523 Mill Street.

Mom's and Dad's address? That was weird. "Why?" she blurted. "Nobody's going to be there."

They turned to her. "How do you know?"

"Because that's my parents' house, and I know they're not home."

"Your parents live there? Your father is William Schroeder?"

Uh-oh. Reporters.

"Which daughter are you?" "How do you feel about your father getting an artificial heart . . . ?" Bob came in and rescued her. "C'mon, Moni, we've got to get going." The reporters tailed them all the way to the house.

Mill Street looked like somebody was throwing a block party in the chilly November night. Cars jammed the roads. The white frame house was lit up with floodlights and TV cameras were set up in the yard. The neighbors were out on their front porches giving their third and fourth interviews to the networks. A van with a satellite antenna was parked next to the house. Soon helicopters were hovering overhead, then landing in the park down the street. It was like a Hollywood movie set, and all the neighbors were extras.

Moni hurried through the crowd. People with microphones were shouting questions. A camera crew was taking pictures of the inside of Cheryl's car and her license plate. Cheryl was in the front yard apologizing to a Jasper *Herald* reporter, trying to explain that Dad had wanted the paper to have an exclusive.

Moni whisked Cheryl in the door. "This is crazy," Moni began. "Up at the gas station—"

"Look, I don't want to hear it," Cheryl said. "Don't tell *me* about 'crazy.'"

Moni went to call Bob's parents. The phone was off the hook, but she picked it up and tried to get a dial tone.

"Moni, don't do that!" Cheryl said. "We—"

RRRRrrrring!

"—took it off the hook."

"Oh."

Cheryl and Glenn peeked through the curtains at the TV crews doing live remotes from the front yard. "This can't be real," Cheryl said. "Let's go to a movie." And they did.

Margaret couldn't reach Terry in Atlanta, so Mel left him a message at his motel to call home. Terry figured something must be up, but every time he phoned the house, he got a busy signal. Oh, my God, was something wrong? He turned on the TV and waited to call again. Was Dad getting worse? Did somebody else get the artificial heart first?

All of a sudden, it was as if the TV announcer had heard Terry's questions. The man was saying that William Schroeder was going to be the world's second artificial heart recipient. His surgery would be on Sunday. Terry couldn't believe it. He dialed Bill's hospital room, but all calls to that number were now being routed through the Audubon switchboard.

"Hello. This is Terry Schroeder calling from Atlanta. I'd like to speak to my mother, Margaret Schroeder."

"I'm sorry, sir. I can't put you through."

"But you don't understand. This is Terry Schroeder. *Terry.* I'm her son."

"I'm *sorry*, sir. Anyone can call and claim to be Terry Schroeder."

"Oh. Well . . . could you please give her a message? Tell her this is Terry. I'm in Atlanta. Ask her to call this number . . ."

He wondered if she would really get the message. He tried Cheryl again. The line was still busy. He couldn't get through at Stan's or Mel's either. Reporters close to deadline were calling every Schroeder in the phone book. A couple of hours later, Margaret finally reached Terry, and they decided that he should fly back to Louisville in the morning. The wedding party in Atlanta had to take up a collection to buy him a plane ticket.

By the time Cheryl and Glenn got home from the movies, the late news was over and most of the reporters had left. But the next morning, they staked out the house, up and down Mill Street and along the side of the house on Sixteenth. It was freezing outside. While Cheryl was getting ready for the trip to Louisville, Glenn started out the back door to scrape off the car windows. All around the house, car doors clicked open.

Oops. He stepped back inside and the car doors closed. He opened the door again. The car doors clicked open. He closed the door again.

This was too funny. "Hey, Cheryl. Watch!" He opened the door one more time. Like magic, all the car doors opened.

Glenn decided to wait until later and use the defroster in the car. "This is crazy," Cheryl said. "*Dad*'s the one getting the operation, not his kids. We're never going to get out of here. I'm calling the police."

Meanwhile, Glenn took out the garbage in record time. When the police arrived, all the car doors opened. The Jasper cop did his best to escort Cheryl and Glenn past the crowd, holding his arms out to either side. Microphones on long poles were dangled over their heads while the reporters threw questions at them like rice at a wedding.

The kids gathered that morning at Mel's farm outside of Jasper, where he and his wife, Patti, lived with their two daughters. They all traded crazy-reporter stories and joked about being celebrities. It was all so unreal, like they were in a movie or something. They formed a caravan of cars and drove to the Louisville airport to get Terry.

By now Terry's shock had turned to excitement. He had never flown before. He went to the Atlanta airport two hours early and bought a newspaper. His own dad was right there on the front page! He had to celebrate. Some men in the airport bar were discussing that guy who was supposed to get an artificial heart the next day.

"Hey, man!" Terry told them. "That's MY dad!" They thought he was nuts until he showed them his IDs. Then they slapped him on the back and bought him beers. The plane ride was terrific, Terry's seatmates were impressed, and the flight attendants wished him the best. When he got off the plane with the Atlanta newspapers under his arm, he had some time to kill, so he bought *The New York Times*, *The Indianapolis Star*, and the Louisville *Courier-Journal*. Dad was on the front page of all of them.

Then Terry spotted his brothers and sisters. "Hey, man," he began, "you wouldn't *believe*—"

"Oh, yeah, we would!" they assured him.

They drove to the hospital, laughing and joking. When they reached Bill's room, it felt even more like being in a movie. Strode, the photographer, met them in the hall and lined them up, first sending in the grandkids to pose with Bill, then the kids, then last, everybody around his bed.

They were shocked when they saw Bill. They'd known that their father was sick, but now he looked more weak and miserable than ever. His color was strange, his skin was cool and damp, and he seemed almost too tired to keep his eyes open. A huge, invisible rock seemed to weigh down his chest as he struggled to breathe. Until that moment, it hadn't sunk in that their father really was dying.

Strode was switching from camera to camera, hopping around to find the best angle. Finally, he perched on a chair in the corner and kept snapping. They stayed only a few minutes to avoid wearing out their dad. When Bill spoke, it was softly and in short phrases. "Take care of Mom," he told them again and again.

They were struggling to hold back tears, and whenever they did lose control, would turn or try to move out of his sight. All it took was one sniffle and like a yawn, it set off everyone who heard it. They were trying very hard to be strong for their dad, who had always been so strong for them. Bill didn't usually express tender feelings, but now tears were slowly spilling down his cheeks. "Take care of Mom," he repeated.

The kids tried their best to say they were proud of him and that they'd be pulling for him. Finally, they ran out of words. A heavy silence hung over them. For a moment there was no sound but the beep of a monitor. Then Stan's six-year-old daughter, Tracey, her chin quivering, piped up in a bright, clear voice: "I'll be *prayin'* for you, Grandpa."

That did it. Everybody gave up trying to hold back. Bill was crying softly, too. Margaret hurried into the hall so he wouldn't hear her weeping. Moni quickly gathered up Tracey and lifted her close to Bill's cheek. "Here, give Grandpa a kiss . . . okay, go on outside now." Then she lifted Abbie. The photographer was clicking away. One by one, they hugged and kissed their father, told him they loved him, and that they'd be waiting for him when he came back with his new heart.

It was Mel's turn. He leaned close. "Hey, Dad." He hadn't expected his voice to be so shaky. "Dad, I planted those fruit trees of yours up at the forty acres yesterday. Now, I expect you to be around to pick the first fruits off of them. You better be there, you hear?"

Bill was so weak he could only nod. "You don't forget that now, okay?" Mel said. "You hang in there. I love you, Dad."

Wiping eyes and blowing noses, they filed out of the room. A nurse escorted them down the hall to a room where a Humana company chef had prepared a magnificent Thanksgiving dinner. Margaret desperately wanted to stay with Bill. But she knew she had to be there for those kids. She didn't want them to guess how worried she was now.

It was the fanciest Thanksgiving meal they had ever seen—turkey with all the trimmings, thick slices of ham, corn, pumpkin pie, red and white wine, champagne, a huge floral centerpiece, and cloth napkins folded so they stood up on each plate. But none of them could imagine getting any food past the lumps in their throats.

Thanksgiving meant Bill banging pots and pans around in the kitchen before anyone else was up, preparing his special turkey dressing the way his mom used to. Thanksgiving was setting up TV trays in the living room or squeezing into a spot on the floor and holding your plate in your lap. It meant Bill presiding, carving the turkey, bragging about his cooking. It meant the guys drifting into the living room to yell at Detroit Lions football games on TV, and the women in the kitchen doing the dishes and talking. It meant playing cards, going visiting, or taking a stroll around the block after they all had stuffed themselves.

Thanksgiving meant family. The *whole* family.

Now they took their places at the long, unfamiliar table. Margaret held out a hand on either side, palms up, and they joined hands to pray. Somehow she found it in herself to say grace the way Bill would have: "Bless us, O Lord, and these thy gifts which we are about to receive through the bounty of Christ." She took a deep breath. "And bless Bill and keep him safe for us. Amen."

At first nobody had much to say, but after a few minutes of

"pass me this" and "pass me that," and grandkids squirming and reaching over each other, the room began to warm with the rhythms of family. Even so, the chef would tease them later that he'd never seen so much of a wonderful dinner go to waste. Margaret slipped out as soon as she could to take some pumpkin pie to Bill. He was too weak to do more than taste it.

Afterward, Margaret and the rest of the family followed nurses Kevan Shaheen and Shirley Moore, the patient coordinators, into the coronary intensive-care unit to Room 8, where Bill would be brought after surgery the next day. Like the seven other intensive-care rooms, it had a sliding glass door that opened directly onto the nurses' station. The room's walls were mauve and beige, and a picture window overlooked a wooded area behind the hospital. It looked pretty empty—they hadn't even brought in a bed yet. Dr. DeVries was waiting there in his green scrubsuit along with Dr. Lansing, Atkins, and Strode, and a video and sound crew.

As the camera whirred, the Schroeders crowded in along one wall, looking dazed by the events of the past twenty-four hours and worried about those to come. "This looks like some kind of family portrait!" DeVries tried to joke. "Um, okay," he said, making motions like a choir director, "why don't we all sing now?"

They all laughed a little nervously.

"Okay," DeVries said, quickly turning serious. "This is Intensive Room Eight, and we've got things kind of scattered around because we're just getting things ready. So, the bed'll be here—" DeVries drew an imaginary line to mark the bed's location. A large console to monitor blood pressure would be on one side, and the heart's drive system would fit approximately where the family was standing.

DeVries told them Bill would remain sedated right after surgery, while the respirator's endotracheal tube was still in his throat. "You'll be able to hold him, talk with him, and that sort of thing. He may or may not be able to answer you back, but don't be afraid to touch him, let him know who you are and that you're glad to have him back, that sort of thing, because he'll probably remember most of that."

Moni asked whether Bill would be kept in isolation, as in the case of heart-transplant patients. No, DeVries explained, because after a human heart transplant, doctors had to combat the body's natural tendency to reject foreign tissue by using drugs that suppressed the immune system, leaving the patient particularly vulnerable to infection. But because human bodies didn't reject synthetic materials, an artificial heart patient didn't need immunosuppressive drugs. Although infection was still a concern, the patient wouldn't have to be isolated.

Margaret and the kids listened, blinking at some of the strange words. They would be allowed to see Bill within hours after his surgery, DeVries said. The operation would last all morning and probably into the afternoon. It might go especially slowly if they had to cut through a lot of scar tissue from Bill's previous surgery, since such scarring tends to bleed more.

"We'll keep you posted during the procedure," Dr. Lansing added. "You'll probably hear that it's over, sometime, I would guess, between two and four o'clock in the afternoon. There's a certain amount of testing before he leaves the operating room, so we will not be in a hurry."

Lansing told them the doctors knew Bill had emphasized that he didn't want to wake up with the endotracheal tube still in his throat, so they'd sedate him until he could breathe without the respirator. "That was essential to him and certainly we will follow his wishes," Lansing said. "His lung function seems good, so there's no reason that the tube wouldn't be out just as soon as possible."

"That's really what concerns him more about the surgery than anything else right now, is that tube in his throat," DeVries said. The family nodded knowingly. Bill might be wide-awake the first time they saw him after the implant, or he might be pretty much out of it, the surgeon advised.

During the operation, the family should remember that "no news is good news," DeVries said. "If we're having trouble in the operating room, and something's not going right, we're going to send out messages immediately and let you know. So if you don't hear from us, things are going smooth, okay?" Kevan, Shirley, and the head nurse, Polly Brown, would leave the operating room periodically to update the family.

Mel asked about the Utahdrive, the large drive system, since none of the family had seen it yet. DeVries stepped out of the room to look for the Utah, but discovered that a technician had temporarily taken it to an upstairs lab. "Well, you'll be able to see plenty of it. It's a pretty large machine."

Mel then asked about the Jarvik heart because they hadn't seen it, either. So DeVries sent Shirley to get one from the nurses' station. She returned holding a funny-looking device made of two baseball-sized plastic chambers with metal bottoms. Each chamber had two white sleeves sticking out on top, and what looked like a rubber hose leading from the bottom. DeVries often used this heart when he gave speeches or interviews about his work.

"There's paw marks on it." He grinned. "This heart's about two years old. See, for example, it's a little loose right there. But this basically is what it will be like."

DeVries pulled the halves apart with a ripping sound. "It's divided into two parts. This is the left ventricle and this is the right ventricle. And it will snap in like this." He pushed the two chambers together again, put one of the hoses in his mouth, and motioned for Terry to stick his finger into one of the sleeves. He could feel the metal valves inside. DeVries puffed on the tube. The valve clicked open and shut. Terry laughed hesitantly.

"Anybody else want to try it?" Moni tried it, then Mel did. "See, that's how it works," DeVries said. "And that's basically how it is. Now, the one that he's going to have in his chest is all wrapped up and sterilized. So it's not in water or anything yet, but it's in the operating room. We actually take three of them, so that we have two backups."

Mel turned the heart over and over in his hands. It looked almost too simple, like a toy. "Those two chambers make up one artificial heart, and it's held together by Velcro," DeVries continued.

"That's it?" Rod asked.

"Yeah," the surgeon said. "Now, after it gets into the body for about a week, the body reacts by forming a scar around it that holds it in actually better than the Velcro. The Velcro is only there to hold it in place for a few days. So that's basically the heart: One's for the right side and one's for the left side. The right side pumps it to the lungs and the left side pumps it around the body. It's about as heavy and as large as your normal heart."

The kids passed it around and tried blowing into the tubes. "You all are going to be experts at it by the time we get through here, you know that?" DeVries said. Everyone laughed a little nervously. "Blood's going through it, right?" someone asked.

"Yeah, blood's going through the valves," DeVries said.

DeVries said he wanted to learn each kid's name, starting with the oldest. Moni raised her hand.

"Monica," DeVries said. "And you're thirty-one." She nodded.

"And you're Mel."

"Right," Mel said. "I'm thirty."

Then they turned to Stan. "You're next, huh?" DeVries asked.

"Yeah, Stan. Twenty-seven." DeVries went on down the line, to Terry, Cheryl, and Rod.

"So Rod's nineteen." DeVries grinned. "Sounds like something on *American Bandstand*, doesn't it?"

They all laughed.

"Okay." DeVries was serious now. "Do you have any other questions about it? Kevan will take you up and show you the drive system. And then when we get everything all hooked up and your dad's on it, we'll bring you in and we'll show you how it works, and you guys will understand that pretty easily and what all the knobs—" He stopped and looked at Margaret. "Do you have a question?"

She hesitated. "No, not really. You've explained it to me. Thoroughly." She paused. "I *hope*," she added.

"Well, yeah, you'll get better at it as you see it and get working with it," DeVries assured her. "Might be a little frightening at first, but it's easier to understand when you get on to it."

Learning to watch over the heart's drive system was like learning to play video games, Lansing added. "They beat you every time to start with, but after you practice a couple of days, you get so you know what the next move is going to be."

Margaret and DeVries returned to Bill's room to go over the consent form a second time, and the kids went with Kevan to see the hefty Utahdrive. It didn't look all that special, kind of like a small washing machine on wheels, with dials, knobs, and square buttons. They didn't really know what to think. They'd all been so caught up in Bill's struggle to get the artificial heart, this was the first time they could begin to think about what it would be like to have him tethered to a machine pumping that strange-looking heart inside. Kevan assured them that before Bill went home they'd have plenty of time to learn how to read the monitors and switch the drive lines to the smaller system.

Margaret told the nurses she'd look at the Utah later; what

mattered now was staying at Bill's side. She didn't care if that thing was as big as a house so long as it kept Bill alive.

Audubon was the second largest of the ninety or so hospitals in the Humana chain. Like other Louisville hospitals at that time of year, Audubon was having a slump in patient admissions, and they were doing some remodeling upstairs, so the entire sixth floor was vacant. During the initial weeks after the first artificial heart implant, Humana would provide rooms for the patient's family on that floor. DeVries and the rest of the artificial heart staff would stay in another wing of the sixth floor for at least the first two weeks. Another room was converted into a temporary headquarters for the uniformed security guards who would keep a twenty-four-hour watch on the hall.

That afternoon the family moved in, spreading out among three empty patient rooms with two beds each, and in one conference room at the end of the hall with a table and chairs. These rooms faced the wooded area behind the hospital, and those of the medical team overlooked the front parking lot. All the rooms were bare, and Kevan was still hunting for curtains and linens. In the meantime, she warned them: "Don't dress in front of the windows."

They thought she was joking. Way up on the sixth floor? So she took them to an unoccupied room next to the doctors', led them to the window, and pointed to the parking lot. Several television zoom lenses were trained on the floor. A few minutes later, when the kids looked out their own windows, they saw a TV camera crew picking its way along a creek.

All through the afternoon, Humana officials brought in more people for the family to meet: the PR staff, some other doctors, nurses, and technicians. They also brought some papers to sign that would release photographs the hospital could use for educational purposes. This was the first time they learned of Humana's arrangement with Black Star. The family were confused by this, but were told it was common procedure. They didn't understand what it meant, but if Humana was going to give Bill an artificial heart, they felt obliged to cooperate. They still had questions about signing those papers, but too many things were happening too fast.

While Margaret and Bill went over the consent form again with Dr. DeVries, the kids settled in upstairs. They tried to pass the time watching basketball games on TV or going to the window to look at the different television vans coming and going, raising satellite dishes, and filming correspondents in front of the hospital. They tried playing cinch and euchre and other card games. But thoughts of their dad were never far away, and as the afternoon wore on, they took turns visiting him for a minute or two. It was all so bewildering. They had no idea what to expect in the coming hours, not to mention the next few days, weeks or months. Even though they were all together, it felt lonely and sometimes scary. There was no other family there to tell them what they were in for.

Dr. Lansing tried to prepare them for the next morning's events. Unless something went wrong in the operating room, they would face three major worries immediately after surgery. First, Bill might bleed more than usual because his previous bypass surgery had left so much scar tissue, which has more blood vessels than normal tissue. The next hurdle would be to prevent postoperative infection. The third potential problem was that a pulmonary embolism, or blood clot, might form in the lungs.

Yeah, right, whatever. But that was all doctor talk, and nobody was listening closely. The doctors were the ones who'd gone to medical school—that kind of stuff was *their* job to worry about. The kids just didn't want their dad to die.

Lansing patiently answered the few questions the family still had; but again it was all so new, they didn't know what to ask. Besides, all they cared about was getting Bill into the OR and safely onto the bypass machine that would take over his heart's job until the new one was sewn in. They could tell he was getting weaker by the hour, now began to worry that he wouldn't live through the night.

Soon it was time for the spouses and grandchildren to head home and carry on with their lives back in Jasper. Just as always, it would be Bill, Margaret, and the kids, traveling together into some unknown place. DeVries dropped by and suggested that the family get out for a while and have some supper. The kids tried to convince Margaret to get out for a while, but she wouldn't leave Bill. So they promised to be back soon, then slipped out a seldom-used exit, piled into one car, and headed out for pizza. The restaurant was packed. A six-foot television screen kept broadcasting updates on the new artificial heart candidate and his family. The Schroeders tried to avoid looking conspicuous. If it got as crazy in Louisville as it had Friday night in Jasper, there was no telling what would happen. They managed to eat and leave without being spotted. Back at the hospital, the kids slipped in briefly to see their parents, then went upstairs for the night.

It was freezing in Bill's room. Because Bill felt hot all the time, and could breathe better in cool air, the thermostat had been set at sixty degrees. Margaret and the nurse, Sandy Chandler, were wearing sweaters. Bill lay propped up at an angle, working harder for each breath, as if that invisible rock were getting heavier. The hours passed so slowly. As darkness fell outside, Margaret knew she was beginning the longest night of her life. She also knew it might be the last one she and Bill would ever spend together.

That evening Father Joe Kirsch, the priest from St. Joseph's, came by and performed the sacrament for the sick, a ritual which by now Bill and Margaret had been through several times before his many surgeries. Tonight, however, was different: She could see with her own eyes that Bill was slipping away from her. She wouldn't leave him, even for a minute. All night long she stayed at his side, holding his hand, soothing his forehead with a washcloth, rubbing his arm or his back. As the hours dragged on, she would climb into bed with him, hug him, snuggle, rub his neck—anything to let him know she was still there. She wished she could do something more to help him.

Members of the medical team slipped in and out of the room, talking quietly. Some began to worry that Bill might not make it until morning. They could do an emergency operation, but they couldn't be sure how close he was to dying; his chances would be better if surgery went as scheduled.

Margaret was afraid that Bill would never hold on that long. *Please, God, after all he's been through, please just let him make it to surgery.* The man who had been so big and strong looked so helpless now.

"Come on, Bill," she said over and over. "You've got to keep breathing. Come on now, honey, come on. Breathe, Bill! Breathe!" She coaxed and coached his every breath. "You've got to fight to stay alive, Bill! Sweetie. Come on now. In—" She begged, threatened, pleaded with him to breathe. Bill would close his eyes and frown, concentrating on each rise and fall of his chest. "Breathe deep, honey! Breathe deep! Come on now. In—" It was as if each were struggling to breathe for the other.

Outside, it was pitch dark. From time to time as the night

wore on, Margaret dropped off into a light sleep while holding his hand.

"Margaret."

"Yes. Yes! I'm right here, Bill. The kids are upstairs. Dr. DeVries is going to give you your new heart in just a little bit. I'm right here, honey," she'd reassure him.

About 3:00 A.M. Bill was mouthing some words over and over. She hugged him close, listening. "What is it, honey?"

"Die," Bill whispered, "die."

Margaret sat bolt upright. "No, you are *not* dying, Bill! You're not going to die. You've just got to keep breathing, is all . . . come on now."

It was as if he were at the bottom of a pond and she was trying to call him to the surface. "Bill! BREATHE!"

"Honey, I'm dying."

Margaret climbed up on the bed and took his face in both her hands. "Bill, you are *not* going to die. You're not going to leave me and the kids. Dr. DeVries is not going to let anything happen to you. Bill. Bill! Do you hear me? Breathe! Don't stop. Come on now, breathe. Please." She took a deep breath.

Sandy, the nurse, was worried, too. She could see he was in trouble. Even if he did make it, there would be more worries: Although the nurses had special training in operating the machinery, they had never assisted in the daily care of an artificial heart patient. It was as if the Schroeders and the medical team were standing alone at the edge of a shadow, poised to walk in together. It was a huge responsibility. And now Bill might not even get a chance to try.

Like a worried mother murmuring a lullaby without noticing, Sandy started humming "Amazing Grace." Back when Bill had felt a little better, she had taken his teasing about her devout Southern Baptist roots and kidded him back about his fondness for old-time hymns. Now, in the deep quiet of the night, she softly sang one of his favorites, more to reassure herself than anyone else.

Bill winced.

"Cut that out," he breathed.

Upstairs, the kids asked the security guards to wake them at 4:00 A.M., about half an hour before Bill would be prepped for surgery. But nobody could sleep anyway.

Moni was exhausted from the long drive and all the emotion of the past forty-eight hours. And the sight of Dad—she hadn't been prepared for that. When the residents at the nursing home looked that bad, death was only hours away. But she'd also seen that Bill's eyes hadn't yet lost a certain look, the look that left when someone felt ready to die. At least he won't go down without a fight, she thought.

Stan lay staring at the ceiling, trying to remember exactly what his father looked like. He was amazed at how hard it was to recall the details of his father's face without a picture of him to look at. How difficult would it be to remember Dad's face if he died?

Rod tossed and turned. Every time he started to doze, someone would be paged over the intercom. "Dr. DeVries, seven one three five." *Oh, God*. Rod could feel his own heart pounding in his ears. Was that for Dad? But several long minutes would pass, and no one came. No phones rang. Throughout the night, there was nothing to do except lie in the darkness and wait, or, if they saw the glint of another pair of eyes, to whisper to a brother or sister: "Are you asleep?"

"No."

"Me either."

Stan walked out to a waiting lounge to get something to drink. Dr. Lansing was there. They talked quietly about nothing in particular. Lansing didn't seem nervous; that was at least some comfort. When Stan came back to the room at about 4:00 A.M., Terry was awake. The two of them decided to go see Dad one more time.

They tiptoed into Bill's room. Margaret was sitting on the bed, wiping Bill's forehead with a wet washcloth and massaging his neck and chest with the other hand. The boys started to tell their dad to hang in there, that everything was going to work out, but when he saw them, he weakly raised a finger to his lips. He was concentrating so hard on staying alive there was nothing he needed to hear from them now. He was reaching somewhere way down deep inside himself. He wouldn't even look at them.

The blood-pressure monitor was triggering again, the only sound in the room, and the readings were coming back very low. The day before, Stan wouldn't have imagined that his dad could look any sicker. But now he looked like a goner. Stan and Terry quickly slipped out and ran up the stairs to warn the other kids that Dad might not make it. The rest went down, two at a time, for one more minute with him. Each time someone came in, Bill put a finger to his lips. The kids knew why. Margaret tugged her sweater around her.

Finally, nurses came to prep Bill for surgery. It was still almost two hours until the operation. The family began the wait of a lifetime; all said the same silent prayer: *Please, God, let him make it to OR*. Wide awake and restless, the kids went down to the lobby, bought a Sunday paper, and spread out on the couch to read it. The family was all over the front page; their names, pictures of Mom and Dad, a diagram of the heart that was going to be put in his chest . . . it didn't seem real. The only thing in the world that mattered right now was for their dad to live long enough to get past those doors to the OR. Just long enough to have a chance.

They'd ask each other, "What time is it *now*?" The answer would always be just five or ten minutes since the last time they had checked. It was getting close to 6:00 A.M., so they went back to the sixth floor. They wanted to be with their parents, but knew that they shouldn't get their father too emotional when he needed every bit of strength he had left. They also decided that the two oldest should go downstairs to be with Mom when they took him to surgery.

Bill was whispering to a nurse, asking if the doctors from Jasper had made it to the hospital. Drs. Dawkins and Salb were summoned from down the hall. Even now, Bill seemed to try to appear stronger in order to impress the doctors. He gave their hands a weak squeeze. "Well, you guys," he murmured, "looks like this is it. And you're the guys who started it. Let's get this thing over with." Dawkins swallowed hard, and Salb just squeezed the hand of his old friend. There was nothing more the doctors could say, so after a moment they wished him well and slipped out.

It was still dark when Bill's stretcher was wheeled into the hall. He was surrounded by doctors, technicians, nurses reading monitors, security guards, and up ahead, Strode and a video crew. Mel and Moni stood at one end of the hall where Bill couldn't see them. Margaret walked alongside him, both her hands on his bare arm. He would have to be wheeled almost the entire length of the hospital.

The group passed the doctors from Jasper, who stood in

silence at the nurses' station, as if paying their last respects. All along the corridor, figures in white uniforms quietly stepped into doorways to watch them go past. Except for the clicking of the video camera, the hall was almost completely silent.

They reached the operating suite and a nurse pushed open the door. Margaret had just enough time to smooth Bill's hair, kiss him, and tell him that she loved him. Strode's camera flashed, and the door swung shut behind Bill's stretcher. Margaret walked back down the corridor with Kevan and Shirley holding her up on either side. Mel and Moni were waiting for her at the end of the hall. It was only then, as they held her, that Margaret let herself cry hard. Now Bill was in the hands of Dr. DeVries and God. She felt an empty relief. Breath by breath, Bill had hung on long enough to get a chance to make that artificial heart work. And if he died in surgery, at least he wouldn't have to suffer anymore.

The rest of the family gathered in one of the rooms upstairs. A little after seven, Dr. DeVries walked in, tall and pale and gangly in his green scrubsuit. All talk in the room stopped.

"Everything seems to be going okay," DeVries said. "In just a few minutes I'm going in, and we'll get started. I'll come back up and see you when we're finished." As DeVries left, they thanked him and said that their prayers would be with him. Then, almost without thinking, they reached for each other's hands and began a group prayer for Bill.

Down in the surgical suite, some two dozen doctors, nurses, and other medical workers assembled; they would be in and out of the OR at various times during the operation. As the anesthesiologist put Bill under, artificial heart technician Brent Mays switched on his portable tape player. DeVries would perform the surgery while listening to Mendelssohn, baroque lute music by Vivaldi, and jazz by Grover Washington. Like some surgeons, DeVries liked to listen to music while operating. He'd finished Barney Clark's implant to the strains of Ravel's "Bolero."

Since there wouldn't be much news at first, the family convinced Margaret to lie down for a couple of hours. The kids were joined by two priests, one who tried to reassure them by talking a lot, and another who comforted them without saying much. The family chatted awhile with the security guards, who advised them to stay on the sixth floor for their own protection. They tried to play cards, but that didn't last long. They talked together and prayed privately. Each spent some quiet time alone with memories of Bill. Maybe he hadn't always approved of everything they'd done. But he'd always stood up for them, and firmly believed in allowing them the freedom to make their own choices and learn from their mistakes. Today, by his own choice, Bill was risking and—they hoped—saving his life in an unforgettable demonstration of that conviction.

Kevan, Shirley, and the other nurses came upstairs every hour or so to give them progress reports. The Louisville newspapers had published a step-by-step description of the operation that morning on the front page. As they reached each stage, Kevan picked up the paper and pointed to the drawings to explain what was happening. At the same time, Humana public-relations officials were feeding this information to 250 reporters at the downtown convention center.

Just before 8:00 A.M., DeVries made the incision down the middle of Bill's chest. An hour and a half later Kevan reported that Dr. DeVries had connected the bypass machine to the major vessels near Bill's heart. Minutes later, she hurried back to the family and reported that Bill was on the bypass machine; it had now taken over for his heart and lungs, pumping the blood and replacing its oxygen.

The kids cheered. Dad had made it! He'd held on until the machines could take over. What a relief! They told each other they knew all along that he could do it.

A few minutes passed, then Kevan was back: DeVries had removed Bill's heart. Now he was sewing in the Dacron cuffs that would connect the Jarvik-7 to the arteries and the natural heart's upper chambers. At each bit of good news, the kids yelled and slapped hands. Dad was looking good. Margaret got up after just a couple of hours' sleep and joined them.

The kids turned on the TVs in three rooms to different channels. The local newscasts were breaking into regular programming to report each update. As they did, the family went from room to room to watch. "It's on in here!" one of them would yell, and they'd all run into that room.

As the day went on, the media seemed to be getting the information as fast as the family. Soon Kevan was no longer waiting for the elevator, but running up the stairs from the second floor to the sixth in order to beat the broadcasts, and sometimes she didn't make it. The kids would wave her back downstairs, saying, "Yeah, yeah. We already know that." It got to be kind of funny. When things were slow, the kids waved to the television crews below, and then went back to see themselves on TV.

Humana sent up box lunches, but nobody felt like eating. Since it was Sunday, there were ball games on TV, which took the kids' minds off things for a moment or two. When they got tired of sitting and waiting, they walked up and down the hall until their legs hurt. Doctors would drop by periodically— Dageforde, Lansing, Rosenbloom, Dawkins, Salb—to assure them that things were going smoothly. Security delivered a telegram from Barney Clark's widow, Una Loy Clark, who'd been trying to phone them all day: OUR LOVE, THOUGHTS, AND PRAYERS ARE WITH YOU. LETTER FOLLOWS.

In the operating room, the green-suited medical team was moving with the synchronized movements of an orchestra, having practiced this many times before. At 12:30 P.M., DeVries finished sewing all four Dacron cuffs, using tiny, meticulous stitches to connect them to the two upper chambers of Bill's natural heart, aorta, and pulmonary vein. After he tested the connections for leaks, DeVries snapped the sleeves of the Jarvik-7 into the cuffs. Next, the surgeon double-checked the heart's two compressed-air tubes, which had been tunneled through an incision near the navel. Then he passed the seven-foot tubes to technicians Larry Hastings, and Brent Mays, who connected them to the Utahdrive. At a signal from DeVries, Larry took a silver-colored key from his pocket, inserted it into a lock on the Utah console, and turned it clockwise as if switching on the ignition of a car. The Utah began a loud, steady thumping and whooshing.

During the next few minutes, the bypass machine was gradually turned down and the Utah was slowly turned up. Everything was going smoothly.

Finally, the nurse monitoring the bypass machine reported, "Bypass off."

Now the artificial heart alone was keeping the patient alive. There was too much going on, too many things to be done, too many readings to monitor for anyone to celebrate at that moment.

The operation proceeded like clockwork. The artificial heart and its pump were working flawlessly. Bill's blood pressure and vital signs were fine. Kevan hurried out to tell the family.

The team kept Bill on the table for another hour to make sure that everything was functioning as it should. About 2:30 P.M., Kevan reported that they were ready to fasten Bill's breastbone back together with wire and sew up the incision. A few minutes later, with the new device ticking in his chest, Bill was swiftly wheeled to his intensive-care room. The room was crammed with monitors, wires, compressed-air lines, and tubes. After the Utahdrive and all the monitors were in place, DeVries leaned way over to Bill's ear. Even though Bill was still sedated, DeVries spoke to him reassuringly. "You did really well. Everything went perfect. You're doing real good, okay?"

The family heard on TV that Bill was in the ICU, and waited anxiously until DeVries and Lansing donned their white coats and hurried up to report the good news themselves.

DeVries came in smiling broadly. "He came through just great! The heart's doing beautifully!" he said. "His blood pressure's one hundred and fifty over sixty, which is just fine, and he's already looking better." The tension building inside the family during the past few hours exploded into a wild round of hugs, cheers, applause, and tears. Dr. DeVries reached out to shake Margaret's hand, and she pulled him way down to give him a big kiss. Then she hugged and kissed Dr. Lansing. These two doctors had given her husband back to her!

"When can we see him?" they all wanted to know.

"In just a couple of hours, but first we want to make sure he's stabilized," DeVries said. Bill should have only a few visitors at first, maybe two or three at a time, he told them.

After the doctors had left to check on their patient again, the family held a long moment of silent thanks. Then they decided that the first ones to go into Bill's room should be Margaret, Mel, and Moni. The rest would watch through the glass door. A number of people came up to congratulate the family. Dr. Robert Jarvik, the heart's designer, introduced himself. He looked about as young as the kids, and seemed just as excited as they were. He told them that Bill's surgery had gone much more easily than Clark's. Peter Heimes, the German-born inventor of the portable drive, also introduced himself. Polly Brown, who had already changed from her surgical scrubsuit back into her street clothes, also congratulated them.

DeVries returned in another hour to say that he and Lansing had asked Bill to open his eyes and squeeze their hands.

Sure enough, Bill did! The family exulted again. The operation had really worked! DeVries said that Bill had been very groggy, but as he began drifting out of the anesthesia, he realized that he still had that awful endotracheal tube in his throat. At that point, DeVries said, Bill's whole body jerked as if he were having a nightmare. He gave the doctors a furious look, then started thrashing around, reaching to yank out that tube himself. DeVries shook his head in disbelief as he recalled: "I swear I gave him enough medication to knock out an elephant, and he's still fighting it! That guy must be strong as a bull! I had no idea—I'm really sorry." But the family had to smile. That was Dad, all right.

DeVries took them down to the coronary intensive-care unit, where Margaret and the two oldest kids had to suit up in special sanitized clothing to protect Bill from infections.

"Bill's alive. He's fine," the nurses told Margaret as they helped her put on a yellow paper gown. Margaret tried to tell herself the same thing, but she felt as if she were in some kind of dream. Bill had almost died; and now they were saying he was going to be all right. The nurses told her to wash her hands with special soap, then put on thin rubber gloves, along with a surgical mask and cap, and disposable covers on her shoes. Mel and Moni did the same. So many people in green, swirling around her like they knew exactly what they were doing. She didn't know what she was supposed to do. She looked through the door into Bill's room: so many little lights flashing, so many numbers blinking, so many needles quivering on the dials. So many machines.

She was scared to go in, but she knew she had to for the kids. She couldn't faint, she couldn't pass out, she couldn't run. Someone slid back the glass door and Margaret stepped in, with Mel and Moni on either side. All of a sudden she heard it: the whole room was going *PUM-pum, PUM-pum, Pum-pum,* like a haunted house. Wires and tubes were hanging down like in some kind of a jungle. There, in the middle of it, lay Bill. He was all white, so white, like he was plain, pure dead, with that machine moving his chest up and down. She didn't know if she was faint or just dizzy. First she recognized the sound of the respirator: *whoosh-shew, whoosh-shew, whoosh-shew.* She'd heard that before. Then she made out the sound of the Utahdrive: *clunkety-whoosh, clunkety-whoosh, clunkety-whoosh,* like loud windshield wipers. Then it began to dawn on her: the clicking of that heart, from all the way across the room. It was almost frantic, like a clock wound a little too tight. And it was coming from inside of Bill.

Oh, my God. Melvin and Moni each put an arm around her. She had to hang on for those kids. The heart technicians, dressed in the same ghostly yellow garb, were saying, "He's okay. He's going to be all right."

But she didn't know what they were saying. It was like the whole room was beating, the whole room was breathing, in and out, opening and closing. The inside of her head was pounding. Or was the pounding outside of her? She didn't know. If she could have done anything, she would have turned and run. She looked back at the door. The kids were behind the glass, smiling and waving. She looked over at Bill, then back at them. She felt like she was in some kind of cage, or a fishbowl.

She was afraid to move. There were words coming out of her mouth. "Are you sure he's all right? Are you sure?" Bill's hair looked slicked back, black against pearly white skin. He had to be dead. "Are you sure?"

"Come over and see him."

She moved closer. She saw two long tubes coming out of Bill's side. Right out of the skin! He was hooked to that big machine! She had never thought it would look like this.

"Margaret, feel his heart," someone said. She reached out for her husband's chest. She still couldn't believe he wasn't dead. Mel and Moni each laid a hand on top of hers. The rest was a blur.

When she came out and sat down, the other kids gathered around her. "Did you see him? Did you see him, Mom?"

She took off the cap and mask and wiped the sweat from her face. "Yeah, I seen him. I guess."

That whole room was still pounding inside of her. She didn't want to tell them she didn't know what was happening in there. She couldn't tell them she was so scared.

"When are you going in again, Mom?"

No. Not again. She couldn't go back in there.

"Well," she said, "how about let's try one of you all going in there next time? You all can take turns."

"Oh, no, Mom," they all said. "Dad'll be looking for you. You've got to go in every time!"

She put her head down and covered her face for a moment.

Every time. Every time. The words were echoing inside her head: every time . . . every time . . . every time.

All around her, the kids were slapping hands and hugging each other, deciding who should go in next. Dad had come through, just as they knew he would.

Dr. DeVries suggested that since Bill would be sedated for several hours, the family should get some dinner and relax. The kids suddenly realized how hungry they were. Margaret didn't want to leave the unit, even though Bill's room had been very scary. But she knew she was outvoted. They went back upstairs to get ready to go.

Someone had left them a phone number for the Louisville *Courier-Journal* in case the family wanted to say anything to the media. They were so excited and proud that they decided to call, just for a minute. Terry wanted the whole world to know how they felt, so he phoned the newsroom. "We're real pleased with the progress thus far," Terry told a reporter. "We're grateful for everyone's support and concern. Our thanks go out to everybody." He declined further comment until later. He got a kick out of that, refusing comment like some kind of political big wheel.

Afterward, Terry decided to make a quick trip to Jasper and back with Rod, Cheryl, and Glenn while the others were eating dinner. Terry had arrived at the hospital from Atlanta with only the clothes he was wearing; Cheryl was going to pick up some clothes for her mother; Rod was getting the jitters from being cooped up in a hospital for so long; and Glenn had to go to work the next day.

Security guards escorted them to their cars, and the younger kids took off for home while Mel, Stan, Moni, and Margaret went to find a restaurant. They settled on a quick meal at Steak N Shake. On the way back, they considered stopping at K mart to get Margaret another blouse, but she wanted to hurry back to the hospital.

As soon as they reached the sixth floor, Margaret called down to check on Bill. The woman who answered said there was no information available at present. That was strange. Oh, well, they'd try again in a few minutes. They all walked over to the windows at the front of the hospital to see if the television crews were still around. There were just as many as before. Mel started toward his room. He rounded a corner and ran into Polly, who was back in her surgical greens again.

"Mel, where's your mother?"

Too late. Margaret had heard. She came into the hall, saw Polly in her scrubsuit, and started backing away.

"What's wrong? WHAT IS WRONG?"

"Now Margaret," Polly began. "Now Margaret, wait a minute . . ."

"POLLY! WHAT'S WRONG?"

"Now calm down, Margaret," she said. "Bill is bleeding internally. We're going to have to open him back up and try to find the source of the hemorrhaging so we can stop it. Now I need you to sign some papers authorizing another operation."

"But they just said he was doing fine!" Margaret was in tears. "Oh, my God, he can't make it through another surgery! He's too weak!" Margaret shook her head. "He's been through too much. There's no way he can make it."

"Now Margaret, just wait a minute . . ." Polly said. Moni and Stan got there just as Polly was saying that there was a good chance they could find the problem right away and correct it. No one was giving up at this point, she told them. But it was clear she couldn't be any more encouraging. Polly motioned for them to follow her.

They suddenly felt completely exhausted, drained, as if someone had shut off the adrenaline that had kept them going for the past seventy-two hours. Their feet and legs felt too heavy to take another step. It was hard to form words.

Mel tried to compose himself and take charge. "Okay," he finally said, "but tell them not to release this to the news media yet. Terry, Rod, and Cheryl went back up to Jasper."

Now Polly looked worried. Humana had been afraid that word of the second surgery would leak out, so they had already announced it to the media.

CHAPTER SIX

The three youngest Schroeders and Glenn were almost home, soaring on adrenaline and wild relief. It was like a
secret mission: Sneak back to Jasper, get clothes for everybody
while all the media were down in Louisville or up at St. Joe's
covering the prayer service for Dad, then whip back to Louisville
before the press knew they'd been there. Even better: Sneak over
to the church and slip in just as the service was ending. Rod and
Cheryl would wait in the car and Terry would stroll up to the
front, ask the priest if he could say a few words, and tell everyone
that Dad was doing great and that the family appreciated their
prayers. Then he'd dash out before anybody could stick a microphone in his face. *I Spy*, Schroeder style!

Glenn took Terry home, left Cheryl at the Mill Street
house, and drove Rod to Lori's. In a few minutes, Terry would
pick up Cheryl, pick up Rod at Lori's, then swing by the prayer
service on the way back to Louisville.

Lori and her folks were watching television when Rod
made his grand entrance.

"Hey, man! How about my dad! Isn't he the greatest? Oh,
man, you just wouldn't believe it down there!"

"Rod," Lori began, "I don't know how to tell you this."

She didn't have to try for very long. Within a moment,
another bulletin was on TV: "Artificial heart recipient William
Schroeder of Jasper, Indiana, has been rushed back into surgery
this evening, after doctors were unable to stop bleeding in his
chest . . ."

Rod couldn't believe it. "What in the hell? We were just
there, just an hour and a half ago! That's impossible!" He tried to
phone Terry and Cheryl, but they were already on their way.

As they drove through Jasper, Terry was rehearsing his
speech. "Hey, I'd like to thank everybody for all the appreciation

that's going on back here. Believe me, he will try for you. Thanks
a lot." The best part of all was that, before long, Dad could come
home and make a speech himself, just like in his old union days.
Hell, he would love to do that.

By the time Terry and Cheryl came up Lori's front steps,
Rod was on his way out the door.

"Let's GO," Rod said. His face was sheet-white.

"But we—"

"C'mon, LET'S GO. Dad's back in surgery."

The porch might as well have fallen in underneath them.
"What the—?"

"It's on TV, man," Rod said. "'Rushed back into surgery
with massive internal bleeding.' We've got to hit it."

"Let's call Mom first," Cheryl said. Terry shook his head,
remembering what happened when he had tried to call from Atlanta. "There's no way we'll ever get through. Maybe we could
call the cops and get a police escort."

Lori called from the living room: "Rod, here it is again!"
She turned up the TV.

"Repeating what we said earlier, artificial heart recipient
William Schroeder of Jasper was sent back into surgery tonight as
doctors try to find the source of internal bleeding . . ."

"Let's just GO," Rod pleaded.

They ran for Terry's car.

The rest of the family had gathered in a tiny waiting room
on the second floor with a couple of nurses. Emergency pages had
gone out to the whole artificial heart team. Dr. DeVries came in
to explain what was happening; he was clearly in a hurry.

"Bill's bleeding pretty badly into his chest," he said
quickly. "We don't know where the blood's coming from, so we've
got to open him back up and find out."

Margaret shook her head. How could Bill possibly live
through one more open-heart operation?

"Now, the source of the bleeding could be very difficult to
find. That could be a real problem," DeVries said. "But hopefully
we can find it right away. There's just no way to predict that. All I
can tell you is we've got to go back in and try."

Margaret looked up at him helplessly. "Well, do what you
have to do," she said, and signed the release. What else could
she say?

DeVries put his hand on her shoulder. "I'll be back as
soon as we finish. Don't worry."

After DeVries swept out the door, Margaret wiped her eyes. "Bill's been through too much," she said over and over. "How can he make it? There's just no way." He'd been so weak to begin with, then all those tests, his teeth, his gallbladder . . . his heart . . .

Moni and Stan were thinking the same thing, but they tried to reassure her. "It's different this time, Mom. Don't you give up on him yet. He doesn't have his old heart. He's got a new one now." But they were trying to convince themselves, too. There would be a long silence, then Stan would say, "He'll make it. He's *got* to." Then another long silence. They were all preparing themselves for the worst.

From time to time, Mel said some words of comfort, but they were mechanical, automatic. He just sat there, numb. He didn't really know, didn't really care whether time was going by fast or slow. After so many long months of watching and hoping, it seemed the bottom had finally dropped out. He felt as if he had somehow simply stopped waiting for the results.

The nurses tried to be encouraging, but there was little they could do besides offer them something to drink or a fresh box of Kleenex. Now Margaret was worried not only about her husband, but also about her three youngest—she knew that as soon as they heard, they'd be flying back down the highway. Everything was happening so fast that no one had thought to monitor the phones upstairs in case they tried to call.

Terry turned on his emergency blinkers and buried the accelerator. A cop was bound to stop them sooner or later. Then they could get an escort. They'd have to travel about seventeen miles of state road to the Ferdinand entrance to I-64. After that, it was a seventy-mile straight shot to Louisville down the interstate. The three of them were in the front seat, trying to keep up each other's spirits. Terry was bearing down on cars ahead of them, flashing his brights, then crossing the double yellow to pass. Just outside Ferdinand, he took a curve too fast and almost lost control of the car. Cheryl and Rod didn't tell him to slow down. Where in the hell were the cops when you *wanted* to be pulled over? Cheryl punched the radio buttons, looking for more news. "Hang on, Dad, hang on," she pleaded over and over. "You can do it, Dad." Strangely, there weren't any more reports about him. Terry turned up the music.

*   *   *

Dr. DeVries spotted the problem as soon as he reopened Bill's chest. Blood was seeping from a line of tiny stitches at the back of the aorta, where one of the Jarvik-7's flexible cuffs had been sewn to it. Polly hurried back to the family to report that they'd found the source of the bleeding.

That bit of news was good, but the family couldn't let themselves get hopeful again. Finding the leak was one thing, but repairing it was another. And after that was fixed, what else would go wrong?

A few minutes later, Polly returned to report that DeVries had wrapped the site in material soaked with a clotting agent. He would hold it there for several minutes, then sew some reinforcements around it, and make sure it didn't bleed anymore.

The door to the conference room opened again. Lansing came in. Like the rest of the staff, he looked drained and weary. They'd spent almost seven hours that morning in the OR, and then had to return that evening for another tense hour of surgery. Lansing assured the family that the bleeding had now stopped. They were just watching for a while to make sure before closing the chest again. They'd suctioned out about eight pints of blood, which had pooled around Bill's lungs and heart, and had given him more than sixteen pints of transfusions, he said. Even with the complication of the second surgery, Bill was already breathing better than he had with his old heart.

However, it was hard to feel relieved. DeVries came in, followed by Strode, both still in scrubsuits. Bill seemed stable now, DeVries said. If he remained stable through the night, he'd probably be out of danger as far as the bleeding was concerned. Strode quietly took pictures of them. DeVries left to check on Bill, but said he'd be back soon to tell them when they could visit again.

Terry made it to Louisville in about an hour without seeing a single cop. He drove to the front of the hospital, where Rod flagged a security guard. "Where's our dad?" he asked.

The guard had been watching for them. "Right this way." He ran up some side stairs and they followed. They raced down the hall and burst into the conference room. There were the others, worn out, just sitting around the table in silence with their heads down. *Oh, God, no!*

Suddenly everybody was talking at once, the three older kids assuring the others that Dad was okay, and the younger ones describing how they'd nearly wrecked on the way back. It began to sink in that they almost lost not one but four Schroeders that night.

"You kids . . ." Margaret said, hugging them close.

"Well, *Mother*," Terry said, "they had us scared half to death!" Rod jumped up and down hysterically, smacking his fist in his palm and yelling, "Yeah! *Yeah!* I *knew* he could make it. *Yeah!* I told you!" He seemed relieved, but somehow more jittery than ever.

Dr. DeVries returned to tell them they could see Bill. This time Margaret and Mel suited up and stepped into his room while the rest stood outside the glass doors. DeVries spoke loudly to Bill, saying that his wife and son were there. "Tell him you're here," DeVries said. "He's sedated, but he can hear you."

"Hi, Dad," Mel tried. "You're looking great."

"Hi, honey. It's Margaret. I love you. The other kids are all outside."

"Bill," DeVries said, "can you move a finger for us and let your family know you're okay?"

Margaret looked over her mask at him. Bill barely opened his eyes and looked into hers. Then he barely lifted his index finger for her to see. Margaret leaned down and kissed him through her mask.

He knew then that he had made it. He knew he had that artificial heart.

By the time Margaret and the kids went back upstairs, it was well after midnight. They'd been up for more than two days and nights, but now they were too wound up, too exhausted, too shaken to sleep. Before they split up into their separate rooms, they promised each other that from now on, however long or short Dad lived, they would take it one day at a time and be grateful for every little moment. For the first time, they all let themselves wonder: "What if that artificial heart doesn't work after all?" For the first time, they realized that everything could go drastically, horribly wrong—in a heartbeat.

CHAPTER SEVEN

Monday, November 26. Nobody had slept well. Some of the family tried to unwind by watching a late-night Woody Allen movie on TV, but their thoughts kept drifting back to Bill. All night they stayed ready to jump if the phone rang, and prayed the whole time that it wouldn't. They slept lightly for a couple of hours, but everyone was up by 7:00 A.M. Breakfast arrived on cafeteria trays, courtesy of Humana. DeVries dropped by early to say that Bill had slept well. The medical team was going to keep him sedated so he could be kept on the respirator for several more hours. The family would probably see him about three times that day. Again, they'd have to take turns suiting up and stepping in his room for just a few minutes at a time.

During their first visit that morning, the Schroeders began to take in more details of Bill's dimly lit room. It looked so different from the first time they had seen it on Saturday. There was no way they could all fit in there now—there was barely enough room for all the nurses, doctors, and technicians. When the family did come in, they had to tiptoe carefully; they were terrified of bumping machines or tripping over the electrical or compressed-air lines.

A seven-foot monitor, about the size of a phone booth, stood in one corner. From top to bottom, dials and digital readouts shifted constantly, and from its middle, the monitor would spit out a wide sheet of graph paper with squiggles of data. IV stands surrounded the bed, supporting bags of various fluids, which ran through tubes down into Bill's body. Beside the bed, smaller monitors with glowing green computer screens measured heart rate, blood pressure, and other vital signs. Next to them, the respirator forced air through the endotracheal tube in Bill's mouth. An enormous number of medical supplies—bottles, gauze, syringes, packets of pills—lay scattered all over the win-

113

dowsill as though someone had just dumped them there. Between the bed and the glass door, the bulky Utahdrive steadily whooshed and thumped. From time to time, indicator lights on the Utah flashed, or beeps sounded from inside it. Technicians would check the readouts and adjust knobs on the Utah's console.

There always seemed to be several people in the room, ghostly figures who were hard to recognize because of the surgical garb and masks that covered much of their faces. For the first several days, Bill would have two nurses and at least one drive technician with him around-the-clock, in addition to doctors coming and going.

Bill had bandages all over him. They covered the site on his neck where a tube supplied medication through a vein; the line of stitches in his chest from the incision; the stitches in his side from the gallbladder surgery; there were more layers of bandages around the drive lines that went into his side, and a splint on his right wrist to secure the IV lines. Wires and tubes were tangled all over him seemingly without rhyme or reason.

The family took turns visiting Bill that morning. He was still sedated, but he could squeeze their hands and open his eyes. Even though he couldn't speak, the furious look in his eyes did his complaining: He hated that respirator tube. He'd made his wishes perfectly clear to the doctors, and they'd promised to respect them. They'd gone back on their word—and Bill didn't take that from *anybody*. The family told DeVries that Bill was angry, but the doctor explained that, just as a precaution, they had to leave the tube in until morning.

When the family tuned in the noontime news, Dr. Lansing was telling the press that yes, the second operation was a major complication, but not a real setback. Yes, he said, it put additional stress on Bill's body, and increased the risk of infection. "Any time you're run over twice by the same automobile, it's going to produce twice as much damage," he said.

Because the second operation had required an unusually high number of blood transfusions, a reporter asked if they were worried that Bill could have received blood contaminated with the AIDS virus.

Lansing gave him a steely look, and replied evenly, "He should be so *lucky* as to develop AIDS three years from now." He explained that AIDS symptoms took years to develop after exposure to the virus—and right now they had no assurances that

Bill would live another day. The family often appreciated Lansing's blunt honesty, but such public pronouncements would cause problems later.

By now Margaret and the kids were dragging from exhaustion. But it seemed that some activity or other was always coming up—another trip to Bill's room, somebody new they needed to meet, papers to be signed, pictures to be taken, decisions to be made. It was as though they were being watched almost constantly. Even when the family retreated to the sixth floor for rest or privacy, the crackling radios of the security guards strolling past reminded them that they were never completely alone.

In fact, the whole world was watching, with reporters from as far away as Brazil and Japan in Louisville vying for interviews. The Schroeders wanted Bill to speak for himself, but the media also wanted to hear from Margaret and the kids. The family talked it over and decided that since the press was bound to catch up with them sooner or later, they might as well get it over with. Humana officials recommended a reporting pool, which would allow two reporters to ask questions of the family in a filmed interview that would be broadcast to the rest of the media.

Getting to conduct the interview firsthand would be a prized assignment for any reporter. The Schroeders had the option of choosing one of the top outfits, like ABC or *The New York Times*, but they picked two young reporters from Jasper, Gabriela Jacobs of the *Herald* and Jon Eckert of radio station WITZ. They figured that helping the hometown press to scoop the national media was just what Bill would do.

The family and Lansing met the interviewers downstairs in the hospital briefing room. Even though the reporters were hometown folks, it was still a scary prospect. What if they said something wrong? How much would the media want to know? What if a tricky question caught the family off guard? It was difficult to know what to say about their feelings. How did people *think* they felt after what they'd just gone through?

"Dad wanted to go through with this and we're behind him one hundred percent," Mel told the interviewers. "We're a little nervous right now. But Dr. Lansing and Dr. DeVries keep telling us that everything is going smoothly. As long as they keep telling us that, we feel a lot better. We've all been worried. But we just take it as it comes. We're all together. We all support each other."

The reporters directed several questions to Margaret, asking her to describe Bill. "He's my helping hand," she answered. "Everything we do, we do together. Always have." She smiled shyly and shrugged. "And plan on still doing it!"

Yes, she told them, her kids had been a great help through the ordeal. "I don't think I could make it each day if they hadn't been with me." As for her feelings about DeVries and the medical staff, she said, "He's in the best hands we feel he could ever be in besides the good Lord above." Mel read a statement he'd prepared and passed around for the rest of the family's approval—just the kind of thing Bill would do. "We thank all our friends, neighbors, relatives, and thousands of people for all your prayers and good wishes, especially all the people of Jasper and the surrounding area . . ."

The media ate it up. This was terrific human-interest stuff. The Schroeders came across as a tightly knit, All-American family from the heartland. They were modern pioneers, supporting each other as they pressed on into the frontiers of science. The interview went smoothly, but the Schroeders were relieved when it was finished so they could get back to see Bill.

They visited him three more times that day. That night the Schroeders were all over the network news again. Gathering around the TVs upstairs, they switched between channels to see themselves on screen. It was like some wild dream, but mostly it was just plain funny. They'd point at the TV and hoot at how silly they all looked. They'd count the media's factual errors and goofs in identifying the family members.

"Oh, my God! Look at Rod's *hair!*"

"I *told* you I didn't want to go on there anyway!" Rod would say in self-defense.

Margaret was still worried to death about Bill, but the kids' laughter was contagious. "You guys . . . !" she'd say, and then cover her mouth to hold back a giggle at a close-up of herself.

Tuesday, November 27. About 5:00 A.M., Dr. DeVries removed the respirator tube from Bill's mouth and fed him ice chips to soothe his throat.

Bill swallowed, then asked, "Is the heart working okay?"

"It's doing beautifully," DeVries answered. "Is there anything else I can get you?"

"A cold beer," Bill quipped.

Everyone burst into laughter, especially DeVries. Later that morning, when the doctor faced the press for the first time since Bill's operation, he couldn't hold back a grin as he reported his patient's first request.

The press loved it. The public loved it. The beer companies loved it. This Bill Schroeder was a regular guy. Yanked back from the edge of death when surgeons cut out his heart and put in an artificial one—and the first thing he wants is a beer. Bill's thirst kept him at the top of the network news and on the front page of newspapers nationwide.

The irony was, Bill didn't even *like* beer.

In fact, he rarely drank any alcohol. But back home asking for a beer was just a good old German Catholic custom. It was a way of telling everybody that he was okay, because those who knew him would see that he still had his old spirit and spunk.

That morning Margaret and the kids saw it for themselves. Bill told them that the artificial heart's ticking felt "very forceful," but he was already getting used to the steady movement and sound inside of him. He also griped about the respirator tube and was already teasing the nurses. Yes, he was still the old Bill.

Afterward, Margaret and the kids were given a "stress class" by Gary Rhine, the medical team's social worker. He had intended to hold the class before the implant, but when Bill's surgery was moved up to Sunday, there wasn't time. The family sat in a circle while Rhine drew some charts and gave a little talk about deep breathing and expressing feelings.

Midway through the class, Dr. Lansing stuck his head in the door. He had a photograph that Strode had taken when Bill was on the bypass machine, while DeVries was sewing in the cuffs to which the artificial heart would be attached. Lansing wanted the family's approval to release it.

Margaret looked at the color picture. There was Bill's old heart lying in a silver pan. Next to the lifeless muscle, on a green-draped table, lay the shiny new Jarvik-7, soon to be put in Bill's chest. Lansing told Margaret that if the picture offended her, Humana wouldn't release it. But, he added, the photo would be useful and educational for the public. He showed her how Bill's heart, which should normally have been plump and firm, had become so thin that it resembled a flimsy leather pouch. And as happens with severe congestive heart failure, the organ had tried to compensate for dwindling muscle power by stretching to

117

nearly twice its normal size. This picture, Lansing said, would dramatically demonstrate how sick Bill had been and how desperately he'd needed the mechanical heart.

Margaret hesitated. What woman wanted to see her husband's heart on TV or in the newspaper? But then Dr. Lansing thought it was a good idea. And she remembered that Bill had said he hoped to help others by going through this operation. She agreed, and the picture was released that afternoon.

Later that day, the doctors started Bill on a low dose of heparin, a blood-thinner, to prevent clots from forming around the heart valves. The doctors seemed to think that Bill was getting better. The most comfort came from Bill himself: He was cracking jokes again, bossing the nurses, lecturing the staff on what was wrong with the hospital food, even complaining about the taste of Louisville's water.

That night Terry and Rod drove back to Jasper so they could be at work Wednesday morning. None of the kids knew how long their parents would need them around, so most of them had arranged to take off only a day or two. Now they had to call their bosses every day or so to rearrange their hours. It would be the beginning of a long series of trips back and forth, of juggling schedules and taking turns being present to support their parents.

Wednesday, November 28. Again, everyone was up early. Dr. DeVries came by before breakfast to report that Bill was doing even better than they had hoped. Margaret could now start feeding him his meals, but because he still hadn't been fitted for dentures, he'd be limited to soft foods.

These early-morning powwows with DeVries became a regular part of the family's daily routine. The surgeon moseyed in wearing a scrubsuit, and they gathered around as he sat down and hunted a table or chair to prop up his long legs. He took time to answer all their questions and outline the coming day's events.

The Schroeders were continually impressed with the surprisingly easygoing, friendly manner of this world-famous surgeon. When he spoke to them, he never hesitated to touch their arms or put a reassuring hand on their shoulders. He talked sports with the Schroeder boys, arguing the merits of Indiana versus Louisville basketball. They often saw him in the hall kidding with the nurses, casually putting an arm around them. In fact, DeVries shared many of their dad's qualities: He was smart, de-

118

termined, hard working, concerned about helping others, and had a great sense of humor.

That morning Mel asked DeVries, "Did you hear the one about the Kentuckian who locked his keys in the car?"

DeVries smiled and answered, "Nope."

"Took him a week to get his family out!"

"Oh, yeah?" the doctor countered. "Well, do you know the best thing to come out of Indiana?"

"Nope," the kids said.

"Interstate Seventy."

It went on like that every day at first. The Schroeders saw more of DeVries than his own seven children did. The doctor was watching over their dad like a new mother, constantly coming in to check on him, always right there if a question arose. They quickly came to feel that DeVries was already part of the family.

The Schroeders in turn were adopted by a larger family. The press reported every detail of Bill's recovery, and people would pick up the newspaper to follow his daily progress, just as they'd check on their favorite ball team or their stocks. The Schroeders were becoming accustomed to the intense interest in Bill's progress. In any case, they were proud of him and happy to see him get the kind of attention he loved. Humana officials began to anticipate what the media wanted to know besides Bill's medical status. Dr. Lansing gave them the anecdotes they wanted, and that morning he even answered a question about what Margaret had fed Bill for breakfast: a little of everything— apple juice, grape juice, milk, Cream of Wheat, and a chocolate milkshake. Then, of course, the press wanted to know if they were going to let Bill have a beer. Probably in a couple of days if he still wanted one, Lansing said.

Meanwhile, because DeVries had FDA approval to do five more implants, the artificial heart team was continuing to search for a third recipient. The day of Bill's surgery, in fact, the screening committee was checking out a heart patient from Tennessee, and another was on his way from Minnesota. But both were sent home after a few days because they weren't sick enough to qualify.

Between visits to Bill's room, the kids relaxed upstairs, opening some cards and letters that had arrived for Bill, and watching the TV crews in the parking lot. Then Stan noticed a Coors beer truck at an intersection near the hospital. "Hey, *that's* what we need," he joked. "Turn this way!" The truck made a left onto the street in front of the hospital.

"Wouldn't it be funny if that truck was coming to the hospital?" Stan said. The truck pulled up into the hospital parking lot. A guy in a uniform jumped out with a package in his hand.

"All right! Must be for us," the Schroeder boys kidded each other. A few minutes later, they heard the jingle of the security guard's keys. "Somebody sent this for your dad," the guard said, holding up a twelve-pack of Coors. The boys popped a couple of brews, toasted their dad, and put the rest of the beer in a refrigerator down the hall. Later they found out it had been sent compliments of a beer distributor.

That afternoon the local airwaves thumped with a tribute to Bill recorded by a couple of deejays from Louisville's WKJJ: a takeoff on Bruce Springsteen's latest hit, "Hungry Heart." The lyrics were changed to ". . . Everybody needs a plastic heart/Replace the old one with some Teflon parts . . ." Station employees also made a seven-foot-tall get-well card for Bill and took it to shopping malls so people could sign it.

The family continued taking turns visiting Bill. They were still dressing in the hospital garb that made them all look alike; newspaper captions constantly confused their identities. By now, nurses had helped Bill sit on the edge of the bed a couple of times and dangle his feet over the side. He was going through the normal stages of recovery from heart surgery right on time, or maybe even a little ahead of schedule.

That evening Bill reached an even more spectacular milestone. DeVries told him they wanted to see if he could stand up. Bill replied that he was tired, so DeVries offered to postpone the try. But Bill couldn't resist the challenge, especially since it came from one of the doctors.

Whether the medical team intended to or not, it seemed that whenever something new or risky was tried, the team attempted it at least once before doing it in front of the family. So Margaret and the kids weren't there, but staffers crowded into Bill's room to watch. DeVries stood in front of his patient. Then he bent over and Bill put his arms around the lanky surgeon's neck. DeVries crouched knee to knee with him. Slowly, carefully, Bill pushed against the surgeon's knees and straightened his own. Bill frowned as he exerted himself. He was wobbly at first. DeVries gingerly took a step back. Strode snapped pictures.

Then Bill was standing by himself. He was attached to a huge machine that was pumping his blood, and he was standing. The staff, usually cool under the intense pressure of a critical-care unit, broke into applause. Some had tears in their eyes. It was almost like the first walk on the moon—a dramatic step by one man, crowning long years of hard work by countless people.

Leaning on his surgeon for support, Bill took another four shuffling steps and was eased into a firm but cushioned chair. He was worn out, but so proud of himself. Damned if he hadn't won his battle after all. He had just taken his first steps toward home.

Back in Jasper, Terry and Rod found they had become celebrities. Terry's meat deliveries took twice as long as usual on Wednesday. Everyone had to stop him, introduce him to bystanders, and ask him the same questions over and over again. Rod's co-workers congratulated him and wished his father good luck. Just about everyone seemed to have his own heart-disease or hospital story to share. It got to be old real fast, but Terry and Rod understood and appreciated the support. After work, Terry and Julie drove back to Louisville to spend the night at the hospital and drive back to Jasper before work the next morning. It was the first real night's sleep Terry had had since leaving for Atlanta.

Thursday, November 29. That morning Margaret, Mel, Cheryl, and Moni sat with Bill during breakfast. As usual, Strode, the photographer, was there with his cameras. Every once in a while, Strode might ask Bill for a wave or a thumbs-up before he snapped a picture. Most of the time, though, Strode stayed in the background, and early on the family learned to ignore him, which was what the photographer wanted. But when he saw the potential for a picture, he was all over the place, leaping onto chairs, beds, or shelves to get the best angle. He'd be so intent, hopping around and sidling past others in the room, that his face would drip with sweat. Bill liked Strode a lot and got a kick out of teasing him, pretending to boss around his "personal photographer," as if Bill were the president.

Now the kids helped Bill into a chair and opened some of his mail for him. The Jasper High class of 1950 had sent a plaque that read: BILL SCHROEDER—A TOUGH OLD NUT. Bill was looking it over when DeVries came by. Mel told the doctor about the previous day's Coors delivery.

DeVries grinned mischievously at Bill. "You still want that beer?"

Bill played along. "Oh, sure."

"Bring one down," the doctor ordered.

Mel brought the beer, and DeVries handed it to his patient. Bill raised the can and took a sip.

"The Coors Cure," Bill joked. Strode snapped away.

When Humana released the pictures that morning, the media couldn't resist them: Photos of the man with an artificial heart guzzling beer were beamed from coast to coast. Even the Humana PR team hadn't expected Bill to become such a folk hero. And it was just the beginning. Ironically, Bill learned later that Coors was nonunion beer, and he was a little perturbed at giving them free advertising.

Meanwhile, the family saw George Atkins, Humana's vice-president in charge of public relations, about as often as they saw Dr. DeVries. George was as tall as DeVries, and a natural with people. The year before he had run in the state Democratic primary for lieutenant governor. George always greeted the Schroeders cheerfully in his booming Kentucky-accented voice. He'd start talking to them like a good friend—which indeed he had become—but eventually they'd hear what was on his mind. His face would turn serious, and he'd clasp his hands together, saying, "Hey, listen, y'all . . ." That day he explained that the national press was still in town, still intensely interested in the story, and he thought it would be nice for the family to make an appearance at the convention center. George never pressured them, but he did do his best to accommodate the media.

Nobody was really eager to face all those reporters. But the Schroeders were beginning to feel an obligation to the press, the public, and to the folks at Humana. If they faced the media at all, they would do it as a family. So Mel told George that Stan, Terry, and Rod were back at work in Jasper, but if they all could take off that afternoon, they'd do it.

Mel checked with his brothers, and all three said they could be there in a couple of hours. After they arrived, the family got into two Louisville police cars behind the hospital, along with Dr. Lansing and Polly Brown. Humana was taking no chances with security, and wanted to be able to return them to the hospital quickly if necessary. The police cars sped off, zigzagging along a shortcut through the back streets of Louisville, flashing their blue lights and turning on the siren whenever they neared busy inter-sections.

The Schroeders couldn't help smiling. This was crazy. A police escort to a press conference where they would be the inter-viewees! This would be with the national media, a couple hun-dred reporters and photographers all staring them down. What if one of them froze in front of all those cameras? "I am *not* ready for this," Stan kept saying. "I didn't even take speech class in high school."

They rounded a corner and suddenly the convention center was right in front of them. An automatic door opened and they were whisked into an underground garage, then up to a door where Robert Irvine and George Atkins were waiting for them. The family followed them through a hallway to a waiting room with drinks and snacks. This was just too weird, like the family were a bunch of rock stars and the PR people were roadies.

Irvine and Lansing quickly briefed them on what to expect. The Schroeders were to look straight ahead as they made their entrance, and ignore any questions that might be shouted at them. They were to walk in single file to a long white table at the front, where there was a place card and a glass of ice water for each family member. Once the press conference was under way, reporters would raise their hands to ask questions. Lansing would call on them and repeat each question for the family, both to clarify the query and to give them a little more time to think. He told Margaret to nod at him when they were ready to quit.

They were all wiping their palms as Irvine took them into a dim hallway next to the briefing-room door and lined them up in order of the place cards, with Margaret in the middle. Irvine opened the door a crack and peeked through. The family could hear a dull rumble as the restless reporters chatted in the huge briefing room. Police detectives and security guards were lined up inside the door in case the family was hassled along the short route to the table.

"Okay," Mel said. "Let's get this over with."

Irvine opened the door and the family filed in behind Lan-sing. The rumble died abruptly, and whispers began. "Sh! There they are! There they are!" At first, all the family saw was one big blinding light—dozens of television camera lights switching on. There seemed to be hundreds of journalists, cameras, and microphones. A few reporters pressed in as close as they could behind the police guard and fired questions at the family.

"I am *totally* not ready for this," Stan said under his breath. "These people are crazy."

They found their places and blinked into the lights bearing down on them. Once the interview got going, it wasn't so bad. Going down the row, they were asked, one by one, to describe their father and the kinds of things he liked to do. Each knew what he or she was going to say but invariably the one before had said it first. By the time the end of the table was reached, Cheryl and Stan were wracking their brains to think of something new to say about their father.

The other questions were pretty predictable. For example, When would the family consider the experiment a success?

"The operation has already been a success," Margaret replied. "Once he went down the aisle to the operating room, I was relieved, because I realized my husband was fading away from me. Now he's back with me again. I feel like I've had another chance with him."

Mel added, "To watch someone having to go through that pain, that living agony . . . A week ago he was in a lot of pain and was short of breath. Now he's the old dad again. We're not thinking of how he's going to be six months from now. We're thinking about tomorrow."

Several minutes later, Margaret nodded at Lansing, but he didn't notice.

Did they feel they could relax now? "I think that as long as Dad's alive, we won't ever feel completely relaxed," Terry said. "We're just glad to have him with us, whether it's for a little while or a long time."

Once more Margaret nodded at Lansing, but again he missed her signal.

The session was confirming what Humana had said about the Schroeders all along. They were a close-knit, loving family— average folks who just wanted their loved one to get well and come home. They could be anybody's family, anybody's next-door neighbor or co-worker, and Bill could be anybody's father or husband. They were ordinary people facing an extraordinary medical crisis hand in hand. A few reporters even got misty-eyed at times.

Finally, Margaret caught Lansing's eye, so he indicated that they had time for one more question. He called on a reporter, who stood up and said he just wanted to thank the family for their bravery and generosity in sharing their experience with the public. He and his colleagues wished them all the best and hoped Bill had a speedy recovery. The family's straightforward answers about their feelings, their devotion to each other, and their dreams for Bill's future had made for a moving interview. As the Schroeders stood up to leave, that roomful of some of the nation's most skeptical reporters broke into applause.

What a relief to have that over! The PR people and Lansing congratulated them. It hadn't been so bad after all. The police cars sped the family right back to Audubon, and as they got out, one of the officers handed them his card and offered his home if they ever needed a place to stay.

Back at the hospital, a steady parade of people continued in and out of Bill's room. Besides the two nurses and at least one heart technician who stayed with him around the clock, a host of doctors from every specialty came in to run their own studies, or just to shake Bill's hand. Peter Heimes, the inventor of the portable pack, was often there, and Strode had a way of showing up unexpectedly. The public-relations people checked in several times a day. Lab technicians were always coming in to draw blood or run a test. Since shifts changed every eight hours, dozens of people went in and out day and night.

Part was due also to Bill's own personality: It wasn't unusual to find a ring of doctors, nurses, and technicians around his bed listening to him tell stories. Staffers who needed a lift would come in, lean on the hefty Utahdrive, and get the patient to cheer *them* up with a salty joke, a terrible pun, or a tall tale about his military days. Sometimes he had the group laughing so loud that a nurse would have to rap on the glass door and ask them to stop disturbing Bill's fellow intensive-care patients. Once again, Bill was master of ceremonies, making speeches and presiding.

He continued to progress wonderfully, though he did have a slight fever. Open-heart patients normally run a temperature for a couple of days, but Bill's had gone on a little longer than usual. That puzzled doctors, but they weren't overly concerned. Bill didn't get much sleep that night because he kept coughing. This was a blessing in disguise: His lungs were clearing up as they should, and he was getting better all the time.

Friday, November 30. Each day marked some dramatic stride forward for Bill and the artificial heart, and Friday was no exception: They were ready to test the Heimes drive. It had been used on laboratory calves. Symbion, the company that manufactured the Jarvik heart, had widely circulated a picture of a calf with a Jarvik-7 grazing while Peter Heimes shouldered the portable drive. But it had never been tested on Barney Clark. If the portable pack worked, it could be the key to helping artificial heart patients live a relatively normal life. It was an extremely exciting possibility.

The test would involve unhooking the drive lines from the Utah, and then quickly hooking them into the Heimes. The ends of the tubes were wrapped in colored tape, one red and one blue. There were corresponding markings on each power source, so the process would be a little like connecting jumper cables—red to red, blue to blue. It was actually quite simple, but scary, because for that brief moment, Bill's life would literally be in the technician's hands. If it worked, Margaret and the kids would be trained to operate it so that they could take care of Bill at home with the machines.

The family wasn't there for the test, but about fifteen members of the medical team crowded into Bill's room. Peter Heimes set the portable pack on a table, and turned it on. The portable drive made a hissing, bubbling sound that was softer than the Utah's. The pumping action of the Heimes drive would be gentler than that of the big machine, an improvement Symbion hoped to implement in the Utah. Heimes reminded Bill that his heart would skip a couple of beats, and that if something went wrong, they'd just plug right back into the Utah.

Bill nodded. Heimes removed the tubes from the big machine, and the Utah's *whoosh-shew* sounded much louder. Heimes quickly stuck the tubes into the portable pack.

They all held their breaths. The steady ticking inside Bill's chest suddenly stopped. Then it started right up again, more gently.

Bill smiled. He'd just taken another step toward home. He'd be able to sling that little pack over his shoulder and go to ball games, visit relatives, maybe even play golf. Hell, at this rate, he'd be dancing at Terry's wedding in March.

Saturday, December 1. Every day seemed to have two weeks' worth of activities crammed into twenty-four hours. The kids and Margaret were often called down to the lobby or an administrator's office to accept some award or another. Trying to answer all their mail was like trying to rake leaves in the middle of autumn; letters were piling up much faster than they could handle them. And they began having visits from celebrities, including Phyllis George Brown, Kentucky Governor Martha Layne Collins, and country singers Ricky Skaggs and Tanya Tucker.

Even though Bill was involved in one of the most extraordinary, high-profile experiments in history, what Margaret recorded in her diary during that first week were the simple, ordinary echoes of home—the kids coming and going, visitors dropping in, sharing meals:

> Moni, Mel, Patti and the girls went to Holy Family Church. Nora and Ralph [her sister and brother-in-law] came about 10:30 A.M. Brought ham, lettuce, bread and things for lunch. She and Ralph got to see Bill while I fed him . . . Stan and Terri brought a big box of cookies.

Margaret was so relieved to have her husband back, taking charge and making decisions again, carrying on like he used to, letting her slip into the background where she felt more comfortable. Pretty soon she could take him home, and they would be a real family again.

Many out-of-town reporters were staying through the weekend to cover Bill's progress. The CBS crew had T-shirts made with a larger-than-life Jarvik heart printed on the front, with Bill's name and the date of his surgery. The back read: AND THE BEAT GOES ON . . . Dr. Jarvik loved the shirts, and gave several to the Schroeders. They put one on Bill. That evening Margaret and the kids proudly wore them to a family seafood restaurant for supper. It was tough getting Margaret to leave the hospital, but she now carried a beeper and kept checking to make sure it was on.

Later Mel and Patti took their girls to see Bill for the first time since his surgery. Children weren't allowed in ICU rooms, so Melanie and Abbie stood outside the glass door and waved. Someone nudged Bill and pointed to his granddaughters. Bill's eyes widened and he smiled.

The girls' lips were moving, but he couldn't hear them.

"Hi, Grandpa," they were saying. "I love you! Look, Grandpa! Look! We love you!" Each girl made the "I love you" sign they'd taught him.

Bill made the same sign back at them, and his chin seemed to quiver a little.

Sunday, December 2. That morning Father Rusty, one of the priests who'd stayed with the family during Bill's operation, celebrated communion with Margaret and Bill. Together they thanked God for his recovery. It was a miracle, really—no other way to describe it. It was simply amazing: Bill was his regular self again, recognizing people outside his door and waving them in for a chat. The doctors upgraded his condition from critical to serious, and said that if he continued this way, he'd be moved out of intensive care in about a week. Even his temperature had dropped back to normal.

As soon as Bill began feeling better, he was eager to get back in control of his life. "You kids go on home now," he insisted. "I'll be all right." Moni decided to leave for Illinois on Monday, and the others continued taking turns coming down from Jasper. Bill felt so good now that he couldn't wait to let the world know how he was doing. The PR folks and the doctors decided to videotape Dr. DeVries asking Bill some questions. DeVries gave the go-ahead for an interview that night.

It would be the public's first glimpse of Bill Schroeder, the man, speaking for himself. As a cameraman, sound man, and Strode took their places, Margaret was right at Bill's side, masked and gowned. Dr. Jarvik was there, too, along with Heimes, who switched Bill to the quieter portable drive for the occasion. DeVries ambled in, wearing his greens. He took off his mask and told Margaret that she no longer had to wear hers because Bill was healing so well.

Bill looked like anyone else in a TV interview, except that he was propped up in bed and had an oxygen tube in his nostrils—and, of course, except for the steady ticking of the mechanical heart and whooshing of the machine that kept it pumping. As the camera rolled, DeVries sat down on the edge of his bed.

Bill asked him politely to get up for a second. "Oh, hey, I'm sorry!" DeVries said, laughing. He had sat on some of Bill's tubes; the two shared a chuckle over that.

The surgeon settled onto the bed more carefully, and began the interview. "You can remember a little bit about how you felt on that last Saturday, and the last couple of weeks before you had the operation," DeVries said. "And you know how you feel now. What does that mean to you?"

Bill smiled, then began in his southern Indiana drawl: "There's just no explanation other than it's just fantastic. It's just a complete turnaround. You can *feel* it."

"In how you feel?" DeVries asked, "Or—?"

"I can breathe!" Bill said incredulously. "When I first come into the hospital, my two sons helped me in, and my wife. And they had to hold me under the arm. I sat down and put my head between my legs, just to help me get my oxygen."

Bill stopped to cough, then pointed to the Utahdrive. "But since my surgery, now, with this machine, and that machine over here"—he pointed to the Heimes drive—"whenever they switch both machines, I can notice one thing. For about a click of a finger, there'll be a pulse missin' and then you pick right up," he said, snapping his fingers.

DeVries said, "You're the only person in the world right now who knows what it feels like to have a machine, an artificial heart, in your chest. You've had the opportunity to feel it with the big drive system and then the small drive system. What does it feel like? I mean, do you have any pain with it, or discomfort with it at all?"

Bill shook his head emphatically. "No pain. No discomfort. I just wish that everybody could—well, for everybody in this room to just put your hand on my chest and you can feel! Just like a threshin' machine! The old-time threshin' machine," he repeated, nodding at the memory of that huge machine in the summer heat on his grandmother's farm. "And," Bill added, opening and closing his fist, "it's just a-pumpin' like everything."

"But it doesn't hurt you at all?" DeVries asked.

Bill shook his head. "No! My breathin' right now, as compared to the time I came in here—" Bill pulled the oxygen tube from his nose and pushed it back over his head, as if pushing back a baseball cap. "I feel like I could take this thing here and just throw it away."

"That's your oxygen tube," DeVries said, reaching to put it back in Bill's nose.

"I breathe so much better!" Bill said.

"What do you look forward to in the next few weeks, months, years? What are your goals?" DeVries asked.

"My goals is—" Bill thought a moment. "Just to be the same way as I was when I was forty years old."

DeVries chuckled.

"I really do," Bill said, breaking into a smile. "I really feel like that I could get out of here and go fishin', watch ball games, and—"

DeVries interrupted: "Last week, before you had this hospital operation, before you had the artificial heart, what did you feel like?"

Bill shook his head. "Oh, I just could barely make it in and out of the house!" The old union negotiator knew he had the floor now. "I *have* to say this. This complete, entire staff of this hospital here—especially good ol' buddy Bill . . ." He reached up and patted the doctor's shoulder.

DeVries grinned and mumbled, "Unsolicited endorsement."

"He has made history!" Bill announced emphatically.

"Well," DeVries said, "I think you had a great part of it."

"And I'm glad to be part of the team," Bill said. "And everybody around here has just been so super. . . . They've got more records—they can tell you, probably, how many rat tracks is going around this building here."

"We don't have rats here!" DeVries said, and everyone laughed. "Let me ask you . . . what does all of this mean to you?"

Bill was winding up for a little speech. "When I came in here, I had about forty days to live. And I know it, because I was gettin' weaker . . . weaker and weaker and weaker." He paused. "Since this operation, I feel like I got ten years goin' right now. I really do."

"Well, we hope you do!" DeVries said, preparing to wrap up the interview. "We're looking forward to you reaching some of your goals: your son getting married, grandchildren being born, and things like that that are important to you. And—"

But Bill wasn't finished yet. He pointed to the Heimes drive, which might make all those things possible. "That little machine right there, they'll try it on me three hours, three and a half hours. It's doin' superbly."

DeVries nodded. "Doing fantastic, isn't it?"

"It's the *biggest* change," Bill said, marveling. He pointed to the Utah. "I could *not* walk around luggin' that thing as a backpack every other day."

"You're not that strong, are you?"

"No, not *yet*," Bill said.

DeVries again tried to bring the interview to a close. "Well, you have the prayers of everybody around, in Jasper and all over the world. And your family's been fantastic. The support you've gotten is unbelievable, all over the world. And I think that's great."

"This whole city of Louisville is just marvelous," Bill said.

"Well, good," DeVries said. "Do you have anything to tell anybody out there?"

"Well," Bill drawled, taking his time, "the only thing I'd like to say is that I wish to thank everybody in my little town of Jasper. The support that they have given me has been just *overwhelming*. You cannot ever imagine what southern hospitality is until you get down there and visit Jasper. You get down there and you tell them that Bill Schroeder lives there. And come down in August! The first week, we call it Strassenfest. Oh, boy, we'll give you the beer!"

"You drank up half the beer there already," his doctor teased. "Okay, thank you for your time and all you've done. This is fantastic for everybody here—"

But Bill still wasn't through. "And my wife, she's got to be the best in the world!" Margaret put her hand on his with an embarrassed smile.

"From day one," Bill continued, "she stood by my side. I told them that no decision was going to be made unless I made the decision, and whatever decision it was, that they would support me. And every one of my kids did. They have. Every one of them supports me one hundred percent."

Bill lifted an index finger to emphasize his final point. After all, the world was watching, and if anyone was entitled to preach a little, Bill was. "Attitude. It's the number one virtue. Everybody that has attitude—they can make it through anything."

"Okay, well, thank you for talking with us," DeVries said. "It's great to be able to work with someone that has the attitudes you do. We look forward to a long and productive time together."

"You're super, Doc," Bill said.

"You are, too," DeVries answered. They shook hands.

The interview was over, but the camera kept rolling. Jarvik shook Bill's hand, then asked, "Aren't you going to tell us a joke?"

Margaret quickly stepped in. "NO!" Not on videotape anyway. Everyone laughed again.

Monday, December 3. Bill insisted to everyone that he'd person-
ally answer each letter he received. Dr. Jarvik tried to explain
that the amount was going to be staggering—from heart patients
and their families, whole classes of schoolchildren, and average
folks around the world who'd never written to a stranger. The
Schroeders were sure Jarvik was exaggerating. On the Monday
following surgery, they figured they were right. Just a few get-well
cards from friends and family had come. On Tuesday there was a
little more mail. On Wednesday Bill received a sackful of letters.
And on Thursday Polly called to say that a cart with Bill's mail on
it, stuffed into three hospital laundry bags, was being sent up.

Every afternoon the Schroeders spent at least two hours
reading letters, always picking out a handful to share with Bill.
They got the usual get-well wishes from friends and relatives, but
there were also notes from long-lost air force pals that usually
began: "You may not remember me, but we were stationed together in . . ." Most amazing of all were the hundreds of letters
from strangers, many of whose lives had been touched somehow
by heart disease or long illness. They'd relate some of their own
struggles, and thank Bill for inspiring them to keep on, like the
man who wrote: "I felt real depressed because of my condition,
but if you can do something like that and still come out with a
positive attitude, then I sure can."

Packages were also coming in by the dozen. Many strangers sent hand-crafted items, like a long placard with SCHROEDER
spelled out in cheery letters, and a musical Teddy bear that
played fourteen Christmas songs as a red plastic heart on its chest
lit up to the beat. During their press conference, the family had
mentioned that Bill was an avid Indiana University fan, so he
received one of practically every IU souvenir, including sweat
pants, posters, hats, an autographed basketball, tickets to the
Indiana-Kentucky game, and a video get-well message from coach
Bobby Knight. Thoughts of Bill taking up Knight's invitation to an
IU game floated through everyone's mind. Pro football and basketball teams sent T-shirts and caps. After Lansing told the press
that Bill was a diabetic who liked milkshakes and popsicles, the
mail room started getting boxes of frozen yogurt and sugarless
fruit bars packed in dry ice. And of course there was beer—

fifteen to twenty cases in all. Many people slipped a dollar inside a get-well card, urging Bill to "have a beer on me!" Bill also received records, tapes, boxing gloves, and fishing rods.

Security guards ran a metal detector over all packages, and opened unusual-looking ones before giving them to the family. Whenever possible, they screened out the occasional letters from zealots condemning Bill for resisting God's will by getting an artificial heart, or for drinking beer.

Several TV news crews sent flowers. Supermarket tabloids sent dozens of roses. Such gifts usually preceded a letter that said that the sender hoped the family enjoyed the flowers, adding, "When you feel like giving an interview, we'd like you to remember us . . ." In Jasper, whenever a neighbor was sick, people collected door-to-door for flowers or donations, but the Schroeders had never seen anything like this.

They had to set aside one of their sixth-floor rooms to store the mail. When that room got full, they piled some of the stuff onto a hospital stretcher and wheeled it downstairs for Mel to haul home in his truck. The Schroeders were completely overwhelmed by the outpouring. None of those well-wishers could ever know how much even the small gesture of sending a card helped them to carry on.

On Monday afternoon, Mel and Margaret were called downstairs to accept radio station WKJJ's seven-foot card, complete with a big heart on it and hundreds of signatures and get-well wishes. Dr. DeVries penned his own message near the top: BILL SCHROEDER—TOOK A LICKING AND KEEPS ON TICKING.

Bill also received congratulatory letters from high-ranking politicians. The staunch Democrat from Jasper had a ready response whenever a letter came from a Republican officeholder. "You know where you can file *that* one," he'd say, pointing to the trash can.

In the meantime, Bill was undergoing experiments, some of them unpleasant and even frightening. Even though many of the tests were uncomfortable and somewhat risky, they were part of the bargain for anyone who signed the consent form. Bill had the legal right to refuse or discontinue any experiment that was too painful or made him feel worse. But in practice, it was a Catch-22. Bill always asked what they wanted to test and why. The doctors would always answer that the test was important because they might discover something that could help him get better. Then again, they might not. Bill also felt a responsibility toward future artificial heart recipients, patients with less severe heart disease, even people suffering other illnesses, who might somehow benefit from the data collected. Besides, Bill owed his life to Dr. DeVries: The family could hardly argue with that kind of reasoning. The least Bill could do was try to help the doctor carry on his research.

That Monday DeVries had the technicians turn down Bill's heart rate from seventy beats a minute to just thirty beats a minute. Bill soon felt as weak and helpless as he had during that long night before the operation. It was a chilling reminder of his dependency on the machine and the technicians who ran it. After several minutes, they turned the rate back up to normal. Later, they briefly increased the rate to about ninety beats per minute to observe his body's reactions to that change. They also tested the effects of three standard drugs to determine their effect on a circulatory system with an artificial heart.

To measure lung output, DeVries put a tight plastic mask over Bill's nose and mouth, promising that the test would run only forty-five minutes. Once they got going, it took longer than expected. At the forty-five-minute mark, Bill motioned to DeVries and pointed at the clock. After an hour, Bill was shaking his fist at the doctor. The test dragged on for almost ninety minutes. Bill was not only exhausted but furious that DeVries hadn't kept his word. Bill sulked the rest of the day.

That night, about 3:00 A.M., Bill woke up, put his hand to his chest, and winced.

"OW!"

The nurses looked up. Bill was breathing harder. "Ow! Oh, God, something's wrong with my heart! Ow! Can't breathe!" The technicians frantically checked the readouts.

"Ohhhh, God. Get a doctor! Hurry!" Bill pleaded.

They paged DeVries, who was sleeping upstairs. Within seconds, he rushed into Bill's room, breathless and ashen-faced. "What's the matter?" he asked.

"Oh, nothing!" Bill said with an innocent shrug. "Just wanted to see if my dog still comes when I call him!"

The bleary-eyed, rumpled surgeon did a double take. "Huh?"

Bill grinned. "Guess that makes us even for this afternoon."

Finally, DeVries shook his head and smiled, too. This guy was definitely going to be a fighter—just the kind to prove that the artificial heart would work.

Tuesday, December 4. Doctors had warned the family that Bill would probably develop "postoperative blues," a form of depression that occurs a few days after heart surgery. It certainly seemed like a normal reaction: You've had your chest cut open and surgery done on your heart. Your breastbone is sore where it's laced back together with wire. You're coughing a lot to rid your lungs of mucus, and each time you do, your ribs tug at your split breastbone. You're still in intensive care. It didn't seem to need a fancy name. You feel *lousy*, not depressed.

At times now, Bill did feel worn out and cranky. He didn't eat well, and didn't feel like talking to anybody. And why not? Everyone who came into his room—and there were dozens each day—asked the same questions. "How are you doing, Bill? How does the heart feel?" After answering twenty times in a morning, he just didn't feel like doing it anymore.

But there was also more tangible evidence that Bill was improving. His bandages were removed and his stitches were taken out. Four thin tubes, which had been left in his chest to monitor his heart and lungs, were removed. Much of the bulky monitoring equipment was removed from his room, and the family set up his seven-foot card in the corner. A triangular bar was hung over Bill's bed so he could pull on it to build up his arm muscles and grasp it to help the nurses lift him out of bed.

Meanwhile, some American Medical Association members criticized DeVries's program, saying the experiments shouldn't be conducted amid the "circuslike trappings" of widespread publicity. It was highly unusual for doctors to criticize a colleague's work so publicly. DeVries endured the criticism because he believed so strongly in the artificial heart. He maintained that often people can learn more from failures than from successes—and if someone could point out his mistakes, he was willing to listen. What he couldn't stand was when so-called experts criticized his work without coming to observe it firsthand.

Wednesday, December 5. Margaret turned on the TV during breakfast so Bill could see the latest reports about his condition.

This morning Lansing told reporters: "I know it's getting boring, but again today I have to say that Mr. Schroeder is looking great."

He certainly was. Bill was in a better mood after a good night's sleep. The doctors decided to increase his heart rate from seventy beats a minute to seventy-five. Because they believed that Barney Clark's seizures had resulted from pumping the heart too fast, they had initially set Bill's rate a little lower. But since Bill was doing so well, and able to be increasingly active, they decided to try speeding up the rate.

As Bill required less concentrated care, the family were allowed to spend more and more time with him, and the rhythms of their daily lives began to echo those back home. Margaret, Bill, and whichever kids were visiting would watch a couple of the soap operas, which Bill had started following when he was too sick to do anything else. However, medical tests and treatments usually interrupted their watching even more often than the commercials.

That morning Mel came by to sit with Bill to give Margaret a rest. He brought his dad a handful of letters and back issues of the Jasper *Herald*. The two of them spent the morning reading and chatting about basketball. Bill looked just like his old self, sitting up in a chair, wearing his glasses and reading the paper. But his son still had many questions about the future. He couldn't shake the memory of the moment when he heard that his dad was back in surgery with internal bleeding, the numbing realization that the artificial heart might fail. After all, part of Mel's engineering training involved fixing the bugs in electromechanical devices. What would Dad want them to do if something happened?

Mel desperately wanted to ask his father about this, just as he used to bring other problems to him. Maybe Bill wanted to talk about it, too, but was waiting for someone else to bring it up the question. But Mel was afraid of upsetting him like the time he'd asked him about finances. Besides, Dad was doing so well. Just get him a little stronger until he could get back on his feet and do for himself . . .

So Mel avoided the questions lingering at the edge of his mind. Instead, he read the sports section to his dad and discussed the upcoming Indiana-Kentucky game. The memory of that morning would later haunt him.

That evening it began snowing hard. The technicians switched Bill to the Heimes drive, and a couple of nurses helped him stand. With Peter Heimes carrying the portable pack, Bill took a few steps to the window to see the snow. Bill looked out at the woods covered in white and didn't say a word. Every simple pleasure had become a miracle he would never have experienced without his new heart. Peter Heimes stepped back as far as the drive lines allowed—enough to give Bill a little room to be alone with his thoughts for a moment.

Maybe he was thinking about how the forty acres must look now, how the gravel road up to the farm would be impossible to drive with all that snow, what kind of animal tracks would be there, how he wanted to get back there by spring. It was difficult to tell how Bill really felt about his chances for the future. He always kept up such an optimistic front, always perked up when he knew doctors were around, always kidded so much with everybody. If Bill ever did worry about that machine, he hid those thoughts somewhere inside.

Turning from the window and leaning on nurses for support, Bill shuffled back across the room to be helped back into bed. Once settled, he asked for a pen and paper to write a note to the staff:

> It comes to the time that I cannot hold off any longer but just to come out and tell the employees in this hospital that they are the *best* employees I have ever in any way encountered toward my recovery from the artificial heart. There are not enough words available to say *thanks* to the entire staff. If all other operations go this good, this hospital staff will have a reputation as the best hospital and staff available in the world. Thanks again and you are the No. 1.
> —Bill Schroeder.

Thursday, December 6. Dr. Dageforde, the cardiologist, dropped by during breakfast to see Bill and Margaret. "How'd you sleep, Bill?" he asked.

"With my eyes closed," Bill shot back. Margaret was so glad to hear those old smart-aleck remarks again. Margaret switched on the TV so they could watch the latest reports about Bill. Dr. Lansing was still briefing the press twice daily, so Bill was all over the news. Critics complained that Humana was getting lot of free advertising through the national media. But at that point the Schroeders didn't care about controversies over ethics, publicity, and for-profit medicine. All they knew for sure was that Bill was getting better, and that he would certainly have died if not for Humana and the artificial heart. If anybody was going to criticize the program, they'd better come talk to Bill Schroeder first. One of his old classmates mailed them a cartoon from a Virginia newspaper with a pretty good likeness of Bill smiling from his hospital bed, wearing an "I ♥ LIFE" button and asking, WHAT DEBATE? That was exactly how the family felt.

All day long, there was more steady progress—more tests, more specialists, more visits from the PR people, more wise-cracks, more mail.

Friday, December 7. Bill was doing so well that the doctors de-cided he was strong enough to ride in a wheelchair to the X-ray department *and* move into a regular patient room. The trip to the first-floor radiology section was a big production, requiring all kinds of planning and coordinating of personnel.

First, Peter Heimes had to hook Bill to the portable pack. Then the nurses had to get him out of bed and into a wheelchair. Bill would be surrounded by an entourage, like he was a VIP— Margaret and the two nurses at his side, a heart technician carry-ing the Heimes drive, a security guard clearing the way ahead, Strode walking backward, snapping pictures.

As he was wheeled out of the ICU, the chatter in the hos-pital corridor came to a halt, and was replaced by whispers. "There's Bill Schroeder!" "There's the guy with the artificial heart!" Doctors and nurses alike looked up from what they were doing and stared. Heart patients strolling the corridor in their bathrobes stopped short. As Bill rode past, people gave him the thumbs-up and told him, "Nice going! Way to go, Bill!" The group picked up several doctors and staffers who tagged along on the way to the elevator.

It was so different from Bill's last trip to the X-ray depart-ment, the day before surgery, which had almost worn him out. Now he was so proud and pleased to be with people again. He smiled all the way, shook hands, invited people to feel his heart. He and Margaret were both sure that one of these days soon, they'd just keep on going right out the hospital door and all the way back to Jasper.

After the tests, Bill's entourage returned to the car-diovascular unit, where he settled into Room 2212, at the end of the hall, right next to the room he'd stayed in before surgery. It was a big move, demonstrating the doctors' confidence in Bill's recovery. The word circulating through the hospital was that Bill might be in the halfway house by Christmas.

With Bill settled in a regular patient room, Polly decided that Margaret had to get out of the hospital where she'd lived for almost a month. So she insisted that they go to a hairdresser together. Polly had a knack for doing things with a flair. If there was an occasion to celebrate, she made sure there was a bottle of champagne around. For this occasion, she gave Terry, Julie, and Rod some money to buy champagne for all the ladies in the beauty salon. She asked the beautician to style Margaret's hair and give her a facial. This was a new experience for Margaret—she'd never bothered with makeup before. Here she was in curlers, sitting under a dryer, sipping champagne, and reading *Time* magazine, which had a picture of her husband's surgeon on the cover. Suddenly she saw a flash and heard a familiar click. Strode, who always seemed to be everywhere, had caught up with her and was snapping away again.

The trip to the hairdresser was a change of pace for her, but there was also another reason for it. The next day the Schroeders were scheduled to tape interviews for three morning talk shows on the networks. Back in Jasper, Mel was making the now-familiar series of phone calls to his brothers and sisters, rounding them up for another trip to Louisville.

Saturday, December 8. The kids arrived at the hospital early in the morning and piled into a van with Margaret and George Atkins for the ride to the convention center, where TV crews were waiting.

The first interview was with Jane Pauley from NBC's *Today Show*. She was a fellow Hoosier, friendly and easy to talk with. Then they went next door for an interview with Ned Potter from CBS. Again, the interview went smoothly, but this stuff was getting old fast. The family had to dress up, pose on couches and chairs, sit under hot lights, and answer the same questions over and over. They'd learned to be careful to give the very same answers in each interview, so that they wouldn't contradict each other. After each interview, there were two minutes of editing, during which they had to sit and talk while the crew took silent shots. The kids were supposed to look interested and glance from the questioner to Mom and back. They felt silly doing that. By the time they trooped in to see Steve Bell from ABC's *Good Morning America*, they were tired and a little bored. They still didn't understand why there was so much interest in what the family had to say—after all, their dad was the one who'd gone through the surgery. Besides, the IU basketball game was on TV in half an hour.

When they all returned to the hospital, Bill was in a grouchy mood. He seemed angry at everybody; no one could do anything right for him. Even the hospital personnel were a little surprised. The family wondered whether he was angry that he hadn't been interviewed. Bill wouldn't discuss it.

Dr. DeVries wasn't at the hospital. Earlier that week, Bill had given the surgeon his complimentary tickets to the IU game. Bill knew that DeVries was a devoted basketball fan, so he'd been glad to do it. Besides, it gave him one more thing to razz the doctor about: swiping choice tickets from a guy on his sickbed. When Bill had given DeVries directions to the game, he kidded him. "Now, you got to go across I-Sixty-four, over into Indiana—hey, you know why the Kentuckians put that bridge there over the Ohio River, don't you? So they could swim across in the shade!"

Now Bill just looked glum. Some of the family went into his room to watch the game. The camera zoomed in on the tall surgeon in the stands, and the announcer made a joke about DeVries stealing his patient's tickets. The kids tried to get their dad to laugh, but he wouldn't say anything. He was also upset because from time to time, he was having trouble breathing. Technicians puzzled over the problem. The feeling must have brought back memories of that miserable, drowning sensation, struggling to suck in enough air; those nights bent over gasping in his easy chair; and that last long night before the implant. No one could figure out what was wrong. Finally, Peter Heimes noticed that one of the flexible drive lines had kinked, partially cutting off the flow of compressed air to the heart.

The discovery jolted everyone. All this space-age technology could be tripped up by something as simple as a crimped tube. Heimes realized they'd have to reinforce the drive lines, make them flexible enough to maneuver but firm enough to avoid being bent. The problem seemed so basic, but it was one of many day-to-day discoveries that would be made while the Schroeders and the medical team made their experimental journey together.

Bill was still grouchy when evening came and Margaret

had some time alone with him. He felt left out: the family doing TV shows, DeVries at the ball game, and here he was, lying in bed with an artificial heart, still weak and sore from surgery.

Margaret insisted that he watch the evening news with her.

"Why would I want to do that?" Bill muttered. Margaret said nothing but flipped to the news and sat down beside him. Bill had no choice but to watch. When a portion of the family's interviews came on, she reached out and took his hand.

There they were, all six kids, telling the whole world what a terrific guy their dad was, and how proud they were of him. Margaret squeezed his hand, kissed his cheek, and said softly, "Now, don't you feel a little foolish about being angry? Those kids really love you! See?" She turned his face toward hers, and saw tears in his eyes.

When DeVries returned from the game, he got a full report from the staff about Bill's bad mood. So he went in to assure Bill that this was normal for any heart patient at his stage of recovery. They spoke for quite a while, just the two of them, and afterward Bill seemed to feel better.

A heart surgeon usually sees a patient for only a brief, intense period—on the operating table and then later for a few days at the most. Then the patient's care is taken over by specialists, such as cardiologists and internists. DeVries, however, was rapidly becoming more than just Bill's surgeon. The two men had already gone through so much together, already worked so hard for each other, that they had quickly grown to be good friends. Bill Strode had spotted the bond developing between surgeon and patient, and his photographs began to capture the mutual admiration and respect that showed in their eyes whenever they looked at each other.

That evening Dr. Salb dropped in for a visit and helped the family open their mail. Some friends from Michigan also drove in to see Bill. The visits did wonders for his spirits, and he joked around and told stories on his old pals until late into the night.

Sunday, December 9. Even though Sundays were usually slower at the hospital, today was busy for Bill and Margaret. All the kids came down, along with Bill's brothers, Jerry and Paul, and their families. It was like a Sunday back at the house on Mill Street, bustling with relatives bringing trays of homemade goodies and catching up on each other. At times, the old sounds of family laughter and news from home almost drowned out the ticking of the Jarvik-7 and the Utah's steady whoosh. For a moment or two, the Schroeders could forget that one of them had a heart made of plastic.

But each time things settled into some sort of routine at the hospital, Bill would do something else spectacular that put him back in the spotlight. That evening, after most of the family had gone back home, he did it again, in one of the most dramatic television interviews in history.

CHAPTER EIGHT

For this interview, people crowded around Bill's bed even more closely than the first time. The interviewers were ABC correspondent George Strait, and Dr. Lawrence K. Altman, medical writer for *The New York Times*. Other media people had gathered in the room: a TV news producer, a cameraman, and a sound woman, and Mark Mayfield, a reporter from *USA Today*. Again, the footage would be pooled for the rest of the media. The heart technicians were there—Heimes, Hastings, and Mays— plus DeVries, Atkins, and Strode with his flash camera. Some family members also squeezed in: Mel, Moni, her husband, Bob, and their two kids sat in the corner. The room quickly grew warm because of all the people and hot lights.

Bill looked apple-cheeked and exuberant, eager to begin. He lay propped up in bed with the Heimes drive resting on the bedside table as it pumped his heart. Margaret sat down next to him, and everybody else took their places.

The cameras switched on, and Altman began. "How do you feel this evening?"

"I feel real good. Real good," Bill drawled. He thought for a moment. "The last couple of days I've felt a little down. But the last two days now, I've come back and picked up, and eating, and feel real good. I feel super."

"You look terrific," Strait said almost incredulously. "A lot of people say this heart will be a success if you should get to go home, or if you're just feeling better today. What about your criteria for success?"

"My criteria for success," Bill said, tapping his chest with his finger, "is what I got right now. That's what my criteria is." He paused. "I only had about forty days to live. But with the new heart, I feel like I got *ten years*. I really do. And I don't see no reason why this thing wouldn't last no ten years. As you go along,

143

it's going to improve. It's just like if I had to have a leg taken off. You can put in a new artificial leg, you know. So you just put in a new artificial heart. That's the way I look at it."

Did the heart cause him pain or discomfort? Altman asked.

"None," Bill said flatly. "The pain was about the same as when I had open-heart surgery, first time around. And I knew what it was like. I knew that the mucus was going to be there, and I was going to have to cough that up. It's just about all gone now. I do very little coughin'." Bill seemed as relaxed as if he was shooting the breeze on his lunch hour.

"I ain't felt no pain since," Bill continued. "As my family and everybody that's in here can attest, I can sit up on the side of the bed, and walk, and carry the 'day-pack,'" he said, nodding toward the Heimes.

"The one thing that I can see now," Bill said, "is that I'm not short of breath like before. I could walk in the house and sit down, and I'd just about had it. Man, it was just like I was goin' to fall *over!*" He shook his head and frowned, remembering.

Strait nodded. They certainly didn't have to prompt this guy or try to draw him out. "Mr. Schroeder," he asked, "I think especially since the first day after the surgery and the 'Coors Cure,' the American public has an idea of what kind of guy you are: kind of a macho guy that likes a beer once in a while. Why don't you tell people what you are really like? Have the news accounts of who you are and what you are been accurate?"

"Okay. I'm the type of a guy that likes a joke. I got a collection of jokes about that thick," Bill said proudly, holding his thumb and forefinger apart almost as far as he could. "Collected it over twenty years of military service, and what-have-you, and cartoons, what-have-you. Everybody's always lookin' forward to my jokes."

Strait asked if Bill had seen news accounts of his hospital stay, and if so, had they been important to his recovery?

"Yeah," Bill said. "I seen a lot of them, and I hope that this is just the beginning, that Dr. DeVries can continue and go on further and get some more. I know that as you go on, things will develop, and things will be a lot better. Things are goin' to be, oh, just super."

Altman then asked what he would tell the next Jarvik-7 recipient to expect.

"I'd probably tell him, if he'd ever had open-heart surgery, it wouldn't be any different," Bill answered. "The only difference is that you got two tubes comin' out of your side. With the improved day-pack, you'd be able to go around nearly eight hours a day, maybe sixteen hours a day, and still live a normal life. There'd be some things they couldn't do, like swimming, things like that. I like fishin' and I like to go watch ball games, things like that, y'know. This will give me time to do it. I don't have to sit at home. I can get outside and do it—and that's what I'd like to do."

Strait mentioned the criticism from the AMA. "Every day Dr. Lansing will come down and tell us how you're doing in a very detailed way. The AMA said releasing that kind of detailed information may not be in the best interest of the patient, that it should be withheld and not told to the American public until it's published in a scientific journal. What do you think about this?"

"I don't think so," Bill said, again just as casually as if simply discussing current events or politics with his pals. Bill said that the sooner they got the information out to the public, the better. That way everybody, including potential artificial heart patients, could form their own opinions.

Strait asked, "Do you think that the release of all of this information hurt you?"

"No." Bill shook his head emphatically. "I don't care if they release every bit of information they got on me. I don't care if they come out and tell the public that I have this, I have that, what-have-you. That doesn't bother me."

Bill began to count on his fingers for emphasis: "All I wanted to do was, number one, to get myself healthy. Number two, I wanted to be able to help other people. And if I can succeed in any of those two, I'll feel like my mission's been accomplished."

For a long moment, there was no sound but the pumping of the Heimes.

Altman asked if Bill had been paying special attention when Barney Clark was hospitalized two years before.

"No, I really wasn't," Bill said. "I didn't take no interest in it, because at that time 'bypass' was all they talked about for me. I didn't know none of this stuff existed, *none* of it." He smiled broadly.

"I'm glad I do *now*," he added. "Surrrre saved me."

Strait asked if his goals had expanded beyond simply staying alive and attending his son's wedding in March.

Bill couldn't keep back a grin at the thought of Terry's wedding. "Well, yes, I look on expectations beyond that," he said and for a moment his eyes seemed to be gazing somewhere far off.

"I can look forward to going out and crackin' my walnuts, pickin' my walnuts out in the wintertime. And do things like, you know, in your winter months. I like to do that. In the fall, I can hunt walnuts, and . . . oh, just about anything." He smiled again. "And fish," he added, "aw, yeah, fish. *Love* to fish."

Strait asked, "Do you feel like you have a new purpose?"

"Yeah." Bill nodded seriously. "I have a real new purpose on life. And that purpose is to be with God. I feel like He was the Number One that saved me."

Bill glanced over at Margaret, then up at DeVries. The instant their eyes met, every line in Bill's face changed. Suddenly he was fighting tears. He took his surgeon's hand, squeezed it, and patted it hard.

Then Bill looked at Margaret again. His chin trembled as he struggled not to cry. He couldn't say anything else. Margaret leaned forward and kissed him. Bill took her hand and turned back to the interviewers, his eyes filled with tears.

"That's my big purpose right here," Bill said in a quavery voice. He swallowed hard. "We've been married for thirty-two years, and I wouldn't take anything in the whole world for her."

He wiped his eyes and said: "Excuse me," and tried to collect himself. He took a deep breath and continued: "I believe I got something to look forward to now. Forty days—I wouldn't even have Christmas. So, I'm just thankful. I've got her, and six healthy children. They're just as healthy as they can be." Margaret dabbed a tissue at the tears spilling along his temples.

"You know," Altman said gently, "it's very touching to hear your feelings now. I think you knew before, many people regard the heart as the seat of emotions—and you have great emotion. I wonder if you could tell the American public what it is like to have an artificial heart and still have emotions?"

Bill smiled. "Well," he said softly. "I don't know if I can tell you that. I think you can probably explain that more by just feelin' what you just now felt. But it does, it just thumps in there. And I can feel it. It doesn't bother my sleep. It doesn't bother me at all. I don't even know that it's there, I've got so used to it. And it really goes—just takin' off like a horse," he said, shaking his head in wonder. "Who knows," he added, trying to lighten up the mood, "maybe I'll be the Bionic Man!"

"I don't think it cost six million dollars, though," Strait said.

"No," Bill laughed, "I don't think so."

Altman asked what concerns Bill had about being discharged from the hospital.

"My concern is going to be that I don't want to go home until I understand this 'output machine' over here, the Utah pack and the big one." Bill gestured toward the Heimes and the unused Utah by his bed, but he'd gotten their names confused. "I want to be able to fully understand. I want to get a van, have a lift put in it, put the machine in it, anchor it, so that I can drive. Or if I don't want to drive, my wife can drive. Whatever."

Strait asked what other preparations were being made for Bill's return home—besides perhaps cutting holes in his shirts for the drive lines.

"Well, the comforts of it doesn't bother me," Bill said with a shrug. "The thing that I want to do is get healthy and get around. As far as having holes in my shirt, that doesn't bother me. I got scars all over me. I've had that leg stripped twice. I've had that arm broken. I've had that wrist broken." He casually held up his hand to show where, as a teenager, a bullet had accidentally grazed it. "I've shot myself here," he said. He pointed to his side. "I've had appendicitis here. I've got a gallbladder out. You name it—I had open-heart history. I got it all."

"What are the little things that you won't be able to do?" Strait asked. "What about taking a shower and taking a bath?"

"That you can do," Bill explained, as if he'd always known. "You can do that with the 'porta-pack' on. In fact, they want you to keep that clean around there," he said, pulling up his pajama top to show where the drive lines entered his abdomen. The site hadn't healed, so it was still covered with sterile gauze. "I don't know if you can visualize it, but this is where the tubes come out. They're pretty durable. But while they grow into the skin, it'll be kept clean thataway."

Altman asked Bill to describe the source of his strong will to live.

Bill answered that as a sergeant in the air force, he'd always tried to instill the right attitude in his men. "With attitude,"

Bill said, "you can just about get anybody through anything. If you're out to set a goal, and you want it done, you're goin' to get it done if you got the attitude. Anybody in this world can do it. They just have to set their mind to it, and go with it, and they're goin' to get it done." He described setting his sights on an elective office in his union, and how he'd achieved that goal, even though his heart problems prevented him from serving out his term.

The reporters thanked him for the interview, saying that it had been a particularly special one.

"Well, I have to thank you for that," Bill said. "I'm not here for praise or glory. I'm just here to get well, and show other people what can be done."

Strait asked whether Bill was bothered by knowing that he could spend the rest of his life tethered to a huge machine.

"No. No, I'm not," Bill said. "I think there's a time gonna come where you won't *be* tethered to a machine. I can remember my dad had sugar diabetes, and lost both legs, was confined to a wheelchair. But you get around. There's a lot of handicapped people worse off than I am. At least, they can't walk, you know. Or bein' blind—what could be worse than bein' blind?"

"Are you worried at all about the machine breaking?" Strait asked.

"No . . . the machine—I wouldn't even be able to guess how many times we've run it, but we've run it on an average of three to four hours a day," he said, referring to the Heimes. "And it's never broke down yet. And besides, there's a backup for that, and a backup for that. So there's always backups."

"Some people have wondered if you feel that a piece of you died when you lost your own heart," Altman said. "Do you have any feelings toward that?"

"No," Bill answered. "In fact, I signed a consent paper that they could use my old heart, and study it, and do whatever they think is necessary to further their study. It's of no value to me. I've got a new one."

Bill was getting tired, but Strait said, "This'll be your big chance: Is there anything here that you want that these people haven't given you?"

Bill started to shake his head "no," but out of the corner of his eye, he caught DeVries grinning at him significantly.

Bill's eyes widened, and he smiled back at the surgeon

with a sly look that said, "ANYTHING, huh?" Everyone started laughing.

"You can't have THAT yet!" DeVries warned.

Bill looked back at the interviewers with a big smile. "Wellll, since you put it *that* way . . . no," he sighed, prompting even more laughs.

"No," he said seriously now, "they've been awful nice to me. Just one super, super-duper crew. They've bent over backwards. There just isn't anything here that they haven't done for me. They're really good. Everything's good."

"In closing," Altman said, "is there anything that we haven't asked you that you want to tell the public, that we weren't smart enough to ask you about?"

"Well," Bill said, "I'm not going to say you're not smart enough, because you're smarter than I am." He paused to think. "But I would say to the people out there in the public: If you have a heart problem, and you need to take care of it, don't wait till it's too late. 'Cause the last tick it does—that's *it*. Get it corrected while you can. At least you're gonna have another—oh, I'd say— ten years."

Strait slipped in a final question about the consent form: "I wonder if it was really possible for you to objectively sign a piece of paper like that when you know yourself that you only have forty days to live. Is it possible, really, to have informed consent when you're under the gun like that?"

"No," Bill said, matter-of-factly. "I had met with Dr. De-Vries on a Thursday, and we discussed it, went home. Then on a Friday evening, with my doctors in my hometown of Jasper, Dr. Phil Dawkins and Dr. J. P. Salb, we went down into the hospital conference room at the doctors' office and laid it on the line. I told them then, I said, 'If there is anything in this world that you people are holdin' back, I want to know it. I want everything up front, laid out, right to the tee, and right now.'

"And they did. I says, 'How many days do I have?' And they told me. So I says, 'Okay.' Now, my children were there, my wife was there, and I said, 'Do you kids got any problems?' They said, 'No.'"

Again, Bill's eyes filled with tears, and his voice went higher as he continued. "So I said, 'Go with it.'"

He swallowed. "So we did."

He took another moment to gather his composure. "And I

said that no matter what happened, if it didn't come out, they would learn something. If it did, that's forty days. What's forty days, you know?"

The only sound was the mechanical whooshing of the Heimes. Bill wanted to make one last point: "You brought the subject up about the American Medical Association and all that. Well, *why* should you prolong something when you know you got a chance, and you can make it? And I feel like I had a chance to make it. I've taken chances all of my life! I believe in them. I was gung-ho for this thing. The only thing that worries me whenever I have surgery is my diabetes—I'm afraid I won't heal. But I have so far.

"Everything was set in place. And I told Dr. DeVries, we called him that night, and he said to come in Sunday. After that, you got to have patience, but we got it going."

"Mr. Schroeder," Strait said. "You're terrific."

"Perfect," Altman said.

Monday, December 10. That morning the whole hospital was buzzing about what Bill had said in the interview. As he and Margaret ate breakfast, they watched themselves again and again on the morning news. It was still strange seeing themselves on TV, but there was Bill, big as life, holding forth as always. Throughout the day, there were more specialists, more tests, and of course, more letters. People all over the country were rooting for Bill. Somebody from California even called to promise a free fishing cruise in the Pacific after Bill was discharged. Bill got to thinking about the van idea, so he instructed Mel to call Paul Uebelhor, a Jasper car dealer and a friend of Bill's, to see what they could work out.

Tuesday, December 11. Like any other recovering heart patient, Bill was slowly increasing his exercise. In the morning, as technician Brent Mays carried the Heimes, Bill walked several yards down the hall to the nurses' station. He had heard that a couple of fellows from Jasper, Woody Erny and Jim Fritch, were in Audubon for coronary bypasses, so he decided to go cheer them up. He figured that no amount of hospital pamphlets, videotapes, or discussions with the doctors would tell them what to expect as well as another patient who'd already been through the procedure.

With the same setup as before—a circle of people around

his wheelchair, Margaret at his side, security guards clearing the way, Strode up ahead—Bill rode up to the fifth floor. Someone opened the door to the Jasper guys' room, and Bill cruised in with the Heimes on his lap.

"Hi, fellas!" Bill said with a broad smile and a wave. "Heard you all were here!"

Woody and Jim looked astonished.

"You guys will do just fine," Bill assured them. "Look, if I can get through *this*," he said, putting a hand over his new heart, "you two can get through anything. Right?" This was the old Bill, lending a hand, being a leader, cheering on somebody else who needed help. "Here! Just feel my heart! Pumpin' like everything, ain't it?"

Bill wasn't tired, so he ordered his entourage on a grand tour of the hospital. Every minute or two they had to stop so people could come up and shake his hand. Bill didn't mind—he loved the attention. It was just like he was glad-handing his way around at a wedding reception. "Feel my heart! It's beatin'! It's doing great! It's okay!" He'd grab people's hands, put them on his chest, and watch the wonder spread across their faces as they felt the heart ticking like a warm wind-up clock.

Then they went to the lobby to see the hospital's Christmas tree. By the time he returned to his room, he was worn out. That evening the staff got him up again for some more walking. Then later that night, Bill saw on TV that surgeons at another of Humana's four Louisville hospitals had implanted an experimental "artificial ear" in a twenty-five-year-old deaf man. The device, a "multichannel cochlear implant," which sometimes restored a crude form of hearing to people with certain types of deafness, was manufactured by Symbion, the same company that made the Jarvik-7. Bill sent the young man a telegram: I WISH YOU THE BEST OF LUCK WITH YOUR ARTIFICIAL EAR. I AM CONFIDENT THAT YOUR PROGRESS WILL GO AS WELL AS MINE. GOD BLESS YOU— BILL SCHROEDER.

Meanwhile, the kids continued taking turns coming down to Louisville. They tried to coordinate their visits so that one or more of them would be there at least three nights during the week plus the weekend. That Tuesday night, Rod and Stan visited their parents.

Wednesday, December 12. Between tests in the morning, Bill was on the phone, talking with relatives and handling family business the way he would from his basement office at home. One phone call in particular left him furious. Eight months before, he'd filed for disability from Social Security but hadn't received a cent. From his union work, Bill knew that his claim shouldn't take more than five months to go through. He'd already called the local Social Security office several times to complain, but always ran into some kind of bureaucratic delay. There was only so much of that he could stand. Bill called again that morning, but ran into more government red tape. He swore that one way or another, he'd get what was coming to him.

Before lunch, the staff got Bill out of bed for more exercise. He walked twice as far as the day before. Then he took off for a wheelchair ride. In the meantime, DeVries got a phone call from Washington, D.C. White House spokesman Larry Speakes asked him if Bill was up to taking a phone call from the president, Ronald Reagan. DeVries said he'd be delighted, that it would probably give Bill a real boost, but added, "I'd better warn you, though, this guy's an ardent, dyed-in-the-wool Democrat, and he'll say whatever's on his mind. You might want to consider that." Speakes brushed off the warning. After all, what would an average citizen say when honored by a phone call from the president of the United States?

When Bill returned from the wheelchair ride, DeVries told him the news.

"Fine with me," Bill said.

The White House was supposed to call at 2:00 P.M., so staffers hooked up a special phone line, and the PR people hastily arranged a television pool. Peter Heimes switched Bill to the quieter portable pack so everyone could hear better. Again, nurses, doctors, and hospital officials were crammed in around Bill's bed, along with Margaret at his side, cameras and mikes squeezed between all the medical equipment, hot, bright lights, and Strode hunting a better angle. Bill lay on his back, propped up just a little.

A camera whirred while everybody made small talk. Two o'clock passed, then it was 2:10. If Bill was nervous, he didn't show it. But Margaret could see that even now he hated to be kept waiting.

The phone rang. Audubon's administrator, Patricia Davis, grabbed it and identified herself. A White House aide asked for Bill, so she passed him the phone.

"Hello, Mr. Schroeder? Sir, this is the White House calling. President Reagan would like to speak with you."

"Okay," Bill said.

Bill put his arm behind his head as if he were relaxing in a lawn chair.

"Okay, one moment please, for the president."

Bill coughed, and an alarm chirped inside the portable pack. Bill looked over at the machine. Peter Heimes checked it, then shook his head to reassure Bill. It wasn't unusual for the alarm to sound when he coughed.

"Mr. Schroeder, the president's on the line. Go ahead, please."

"Mr. Schroeder!" the famous voice said.

"*Yes*, sir," Bill responded, as if greeting an acquaintance he hadn't seen in a while.

"I just wanted to call to say hello and to wish you the best," the president said. "You certainly have impressed us all with your remarkable recovery. And we admire your strength and courage. Nancy and I have just been two of a great many people who've been keeping score on you, and saying a prayer."

"Wellll," Bill drawled. "I sure appreciate that. And I thank you for it, and uh—"

"Well," Reagan said, "I understand that while you've been in the hospital you've taught the doctors a thing or two about 'medicinal' liquids! There's not a one of us that doesn't know what it's like to relax with a beer at the end of the day."

Bill was a little surprised, but he smiled. "Well, that's one of those common remarks I make. But I just want a sip now and then. That's it. But uh—"

Reagan interrupted him again. "I know they've got you on a tight schedule, and I don't want to tire you out, but I'm delighted that your new heart is pumping away, and that you're getting in shape to be able to leave the hospital. Nancy and I join your family and friends in wishing you the very best in the days to come."

"I just wish that more people could take advantage of this," Bill said. "It's workin' terrific. It's just super. I'm up walkin' around, and ridin' all over the place. It's really grand."

Bill paused. "But I got one question that I would like to ask you." He looked up at Margaret with a mischievous grin.

Oh, no, Bill. Don't you dare!

"All right," the president said amiably.

Margaret's eyes opened wide and she tried to catch Bill's attention, but there was no stopping him now.

"I got a Social Security problem," Bill said, and let that sink in for a moment. "And my problem is that I filed for Social Security in March of 1984 . . ."

"Well . . . now, wait a minute. I'm having a little trouble hearing you there," the president said. "It . . . you . . . this has to do with Social Security?"

"Yes, sir."

"And . . . and . . . what's the, what's the question again?"

"Okay." Bill was ready to go back to the beginning and explain all day if he had to. "I filed in March of 1984 with Social Security . . ."

"Yeah."

"And I'm just gettin' a runaround! I'm just not gettin' *anything* at all. And I just called them people today, and I just keep on callin' and keep on callin'. I don't get *anywhere!*"

"Bill," the president answered, "I will get into it and find out what the situation is."

"Okay." Bill nodded.

"All right," Reagan said with a chuckle.

"I'd sure appreciate it," Bill said.

"Well, I'll get on it right away," Reagan assured him.

"Thank you, Mr. President."

"All right."

"All right, Bill said. "'Bye."

"God bless you, and good health."

"Yeah, thank you," Bill said.

"All right," Reagan repeated.

"All right," Bill said again.

"'Bye."

"'Bye."

Bill hung up with the satisfied smile he always had after he'd straightened something out. Everyone clapped and howled with laughter. Bill shrugged. "They always say, 'The buck stops here.' And that's exactly where it's gonna stop. He said, 'I'll get into it right away and I'll take care of it.'" This was nothing new to Bill. He was used to going over people's heads if that's what it took.

The media went wild. Bill had done it again: the Average

American who upstages the president's congratulatory phone call with gripes about a bureaucratic runaround; the little guy who reaches out and puts the touch on the chief executive—three weeks after doctors replace his heart with a plastic one. Even the Humana PR people shook their heads in disbelief. They never dreamed that Bill would grab headlines for so long. And to think that he bent the presidential ear about Social Security, of all things! Later that afternoon another White House aide called George Atkins, ready to ream out Humana for illegally recording the president's conversation. Atkins explained politely that he had cleared it with another aide, so they could forget a lawsuit.

President Reagan kept his word. Within a couple of hours, Social Security officials called Bill to investigate the specifics of his complaint. Bill relished making them take down every detail of his case. For this lifelong Democrat, it was a sweet victory.

Back home, the kids heard about Bill's latest coup from the news media or from friends who offered congratulations. Stan happened to be at a bar in Jasper when his father's face appeared on the overhead TV screen. Someone turned it up, and the whole place went silent. There was ol' Wild Bill himself, griping to the president of the United States. Stan laughed so hard he nearly choked on his beer. Everybody cheered and slapped palms, and the bartender declared the next round of drinks on the house.

That evening Mel and Terry rode to Louisville with Jasper car dealer Paul Uebelhor. While Bill and Margaret looked over brochures about vans with Paul, the boys chatted with Larry Hastings, the technician. Hastings was an easygoing young guy, laid back in a Western denim-and-cowboy-boots way. Hastings switched Bill to the Heimes for a while; because the portable pack had never been tried in humans before, FDA guidelines allowed the medical team to use it only a few hours a day until they'd gathered more data on its performance.

"Hey," said Hastings, "I've got to go upstairs to the lab for a little bit. You guys want to come up and learn how to switch the drive lines?"

Mel and Terry figured it would be worth a look, so they went along to the makeshift lab on the sixth floor. Hastings hauled out an extra Utahdrive, and proceeded to demonstrate how to connect and disconnect the two hoses that supplied compressed air to the Jarvik heart. The end of each hose was marked with red or blue tape, corresponding to markers over the holes on each power source where the hoses were inserted. The red hose powered the left ventricle, which pumped blood to the body; the blue powered the right ventricle, which sent blood to the lungs. The blue hose had to be switched before the red one because otherwise blood might back up into the lungs. The changeover involved turning on the Heimes, reaching around to the back of the Utah over other cables and hoses, grabbing the connectors, pressing a release switch on them, pulling out the hoses, then shifting them to corresponding connectors on the Heimes. Larry advised them that the important thing was not speed but smoothness. It should only take a couple of seconds. One-thousand-one, one-thousand-two, and it was over. Just don't be nervous, he said.

Sure. That was easy to say, but how could you *not* be nervous when you literally held your father's life in the palms of your hands? The boys were nevertheless determined to learn because it would mean another step homeward for Dad.

Mel and Terry knelt between the Utah and the Heimes, and practiced until they could make the switch in one quick motion: blue to blue, red to red. After a while, they felt a little better about trying it on their father sometime. But those two seconds when the hoses were disconnected still seemed more like two minutes. Maybe they'd try it for real after Dad moved to the halfway house.

They went back to see Bill again, and Larry casually mentioned that Mel and Terry did just fine learning to switch the hoses. A couple of hours later, it was time to reconnect Bill to the Utah.

Larry grinned. "Hey, Bill," he said, "how about if we let Mel try the real thing?"

Mel was shocked. "Now?" he asked, hoping he didn't sound nervous.

"Sure! Why not?" Bill said with a wave of his hand.

Mel gulped. "Okay, Dad. Uh, okay, sure."

Larry turned on the Utah, and Mel knelt between the machines. He took a deep breath. Okay. His hands were shaking as he practiced moving imaginary drive lines back and forth: Heimes to Utah, Heimes to Utah, Heimes to Utah.

"Uh, okay, Dad," Mel said. "Ready?"

Bill shrugged as if to say, "Anytime now."

"Okay." Mel took another deep breath. "Here goes."

Grab connectors, release switch. Now, quickly, smoothly: blue to blue, red to red. There.

Mel looked up. Bill's head was thrown back, his eyes were closed, his mouth had dropped open, and his tongue hung out. Mel's jaw dropped, and his own heart skipped a couple of beats.

For a moment, they all just stared. What could possibly have gone wrong?

Finally, Bill cracked a grin, delighted with himself.

"You son-of-a-bitch!" cried his shaken son. "Don't you *ever* do that again!"

However, after Mel caught his breath, he, too, had to laugh. No doubt about it: Bill was still the same old dad, through and through; he was on top of the world, and getting better all the time.

Even so, Margaret could see that Bill was exhausted from all the day's excitement. And she could tell that, for some reason, he felt hot. So she sat up with him until after midnight when he finally fell asleep.

Thursday, December 13. Bill was still worn out. He sat up in a chair for breakfast and to have a sponge bath, but then got back in bed to rest. A physical therapist came to make him exercise his arms and legs as he lay in bed. Lab technicians arrived to draw blood. The rest of the morning, Margaret tried to keep intrusions to a minimum so he could get some sleep.

Then the Social Security office called with a familiar message: "The check's in the mail."

Air mail, as a matter of fact—Bill's first disability check was being flown to Louisville that morning. Sure enough, right after lunch, Bill was visited by the deputy chief of the Social Security Administration's Systems Management Branch in Philadelphia and by the assistant district manager for the agency's office in New Albany, Indiana, just across the river. Apparently it took two federal bureaucrats to deliver one envelope containing Bill's disability payments for the past four months. Bill cheerfully accepted it and mugged for photographs.

Bill would be the lead story again on the network news that evening. Once more he'd done the impossible—not only fighting off certain death but, maybe even more difficult, cutting through a tangle of government red tape with just one phone call. That evening Johnny Carson would joke in his opening monologue that thousands of people who couldn't get their Social Security checks were signing up to get an artificial heart. It was beginning to seem like there was nothing this Bill Schroeder couldn't do. The doctors were even talking about discharging him in a couple of weeks.

That afternoon Bill took another wheelchair ride throughout the hospital, inviting everybody to feel his new heart, accepting congratulations, and cracking jokes. Once again, he was the life of the party.

Just before supper, Dr. DeVries dropped by Bill's room. Nobody was prouder of Bill's feisty phone conversation with the president than his surgeon. Bill was doing so well that DeVries was moving back home, a twenty- to thirty-minute drive away. In fact, the surgeon's wife was flying to Utah that night to visit their eldest son in college, so DeVries was preparing to spend the weekend looking after the six children still at home. The doctor patted Bill's shoulder to congratulate him once more and said he'd be back in the morning.

Supper trays arrived. As usual, Bill sat up on the edge of the bed to eat, with Margaret facing him across the bedside table. Bill was tired, but he was looking forward to calling some relatives after a while. Throughout supper, he and Margaret talked about nothing in particular. Bill was saying something as he lifted a forkful of peaches.

Then he stopped.

Margaret glanced up. Bill's hand had frozen in midair, and he was looking straight ahead, eyes wide and staring, as if he were seeing a ghost.

"Bill!" Margaret cried. "What's the matter?"

His eyes turned up toward the ceiling and his head began to sway. Margaret reached for him with both hands over her tray, then shoved the table aside and screamed.

"BILL! Oh, my God! BILL! WHAT'S WRONG WITH YOU, HONEY?"

The nurse was there in an instant. Bill's whole body went limp, so heavy that it took both Margaret and the nurse to get him back in bed. They put out a call for immediate help—and suddenly there were nurses everywhere. The entire artificial heart team was being paged. Margaret was so frightened that she wouldn't let go of Bill while they worked on him. Dr. Albert Hoskins, the internist, arrived within seconds and started the IV lines. "What's wrong with him?" Margaret asked frantically.

Hoskins looked up briefly and said, "I think he's had a stroke."

A stroke? Margaret wondered. *Well, what is THAT?* Everyone was too busy to explain. Margaret held on to Bill until they took him back to the ICU. Once again, he was out of her hands as the doctors took over. Polly Brown, who'd been out to dinner with friends, soon arrived to comfort her.

Margaret stood shivering outside the glass door. Laura Wood put an arm around her while she tried to explain what happened. Margaret just kept shaking her head. All she knew was that Bill had been just fine one minute, then suddenly, he looked terrible.

DeVries sped back to the hospital and rushed in to check on Bill. When he came back out, Margaret searched his eyes before he spoke. His face was as white as a sheet. Margaret's knees gave way. DeVries and Laura Wood each put a hand on Margaret's shoulders to steady her.

"Margaret," DeVries said gently, "we think that Bill has had a stroke, but it looks like he's going to pull through." What they wouldn't know for a while, he said, was how much damage the stroke had done, or whether Bill would ever be the same again.

DeVries explained that the stroke had damaged part of Bill's brain by depriving it of oxygen. There were different kinds of strokes, he said, and it was still impossible to tell what kind Bill had suffered. They did know that it had left him completely unconscious for almost an hour and had paralyzed his right arm and leg. The paralysis might only be temporary, but then again, it might not. Many stroke victims could recover fully and resume normal lives; but some did not. Some people lost speech, memory, control of their arms and legs or other bodily functions, depending on what part of the brain was damaged.

Margaret was trying hard to understand, but nothing was making sense. All these words were raining down on her, some soaking through and others sliding off. All she wanted to know was whether her husband was going to be okay. Her mind kept going back to that moment: Bill staring ahead, his hand holding up his fork in front of him.

Dr. DeVries explained that they couldn't be sure of the cause of the stroke just yet, but a CAT scan should give them an idea. The stroke might have been caused by a hemorrhage, meaning that tiny blood vessels had broken and bled into the brain tissue—always a risk in a diabetic because the smallest blood vessels tend to constrict and break. Or it could have been caused by an embolism that occurred when a tiny clot lodged in the brain and blocked the blood flow.

"Embolism." Margaret had heard that word somewhere before. But what did it mean? None of these words made any sense. He'd been just fine, they were eating dinner, and then . . .

Had *she* done something wrong? Maybe this wouldn't have happened if she hadn't let them push him so much in physical therapy. Maybe if she hadn't let him have so many visitors. Maybe if he hadn't had all that excitement. Maybe . . .

DeVries was saying that it would be a while before they knew whether the damage was permanent. The next forty-eight hours would be crucial: If Bill showed a strong improvement, he might do fairly well, maybe even recover completely—or almost completely.

"So what you're telling me," she said finally, "is that you just don't know anything right now. Is that it?"

"That's right," DeVries said. "We'll just have to wait and see."

Wait-and-see. Wait-and-see. It still didn't make any sense. Margaret kept peering in the door of Bill's room, wishing she could be with her husband. DeVries told her they both needed rest right now. Nothing could be done until several hours later when Bill woke up, and they'd be sure to call her if there was any change.

Polly took Margaret down the hall to her office to call the kids. Margaret reluctantly put her hand on the phone, then hesitated. She still didn't understand what a stroke was—how was she supposed to explain it to her family? She couldn't reach Mel, so she called Terry and told him what the doctors had said. Terry said he'd try to round up the others, and they'd be there as soon as possible. Once again, the family hurriedly packed clothes, made arrangements to leave their homes and jobs behind. And once again, their loved ones lay awake that night, wondering what was happening at the hospital, how long they'd have to go it alone this time. Sometimes the Schroeders returned from the hospital cherishing their own families more than ever. Sometimes when they came home, they seemed distant, with a load of worry and weariness that no one could lift from their shoulders.

The PR officials immediately scheduled a 9:30 P.M. press briefing to report a change in Bill's condition. Now the heart institute's phones were ringing off the hook, mostly from reporters asking what had happened. Polly Brown sat Margaret down at a phone and instructed her to say, "Humana Heart Institute, please hold" until Polly got around to those callers. Margaret did as she was told, answering one reporter after another—all of whom were unaware that they were missing a chance to interview the patient's wife. Everything was happening so fast. Margaret was so frightened for Bill, so frustrated not to be with him. But Polly's move had been shrewd; at the very time when Margaret felt most useless, it was at least some comfort to be doing *something*.

Kevan Shaheen arrived and took Margaret upstairs to get rooms ready for the family. But since the kids were no longer living at the hospital, some of the beds had been pressed into service elsewhere in the building. As Kevan and Margaret dragged in mattresses so the kids could sleep on the floor, Kevan did her best to answer Margaret's questions.

A CAT scan of Bill's brain showed several dark spots, indicating that the stroke was massive. Several tiny clots, or emboli, had settled in the brain's lower left portion, responsible for speech, memory, and limb movements.

It had been an embolic stroke after all. DeVries had dreaded this news because he figured that the source of the stroke was almost certainly the Jarvik heart itself. Clots had probably formed on the valves, broken loose, and traveled to Bill's brain. DeVries had given Bill a combination of blood-thinning drugs in hopes of preventing just such an event without causing the internal bleeding problems Barney Clark had suffered. Now it seemed that in Bill's case, DeVries had gone too far in the other direction. The surgeon realized that the right balance of anticlotting drugs for his next artificial heart patient would have to fall somewhere in between.

It was an extremely important discovery. DeVries had publicly maintained that the only way to make such discoveries was to test the heart in humans, a process that would involve learning from mistakes. That was fine in theory; in practice, it was a gruesome way to learn. DeVries had tried to keep his professional distance from Bill and the family, but he was clearly shaken now.

Within a couple of hours, Dr. Lansing came by to tell Margaret that Bill seemed to be a little better. Lansing was on his way to another news conference, saying that they had to report the bad news as well as the good. Margaret nodded, but it still didn't make sense. How could he brief the media about Bill's stroke when they couldn't even tell *her* exactly what had happened?

Meanwhile, nurses were stunned to see that Bill was already waking up. He was even trying to talk, although his words were garbled. He was already moving all of his limbs again. That rarely happened so quickly in someone with such a massive stroke.

In fact, a stroke of that severity might well have killed a person with a normal heart. But Bill's artificial heart kept pumping blindly, oblivious to the fact that anything was wrong, nourishing the injured brain more efficiently than a human heart ever could.

Nurses monitoring Bill through the night were astounded to see him bounce back so fast. They had expected to chart changes in his condition every few hours or so, but he was improving so rapidly they were making notes every few minutes. He even smiled crookedly when Lansing made a joke. From a purely clinical standpoint, Bill was doing amazingly well.

However, when Mel, Stan, and Terry arrived about 1:00 A.M. and went into the ICU with Margaret, they were frightened. Bill looked confused and scared to death. The right side of his face drooped. He stared into their eyes and frowned as he tried to talk, but he could only make moaning, whimpering noises. He was teary-eyed and cried at every little thing. Margaret and the boys tried desperately to guess what he was struggling to tell them, but they couldn't, so Bill would cry some more. By now, Strode had arrived and was discreetly taking pictures.

Friday, December 14. Early the next morning, Lansing went on TV to announce that Bill was recovering "brilliantly" from the stroke. "I'm very much encouraged at how much recovery there's been within a few hours, so it is on that basis that I am telling you that at the moment it is not a disaster," Lansing said. "If he continues as he is, with his particular spirit and family support, he will make a rapid recovery."

It was beginning to seem as if the doctors and the family were speaking different languages. When Margaret and the boys saw Bill later that morning, he looked just as bad as before. If this was a brilliant recovery, they'd sure hate to see him in bad shape. The rest of the kids soon arrived, encouraged by news reports, only to be disheartened by the grim reality before their eyes. Throughout the day, newspaper headlines and television reports continued to be maddeningly contradictory.

The family's confusion was reflected in that day's entry in the diary Mel kept during the first weeks after Bill's surgery:

. . . Dad was awake and moving. He was saying words, but hard to understand. We didn't want to arouse him so we didn't stay too long. Everyone was saying he was doing much better. A Dr. Fox [the neurologist] was checking Dad out to see how he was doing. We talked with Fox. He said everything was going well. They were going to take another brain scan and an ultrasound on his veins in his neck to see if there was any blockage . . . [Terry and Cheryl arrived] and all of us went with Donna Hazle to meet two individuals from Knights of Columbus which wanted to present cards from fellow brothers. We took pictures and got back. Mom and Rod was looking for us. We all went to see Dad. He was awake and we gave him our encouragement. Mom stayed—everyone else went upstairs.

Ordered lunch and sat around. Restless. Went back downstairs around lunch to get Mom. Dad was sleeping but just woke up and all the boys went in to see him. He tried to talk, but hard to understand. We were tiring him out because we couldn't understand him and he was frustrated. He was emotional as well.

They were going to take Dad down to X-ray so we left. We didn't know what to expect from a stroke. Docs said everything was good, but after seeing Dad when he was up and talking—and now, we didn't feel very good about the way he looked . . .

Everyone was sleepy, so several took naps. Got mail and everyone helped open it. . . . There was a lady from local government employee union that wanted to give us a check. Stan, Terry, Rod and me went downstairs to meet her.

. . . We checked on Dad. Still sleeping . . .

And Margaret wrote in hers:

Friday, Dec. 14. Such a day. I sat with Bill for a couple hours. He sleeps all the time. He squeezed my hand this morning and tried to talk to me about his Social Security check.

Every time I go down there he is asleep. They tell us he is doing fine. I don't know. I wonder if he will ever be OK again. I love him so much. He looks so helpless.

I fell asleep some today. I tried to pass the day. We went to K mart tonight. He just sleeps on.

[My sister] Nora called me. Am going to bed now. Hope he's better tomorrow.

Saturday, December 15. For Margaret and the kids, another day of wait-and-see. Bill seemed no better at all. When Terry switched on the special telephone hookup so Bill could hear a radio broadcast of the basketball game between the Jasper Wildcats and Southridge High, he just stared, expressionless. Terry tried to talk to him about the game, but Bill kept struggling to say things until he got frustrated and began to cry.

On the TV news that day, Lansing said that although Bill was recovering well, the stroke had had a "sobering influence" that "was perhaps needed." It was "very beneficial . . . a slap in the face . . . because it brought us back to realism," he said. Lansing also used the event to underscore the experimental nature of the artificial heart program by comparing Barney Clark's setbacks—and now Bill's stroke—to the World Series. "Even if you lost the first two games, you wouldn't pack up and go home," Lansing told reporters.

"There are seven games in the World Series. There are seven implants planned. We may have had an error in the first game and an error in the second game. We haven't lost the second game yet, but we're still in only the second game. The purpose of this whole thing is to find out answers to questions . . ."

When DeVries faced the media that afternoon, he contradicted Lansing on some points. Lansing had said the stroke might have been caused by plaque breaking off an arterial wall, rather than by clots from the heart. But DeVries maintained that chances were 95 percent that clots from the heart caused the stroke. Bill was also experiencing some edema, or fluid buildup, in his tissues, and the doctors differed on the cause of that also. Lansing blamed the edema insufficient protein in Bill's diet, but

DeVries insisted that it was just the normal postoperative swelling that often occurs after surgery.

The Schroeders were learning to expect different opinions and explanations about Bill's condition, depending on who was doing the talking. They were also becoming skeptical about everything the media reported. And as for the experimental nature of the program, well, that was fine in theory, but they were talking about somebody's husband and father here. They couldn't imagine anybody really considered Bill a guinea pig.

CHAPTER NINE

Sunday, December 16. Bill seemed no better. In the morning Strode came to take a few pictures of Bill sitting up in bed, but he couldn't get him to smile. "Come on, Bill," a nurse urged, "give us the thumbs-up now." Bill finally responded with a half-hearted gesture, and Humana released the photo of Bill giving the thumbs-up.

Actually, Bill was anything but chipper. He was sleeping almost all day and night—or at least keeping his eyes closed. When he was awake, Bill looked sad and listless, as if he really didn't care whether he got better or not. He didn't even try to talk, and a feeding tube had been placed in his nose to supplement his nutrition. When they got him up to sit in a chair for a while, he complained with angry groans.

The family felt so confused. That man in intensive care was Bill Schroeder, but at the same time, he wasn't. They didn't know what to hope for or even how to console each other because everything was so uncertain. The doctors kept saying Bill was doing well, considering the extent of his injury. Maybe that meant he could fight back and be the same old dad again, but maybe he'd just live the rest of his life like that. No one had any answers.

On the TV news that evening Lansing would worry aloud to reporters about what he called Bill's "withdrawal." The doctor said: "He just sort of lies with his eyes closed most of the time unless we talk to him, stimulate him or test him for something . . . it's almost like an ostrich type of approach." Bill seemed to have lost his appetite for many things—maybe even for life itself, he told reporters. Although depression and feelings of indifference were common in stroke patients, Lansing said, "I would get concerned if over the next two or three days we can't shake him out of this."

Great. It was hard enough for the family to see their husband and father like that. Now to hear such discouraging comments secondhand from a doctor on TV—to have the whole world hear them, in fact—just made it harder. All they had heard any of the doctors say was that they just didn't know how Bill was going to be and wouldn't know for several days.

That afternoon some of the family and their kids went to see Bill. He seemed to wake up a little more when told that his grandchildren were there, but he said nothing. The family took Margaret out for a little Christmas shopping, but she kept thinking about how Bill would have especially loved to take the grandchildren himself, maybe even tell them how he used to play Santa back at Sakel's drive-in. And, she wondered, what in the world should she give him for Christmas now?

By now the staff not only worried about Bill, but also about Margaret. She was at Bill's side almost constantly, and had virtually lived in the hospital for more than a month. The intense stress had been unrelenting, and she had to be on the verge of exhaustion. Anyone in such a situation could literally become sick with worry. They knew also that Margaret herself had a delicate heart.

Since the family had to return home that night, nurse Laura Wood invited Margaret to spend the night at her house. The kids urged their mother to go, then privately asked Laura to persist in her invitations. Margaret finally accepted, provided that she could carry a beeper. Laura had grown up "country" too, in rural Kentucky, so she and Margaret had lots to share. They had a good time at Laura's, but all night long Margaret's thoughts kept flitting back to the hospital.

Monday, December 17. Margaret and Laura returned early in the morning to a surprise: Bill was much better. He was wide awake, and when Margaret came in he smiled crookedly, took her hand, and wouldn't let go. The nurses told her that he had managed to pull out his feeding tube, which he'd had for a day or so, and the doctors said it was okay to try leaving it out. To Margaret's delighted amazement, Bill let her feed him breakfast and eagerly finished it off. Dr. Lonnie Mudd, the psychiatrist, came to evaluate Bill's depression. Mudd told Margaret that Bill probably didn't need antidepressant drugs, just more time and TLC. Margaret figured that the doctors had been right after all. Maybe Bill was going to get better; it would just take longer than she expected.

In fact, the doctors felt Bill had improved enough to be moved from intensive care back to a regular room. The family wasn't so sure—it had been only four days since the stroke—but the medical team told them that the move might lift Bill's spirits because it would show their confidence in his recovery. Margaret was nervous about his moving to a room staffed by fewer nurses, but the decision was already made.

That morning Bill's entourage gathered for the wheelchair ride down the hall to his old room. Since Bill was doing so well, they made a quick detour on the way, taking an elevator to the first-floor lobby to show him the hospital's Christmas tree. They arrived just as some third-graders from a Catholic elementary school began to sing carols.

Christmas! Bill's eyes widened and he managed a smile. His lips moved, and a soft, pinched voice came out. Margaret leaned close. He was trying to sing "Silent Night" with the children. When the song was over, Margaret took him back upstairs and settled him in his old room at the end of the hall.

Back in Jasper, the kids talked about their father's setback with several friends whose relatives had also suffered a stroke. The story of their slow progress sounded a lot like their dad's. The family all began to understand that it would be a long, long road. Whenever people learned who the kids' father was, they were always eager to share their own stories of heart disease or stroke or of a loved one's long illness. It helped to compare notes with other people who had been through it, often more than it did to talk with the doctors.

Cheryl called her mom in the afternoon, and she confirmed that Bill indeed seemed better. Lansing had given the press the same news earlier in the day: "Anybody who makes that much progress in that short period of time is likely to make even more progress in the future. I have seen people look infinitely worse than Mr. Schroeder who recovered completely."

When the kids got home from work that day, however, they were shocked to hear another doctor on TV saying something completely different. Humana officials had put consulting neurologist Dr. Gary Fox before the press for the first time, and his assessment of Bill's condition was much more pessimistic than

Lansing's. Fox had examined Bill shortly after the stroke on Thursday, then on Friday, and again on Monday morning.

"He had essentially no recall for what happened over the weekend," Fox told reporters Monday afternoon. "He thinks it's still Friday; it's very difficult to assess at this point." The dark-haired, tanned neurologist said that Bill's responses were all very slow and "he had difficulty at times recognizing members of the family."

The kids were confused, then outraged. Where in the hell did this guy get off saying that kind of thing? They knew that Dad had recognized them just fine any time they'd been there since the stroke. Even if this doctor was correct somehow, why hadn't Mom been told before he went to tell the media? Margaret agreed. That doctor didn't have any bedside manners at all, she thought.

When Mel called the hospital that night to find out what was going on, Stan told him to ignore the news reports; Dad was just the same as when the kids last visited. They decided to complain to the medical team and insist that the doctors at least tell Margaret before saying anything like that on TV again. When the Schroeders confronted DeVries with Fox's comments, he just wrote off the differing assessments as part of a system of checks and balances. He assured them that it was good to have doctors on both sides of the fence, to challenge each other's ideas in an effort to find the truth.

Maybe. A healthy difference of opinion might be good for the artificial heart program, but it was small consolation for the patient's worried family.

Tuesday, December 18. Bill seemed a little better. The family was learning that with stroke patients, you must measure progress in baby steps and celebrate every little achievement. One of Bill's therapists had him hold a pen and try to sign his name. He couldn't write, but did make an X. The therapist also brought him a green balloon. Batting the balloon back and forth with Bill would help him regain his eye-hand coordination. Cheryl drove down to spend a few days helping her parents, and that afternoon, she and Bill played with the balloon for a long time.

In the days following Bill's stroke, the doctors ordered even more tests. They were still unsure how much Bill would recover, or whether, as they put it, he might "stroke" again. Some nuclear-medicine specialists from Vanderbilt University in

Nashville, Tennessee, arrived. They were colleagues of Dr. David Rollo, a Humana vice-president who taught part time at Vanderbilt, and would perform an experimental radioisotope test on Bill. Staffers explained to Margaret that the test would involve removing some of Bill's blood, separating out the platelets and treating them with radioactive material, putting them back in his body and observing them with a special camera. The researchers could then try to track the treated platelets through Bill's bloodstream. The platelets should stick to fresh blood clots, which would show whether any more clots had formed on the heart's metal valves. If clots were present, the doctors would try to prevent another stroke by treating Bill with clot-dissolving drugs. As a last resort, surgeons might have to go back in and replace all or part of the Jarvik-7.

They told Margaret that this was not a standard test, but there was only a slight risk involved, as far as they knew. And even if no clots showed up, they said, the doctors would gain useful scientific information.

Margaret was asked to sign a consent form authorizing the test. But it all sounded so weird to her. Take Bill's blood out of his body, make it radioactive, then put it back in to see what it does? If the test was experimental, there was no guarantee that it would even work. She began to wonder what the doctors considered more important—getting Bill better or finding out the answers to some scientist's questions? She couldn't see putting Bill through a test like that if it wasn't absolutely necessary. It was another one of those situations where you were damned if you did, and damned if you didn't. The doctors wouldn't force you to go through with it, but they'd say the test was important and might help Bill or someone else.

Margaret was on the spot. It was so hard to make such a choice for a husband who always knew what to ask, always made his own decisions, always seemed to know what to do. She hated to question the judgment of the Humana staff—even when she talked to the doctors from Jasper, she was still a little tongue-tied. The one person in the world she wanted to talk to about all this, more than any doctor or nurse, was Bill himself. A while back, when the doctors had asked her opinion, she looked to Bill for cues. But now she had to step into his place and ask herself what he'd do, until he could get back on his feet.

So Margaret stood her ground, saying she wanted to talk to

Dr. DeVries or Dr. Lansing. Since DeVries wasn't available, they called the convention center and got Lansing out of a press conference to answer her questions over the phone. Lansing assured her that the test was important, and that although it was experimental, it carried minimal risks. After they talked awhile, she apologized for holding things up, but Lansing said he was glad she asked because she needed to understand what was happening. She signed the form, hoping she was doing the right thing, and stayed with Bill throughout the test.

The test left Bill exhausted. When he and Margaret returned to his room, they discovered that while they were gone, a man from New Jersey had dropped by and left Bill a gold watch as a present. The Schroeders never learned his name. Bill wore the watch and wouldn't let anyone remove it. Meanwhile, more letters were pouring in. Hundreds of people had simply added the Schroeders to their Christmas card list. In addition, many stroke patients and their families wrote notes of encouragement and shared stories of their own struggles.

Thursday, December 19. Representatives from Jasper's WITZ radio station and the *Herald* brought even more good wishes from home. The newspaper people had a sack of mail for the family and a big Christmas card with more than six thousand signatures. The PR folks suggested it might be nice if Margaret and the kids opened some of the cards for a TV crew. So they made a brief appearance before the cameras.

Bill seemed somewhat better. He sat in his chair a few times that day and the next. But he rarely spoke unless he was spoken to, or something made him uncomfortable. He was still hard to understand, although he seemed to have less trouble talking in the mornings, as if somehow he got recharged overnight, but wore down as the day went on.

That evening Mel wrote:

> Went in and seen Dad. He knew me right away. . . .
> I sat with him. He didn't talk very much and when he did it
> was slightly over a whisper—hard to understand. He would
> hit the triangle bar he used to help lift him, and watch it as
> though a child admiring a plaything hanging above a crib. I
> hadn't seen him that awake before. He looked pretty good
> but still had a long way to go. Physically pretty good, men-

tally a little lacking. Seemed like he had periods where he was in a different world away from reality . . .

Saturday, December 22. Another encouraging day. Bill murmured to Margaret that he hadn't slept well the night before. Dr. Salb came by, and Bill recognized him instantly. They watched a videotape of a recent basketball game between Jasper and their arch-rival, Huntingburg. At times, Bill seemed more interested than he had been the week before. He sat up in his chair, and held his granddaughters, Melanie and Abbie, on his lap. When they gave him the "I love you" sign, he'd do it back. He tried to tell them things, but they couldn't understand his garbled words.

Another videotape arrived, this one from IU basketball coach Bobby Knight. The family played it for Bill twice that day. He smiled when Knight appeared on the screen, and when the coach looked into the camera and said, "Give 'em hell, Bill!" Bill smiled again and made a fist at the TV.

Cheryl and Glenn came down to Louisville, along with Rod and Lori. A local seafood restaurant, the Red Lobster, catered a huge feast of shrimp and lobster for the family at the hospital, and waited on them hand and foot. Since Bill wasn't strong enough to make the trip down the hall, the family gathered in his room after supper while Margaret fed him some lobster, which he seemed to enjoy.

That evening Terry tried to rouse his dad to watch the IU game on TV, but Bill slept through the first half. When Rod came into the room at half time, Bill woke up and watched the rest of the game with his sons.

Sunday, December 23. The effects of the stroke were still very confusing. It was as if each time Bill fell asleep, the cards were reshuffled and dealt again. He might act one way before his nap, and then be completely different when he woke up. The kids never knew what to expect from one visit to the next. He might be able to feed himself with a fork at the beginning of a meal, but then his hand would get weak and tired before he finished. At times, usually in the mornings, he could speak clearly enough to have a fairly normal conversation. Sometimes he made perfect sense; at others he might say "No" when he meant "Yes," or he would refer to his finger as his toe. And sometimes it seemed as if his thoughts stayed in some shadowy place that only he could see.

173

This Sunday Bill had a good day. He sat up awhile and played with the balloon. Later he got out of bed and took a few steps. He often whispered to Margaret and even tried to whistle a tune. When some of the kids came, he smiled and took their hands. When a couple of Bill's old co-workers dropped by, he knew them right away.

The next day, Monday, was bad. It seemed that all Bill could do was sleep or cry. He wouldn't even try to speak to Margaret, the kids or the staff. He moaned and groaned through his exercise session, resisting all the way as the physical therapist tried to get him to lift one-pound weights. Afterward he seemed completely exhausted. Now Margaret was not only worried about Bill, but confused as to why he was being pushed to exercise when he was too tired.

That morning George Atkins, the Humana vice-president for public relations, dropped by. He and Margaret talked awhile, then George clapped his hands together and began. "Hey, listen . . ." Humana was still giving regular press briefings about Bill, and now the media were eager for a Christmas Eve statement from him, he said.

How Bill would have loved to deliver that kind of message himself! But Margaret knew that he couldn't now, and wouldn't want to be seen in his present condition—maybe later when he felt better and his speech had improved. George said he certainly understood. But maybe, he suggested, she would be willing to speak briefly to the press on Bill's behalf?

At first, the idea sounded crazy. What would she want with all those cameras, microphones, bright lights, and strangers asking *her* questions? She'd always preferred Bill to have the spotlight, while she gave him a smile and a thumbs-up from the quiet safety of the shadows. But her husband couldn't face the cameras now; she would have to step between him and the media until he got better. It would be scary, but so many people were pulling for Bill, and he would want them to know that he appreciated it. She knew he was grateful also to the folks at Humana who had worked so hard to save his life. Two months earlier, wild horses couldn't have dragged her in front of one reporter with a microphone— much less dozens—and TV cameras besides. Now, somehow, it just seemed to be the thing to do.

Okay, she told George, she'd do it.

Moni was visiting, so she and Polly Brown accompanied

Margaret to the press conference that afternoon. George suggested that they take along an example of the gifts Bill had received. They brought "Schroeder Bear," an electronic toy bear with a plastic heart that played Christmas carols. If they ran out of things to say, they could kill some time by having the bear play tunes for the press.

Another PR official, Bob Irvine, escorted them to the convention center, and George introduced them at the podium. The huge room still had lots of reporters, cameras, and lights. *Why did I ever say I would do this?* Margaret wondered. George turned to her. *Too late now.* She stepped onto the podium and pulled the microphone down to her level. Moni stood beside her, holding Schroeder Bear. Margaret tried to keep her hands from shaking as she unfolded her handwritten speech.

"I came here today to wish each and every one of you a Merry Christmas." She paused, and managed a smile.

"And," she continued emphatically, "to let you know that Bill is recovering—but very slowly. And at this time we feel it's not appropriate for him to meet the press. But we thank you for your patience. We hope that you understand our feelings."

George asked if she'd answer some questions. She couldn't say no—right there in front of all those people. So, as the cameras rolled, Margaret faced difficult, disturbing questions from strangers.

How did she feel when Bill had his stroke?

She thought for a moment. "I never had seen anyone that had a stroke," she said. "I didn't know anything about a stroke . . . so it really was depressing at the time."

Was she optimistic that Bill would improve?

"Well," she answered, "he's not going to get better overnight—I know that now. But at first I thought, 'Tomorrow he'll be better.'" She knew that Bill might see her on TV, so she made sure that he would know she had complete confidence in him.

Had Bill been able to talk to her?

"As far as him communicating with me, I can communicate with him. I think all of us do. He knows every one of us and tells us things and we can understand him. . . . It's not like he's just lying there staring or something. He's getting better every day." All she could do was just be honest—that's what Bill would do.

Finally, someone asked about the bear, which was a relief. Moni switched it on, and the bear played some Christmas songs.

George declared the briefing over. On the return trip, he and Polly congratulated Margaret and Moni on another great job, but all they cared about was getting back to Bill. When they arrived, he was asleep; and when he finally woke up, he was no better.

Tuesday, December 25. "Merry Christmas, Dad." All the kids and their families had come to the hospital for this day. Once again, they had no idea how their dad would be when he woke up. When they saw him that morning, Bill was wide awake. His face brightened, and he whispered back, "Merry Christmas."

He knew. He *had* to know. He had made it to Christmas.

Bill seemed so well rested that morning that the kids laced up some boxing gloves on his hands—a gift from a sporting-goods company. Mel pretended to box with him, and Bill hit back with some surprisingly strong punches.

Terry cheered him on: "Right cross, Dad! Give him a right cross!" Bill did just that. Once, Mel's hand slipped and accidentally tapped his dad's nose. Then Bill really started throwing punches. He and the whole family were laughing. Margaret and the kids were encouraged—maybe it would just take a little longer for Bill to be his old self again.

While the family went upstairs to settle in and get ready for lunch, hospital staffers switched Bill onto the Heimes, changed his pajama top to a pullover shirt, helped him put his IU cap on his head, and took him by wheelchair to a conference room where Humana had laid out another lavish spread. The Schroeders were called down to the room, and as they trooped in, starting with the grandkids, they sang, "We Wish You a Merry Christmas."

Bill was so touched that he cried. He kept reaching for everyone's hand, kissing them, and telling them "Merry Christmas." As each family member brought him a loosely wrapped present, Bill eagerly opened the packages, smiled at each one, and whispered how much he liked them: an electric razor from Margaret, a box of fishing tackle from technician Larry Hastings, a portable cassette recorder from the kids. Strode was there, too, snapping pictures.

Then they sat down to a delicious dinner of shrimp on ice, baked ham, asparagus, baked potatoes, and wine. Bill was able to feed himself most of the meal; he even pushed Margaret's hand away sometimes when she tried to help. Melanie, Abbie, and

Tracey couldn't sit still long what with all the excitement, and soon gathered around their grandpa, jumping up and down, vying for his attention, and talking to him about their presents. Bill was surrounded by everything that meant Christmas—the loving smiles of his wife and kids, the breathless chatter of grandchildren, the family's gifts to each other, the happy mess of scattered wrapping paper and ribbons, the hugs and the teasing, the togetherness. Bill put down his fork, covered his eyes, and wept again. As the girls stroked his arm and tried to cheer him up, Strode took a picture.

After the meal, Bill held his grandchildren on his lap and hugged them. Then Strode gathered them together for some family portraits. More hospital staffers dropped in; they were now becoming like another family to the Schroeders. Bill was so happy to see everyone together, but he was beginning to get tired. Then DeVries and his wife, Karen, dropped by.

When Bill looked up and saw DeVries, he seemed to snap wide-awake. The lanky surgeon and his wife knelt in front of Bill's wheelchair to talk with him.

Forty days. Christmas.

Bill started to cry again. He took the surgeon's hand in both of his, and looked into his eyes intently.

"Thank you," Bill said slowly. "Thank you for giving me this day."

CHAPTER TEN

Days began blurring into weeks. As it became clear that Bill's recovery would take longer than expected, the medical team set up a weekday schedule for him. From early morning until after-supper visiting hours, Bill's day was packed with physical therapy, occupational therapy, speech therapy, doctors' examinations, tests, and treatments. The stroke had turned each of those activities into a tedious, minute-by-minute struggle for everyone, but especially for Bill. In fact, it was as if he were still working a grueling eight-to-five job, five days a week—and there could be no doubt that this was the hardest job he'd ever had.

A typical day began about 7:00 A.M. when Margaret came downstairs to Bill's room. She didn't have to get there so early, but she'd learned that in a hospital, you have to fit into the doctors' schedule if you want to see them. She could be fairly sure of catching them during early-morning rounds. The parade started about 7:30 A.M. One by one, the doctors would come in and ask the nurse for Bill's chart, note each new physical change, talk briefly to Margaret, write another prescription or order new tests, and leave after a few minutes.

Margaret's mind was always full of worries, but at first she hesitated to ask the doctors many questions. After all, they ought to know what they were doing, and certainly didn't have time to teach her everything they'd learned in medical school. Besides, Bill had always been the one to talk with the physicians. However, as Bill's hospital stay dragged on, Margaret tried to guess what he would want to know from the doctors and she worked up the courage to ask. Still, their replies often raised more questions than they answered—and it seemed that she could never remember what she should have asked until after the doctors had gone. She soon found it helpful to keep a running list of questions, jotting them as they occurred to her, just as Bill had always done. But she faced the additional problem of gathering information from seven or eight different physicians at once instead of from only one or two.

In addition to DeVries, several of his associates would look in on Bill. Many other physicians also donated their time and services: The internist, Dr. Hoskins, followed Bill's general medical condition, monitoring such problems as his diabetes. Dr. Julio Melo, another internist, was responsible for monitoring and treating signs of infection. The psychiatrist, Dr. Mudd, assessed Bill's mental state and spirits. Dr. Fox regularly examined his neurological condition. Drs. Yong K. Liu and Daniel C. Scullin, both hematologists, saw Bill each day, gathering a variety of data about his blood. Dr. Stephan Johnson, a pathologist, regularly analyzed samples of blood and tissue cultures. The longer Bill stayed in the hospital, the more specialists came to see him, often bringing along colleagues—not only local doctors, but from all over the world. Others came at DeVries's request to perform specialized tests on Bill and the artificial heart.

Many times when Margaret put the same question to several specialists, they'd all give different answers. It was like the old story of the blind men and the elephant. One might tell her it was very important to run a particular experimental test; the next might say the test wasn't all that crucial. One might say that a slight infection of the area around Bill's drive lines could cause real problems; the next doctor would tell her this was nothing to worry about. Maybe, as Dr. DeVries had said, it was helpful to hear the differing opinions of several doctors. But at times it got downright confusing. Each doctor's observations provided only one piece of the puzzle, and some pieces didn't seem to fit anywhere.

While the doctors were making their rounds, Margaret and the nurses would help Bill into a chair for a while. Like his wheelchair rides, getting out of bed had to be carefully coordinated, partly because of the layout of equipment in Bill's room. To his left, the Utahdrive was squeezed into the tight space between his bed and the wall. On his right stood two IV holders supporting the bags of anticoagulants and antibiotics that dripped through tubes into his veins. Beyond the IV stands was Bill's cardiac chair, which had a firm, sculpted cushion to support his back.

Bill always got out on the right side, which meant that the Utah had to be moved around to the foot of the bed because the drive lines wouldn't reach all the way to his chair. On the floor beneath the Utah and under the bed lay a mass of electrical wires and hoses, which also had to be moved carefully and simultaneously to clear a path for the bulky drive system.

With the Utah in place, one helper lifted Bill's shoulders, taking care that the drive lines didn't catch on anything. The other grasped Bill's feet and swung them out of bed, or, if Bill felt strong and eager to get up, he would swing his legs around by himself and dangle his feet. Margaret made sure he had on his slippers, and then someone stood in front of Bill, knee to knee. Bill would clasp his hands around that person's neck. As one helper kept the IVs from tangling or slipping out of Bill's arms, another made sure the drive lines were okay. The third would say, "One-two-three, go!" and help Bill stand up, trying to help him balance on his own. Then they all moved the drive tubes and IV lines in unison as Bill shuffled the few steps across the room. He'd slowly turn around so his back was to the chair, then they'd ease him onto the seat. When it was time to return to bed, the whole process was reversed.

This might take as little as one minute or as long as five minutes depending on how strong Bill was, and whether he was roused from bed against his wishes. Sometimes he needed very little support, but at other times he'd moan and groan and could barely stand without assistance. From one day to the next, his reaction was impossible to predict.

After Bill was settled in the chair, breakfast trays arrived for him and Margaret. This was usually the easiest meal for Bill to manage, but no meal was ever quick. He had to concentrate intently just to grasp his fork and scoop up a bite. Then he'd try to keep the food balanced on the fork long enough to raise it to his mouth. Often he'd drop it and have to start all over again. It took an enormous amount of patience, not only for Bill, but for the whole family who watched him struggle. They could only imagine how frustrating it must be, especially for someone who loved cooking and eating the way he did.

The physical therapy staff insisted that Bill had to learn to feed himself properly. That meant Margaret had to restrain herself from helping him, and settle for sitting beside him and coaching. Whenever he got disgusted and gave up, she'd persuade him to try one more time, reminding him of his goals of getting well enough to go home, to visit the forty acres, or whatever she could think of. He'd struggle with the meal as long as they both could stand it—sometimes it took nearly an hour—but if he still hadn't eaten enough by that time, she'd feed him herself. And this sometimes led to confrontations with the hospital staff.

They warned her that she wasn't doing Bill a bit of good to baby him. Stroke patients, they said, must be pushed hard to relearn simple skills; otherwise they become increasingly dependent. Margaret told them that she certainly did want him to regain those skills. But it was also clear that Bill needed proper nutrition to build up his strength and to keep his diabetes under control. If it came down to a question of nourishing him now or rehabilitating him in the long run, Margaret figured she'd better make sure he was nourished.

Even though the methods had been refined through years of research and practice, they were hard for Margaret to watch. The therapists insisted, for example, that Bill grasp his fork just so. But she could see that it took more energy to hold his fork that way, and he already seemed exhausted all the time. If Bill could eat more easily by holding the fork with his fist, well, what was so bad about that? It was like the painful process in the movie *The Miracle Worker*, where Helen Keller goes through childhood doing things her own way until a new teacher, Annie Sullivan, forces her to start all over.

But Bill wasn't a young child. He was a man who'd been dying until he got an artificial heart. Margaret had experienced enough jolts by now to know that something could go wrong at any moment. If, as DeVries himself had said, the heart might last only two years or so, why should Bill be put through such misery in order to learn skills he might never live to use? Just get him well enough to go home and share a little more time with his family. The issue of how much and how fast the staff was pushing Bill disturbed the whole family, and often Margaret and the therapists took turns unraveling what the other had just done.

After breakfast, Margaret and the nurse helped Bill clean up for the day. Sometimes Margaret gave him a sponge bath, but usually he had a shower. The bathroom was too small to accommodate the Utah, so Margaret and a nurse or a physical therapist usually took him down the hall to a larger shower stall adjoining the intensive-care unit. For this excursion, the Utah had to be unplugged from the wall's electrical and compressed-air outlets. A primary air tank would activate automatically, supplying compressed air for up to an hour, and the electrical system would switch over to a battery good for seventy-two hours. When the reserve tank was in use, a yellow light on the console would blink and emit beeps every few minutes as a reminder. If the reserve tank ran out, the Utah automatically switched over to a second reserve tank, which could also be replaced if necessary. Margaret learned to switch the tanks herself. This involved reaching inside the cabinet under the Utah's console, shutting off the air valves inside, freeing the tank from its coupling with a wrench, then putting in a new one and securing it. Although the procedure wasn't very complicated, it could be difficult if you hadn't done it in a while, so Margaret stayed in practice, just in case.

When Bill was out of bed and the Utah was set to go, his entourage would assemble. Sometimes this involved a wait, if, for example, they had to round up an extra nurse or track down a security guard. In the meantime, Margaret combed Bill's hair and made sure he was presentable in his bathrobe and slippers. Then Bill stood up and leaned on one end of the Utah, pushing it like a shopping cart, as a nurse or physical therapist guided the front end into the hall. Margaret walked alongside, sleeves rolled up and arms full of soap, shampoo, towels, and washcloths. A nurse followed behind, loosely holding a hand at Bill's back, encouraging him to walk on his own, but staying close in case he lost his balance. The security guard led the way. When they reached the bathroom, a nurse plugged the Utah back into an electrical outlet and a large compressed-air tank there. The seven-foot drive lines reached into the shower stall. The nurse and Margaret helped get Bill undressed and into the shower. Anybody who has ever checked into a hospital knows that modesty is something you can't bring with you. But it must have been weird for Bill to have so many people helping him to the shower. Even Strode came along once and took pictures of Bill peeping around the shower curtain.

Using a green liquid antiseptic and a washcloth, Margaret would carefully swab the area where the drive lines were connected to his body, an extremely important ritual to help prevent infection. Then she lathered up the washcloth so he could wash himself, and gave him a hand-held shower head to rinse off. When Bill felt good, he could do a lot for himself with minimal supervision from Margaret. Usually he could even shave himself by holding the rechargeable razor still while he slowly moved his face against it.

Bill really liked taking showers, perhaps because he could be pretty much in control of things for a change. He loved the fresh feel of the water hitting his skin—but what he enjoyed even more was suddenly turning the sprayer to hose down the nurses. Bill would laugh so hard that everyone else had to laugh, too. He was still the same old jokester, just like when he used to spray pranksters on Devil's Night in Michigan.

By the time Bill had been dried off, dressed, and taken back to his room, it would be midmorning—and he already looked worn out. He was helped back into bed for a nap, which provided a welcome break for Margaret and the nurse. But many times the nap would only last a half hour or so before the occupational therapist knocked on the door. Again, Bill would be roused from sleep and assisted into the chair. The occupational therapist tried to help Bill's eye-hand coordination by having him work puzzles, or test his dexterity at dropping various pegs into similarly shaped holes.

By the time OT ended, Bill seemed weary but his day was far from over. About noon, the speech therapist was at the door. It was hard for Margaret to imagine how frustrating it must be for Bill to know what he wanted to say but not be able to get the words out. He'd always had a quick comeback or a new joke to tell, always razzed anyone and everyone, and never hesitated to speak his mind—as the whole world knew after Bill's chat with the president. Now he was reduced to thinking out every tiny step to form each word before he even tried to say it.

By mid-January, Bill could answer questions with one- or two-word responses. But the possibility of having a full-fledged conversation with him was gone. If people took the time to listen patiently and concentrate, Bill could still communicate enough to let them know what he wanted. Margaret learned better than anyone to figure out what he said. Sometimes when the Schroeder kids visited, they'd look at their father in confusion as he murmured something unintelligible.

Margaret would jump up and say, "Okay, honey, I'll get you one."

"What are you doing, Mom?"

"You heard him. He wants a glass of water."

The kids would look at each other in amazement as Bill gratefully took a sip. It sure hadn't *sounded* like he was asking for water. But Margaret knew Bill better than anyone. And she sat with him, day after day, figuring out what he was trying to say.

The kids would concentrate hard as Bill slowly struggled to make sounds come out and gave them a hopeful, expectant look, as if to say, "You understand?"

"I'm sorry, Dad, I didn't get it. Say it again. Real slow this time."

He'd work at it again and again. Sometimes they'd try to guess, as if playing Twenty Questions. Or, sometimes, like many stroke patients, Bill would still say one thing, when he meant something completely different.

Since the speech therapist required Bill's full concentration, Margaret often slipped upstairs to put her feet up for a while. Her arthritis still flared up frequently. This would make her feet swell if she stood for more than an hour. He hands were unable even to twist off the cap on a soft drink. But she felt that those problems were nothing compared to Bill's; she'd worry about them later. She'd take all her medicines for the arthritis and heart condition, open some mail, and be back downstairs by the time the half-hour speech-therapy session ended.

By now Bill would be drained mentally as well as physically. He'd been up for about five hours with only a half-hour nap, and he looked wearier than ever. Lunch was supposed to arrive about then, but nearly every day it seemed that something else would throw off the whole schedule. Between all the regularly scheduled activities, dozens of tests had to be squeezed in as the doctors ordered them—EEGs, X rays, blood work, exams by some new specialist, and the like. The tests had priority, so the rest of Bill's day had to be hastily rearranged. But then, too, how many times have you been told to be ready for an X ray at 2:00 P.M., only to have them come for you an hour later?

Ideally, Bill's schedule called for him to nap for about an hour after lunch. Then the physical therapists returned to take him downstairs for an exercise session. Again, this was a big production. It meant getting Bill out of bed, readying the machinery, gathering his entourage, sending the security guard ahead to hold the elevator. They usually brought along a wheelchair in case Bill started to falter. Whenever he left the room, Margaret insisted that he look presentable, as if they were going out to eat or to church. After all, Bill did have a following: Everyone in the halls either knew him or wanted to be introduced. And unless he was completely exhausted, he enjoyed getting out, waving at people, and just being around them.

In physical therapy, Bill's favorite activity was riding an exercise bike which faced a big picture window overlooking the wooded area behind the hospital. On good days, he'd show off by pedaling faster or with no hands whenever anyone was watching. He was also put through a grueling series of walking and stair-climbing exercises. Even when Bill grew tired, the therapists kept urging him to take a few more steps. Bill would give Margaret a helpless look, as if pleading with her to make them stop. Margaret had to bite her tongue to keep from assuring him that he could stop to rest. She was torn between staying there and seeing him look so miserable and wondering what would happen if she left. The therapists kept pushing him to take "just two more steps, Bill, and that'll be enough." But if he complied, they sometimes said, "Okay, you did so well, let's try two more." It just seemed to go on and on until Margaret couldn't blame Bill if he never believed another word the therapists said.

Besides, even if the rehab staff did know how to help stroke patients, they apparently had forgotten that this one had an artificial heart. Maybe they *didn't* know all there was to know about helping someone like Bill, Margaret thought. Maybe, like everyone else in the artificial heart program, they had to learn as they went along.

The whole Schroeder family also had to wonder on a deeper level about why Bill was being pushed. Was he under special pressure because he was in the middle of this high-profile medical project? Was the staff trying, perhaps unconsciously, to make him some kind of "star patient," to show off how well someone with an artificial heart could recover from a stroke? Or, even more disturbing, were the doctors eager to move him out of the hospital so they could start over with a new Jarvik-7 recipient? The staff could have shown the family study after study or a stack of medical textbooks that said that stroke patients needed that kind of urging, but such questions still bothered them.

After physical therapy, Bill & Company would return to his room around the 3:00 P.M. shift change, when the departing nurse briefed the incoming nurse about what had happened that day and what needed to be done on the next shift. The security

guards always made a point of coming in to say hello to Bill
before taking up their post outside his room. Bill especially enjoyed visits from them, and always shook their hands and called
them "My Protectors." By this point in the day, Bill required
even more help to get back in bed, and he usually fell asleep
quickly. About an hour later, supper trays arrived. By now Bill
would be difficult to wake, and Margaret had to help him a lot
with his meal.

In fact, he was so tired all the time that his family wondered whether the artificial heart or his medications might somehow be contributing to the fatigue. When they asked Dr. DeVries,
he said that stroke patients were often easily fatigued. Besides,
the Jarvik heart was pumping the same amount of blood at the
same rate that a normal heart would in a man his age. However,
what Margaret saw with her own eyes still raised questions.

After supper, Margaret and the nurses once more helped
Bill out of bed and into the chair. He almost always had a few
visitors then—family, friends, sometimes a local celebrity or two.
The Schroeder kids still took turns driving the ninety miles to the
hospital and back. Every day at least one of them would call, and
Margaret would describe Bill's condition, based on information
she had gathered from the doctors and from what she had observed firsthand. The kids had generally stopped listening to news
accounts or reading the papers because so many reports were upsetting, inconclusive, or just plain inaccurate. Instead, they relied on the information from their mom. Even then, it was hard to
keep up with how their father was doing. Sometimes, as word was
relayed from one family member to another, details were changed
inadvertently or left out entirely, as in the game Telephone. They
were torn between wanting to be there to support their parents
and carrying on with their own lives, as they knew Margaret and
Bill also wanted them to do.

From Margaret's diary:

Jan. 19. Mel called and I let him talk to Bill and he started
crying and wanting to see the grandchildren. Mel couldn't
stand that so he gathered them up and here he came. Bill
cheered up and went to PT.

Sometimes Margaret would call one of them and pour out
the frustrations and worries that had built up inside her through-

out the day. Maybe Bill seemed more tired and depressed than usual, or he wouldn't talk to her at all, or he refused to eat. If the day had gone badly, she faced the dilemma of deciding whether she should ask the kids to drive down or hold off until things got worse.

On the other hand, visiting hours—in the evening and all weekend—often brought good times. Whenever the kids visited, they'd sit close to their dad, hold his hand, and remind him that they were behind him 100 percent. They'd catch him up on what was happening in their lives, and often brought along snapshots of the latest wedding or family gathering. Sometimes they'd get him into a card game, which he really enjoyed. Bill's dexterity was improving enough so that he could fan out the cards in his hand, and play a card when his turn rolled around. His short-term memory might have been impaired, but he never forgot the object of the game, and always tried hard to win. At times, to tease the kids, he'd even try to cheat. But on bad days when he didn't feel well, he might sleep throughout their visit. They never really knew what to expect until they arrived.

Sometimes the kids took off work to stay at the hospital for a day or so just to give their mother a few hours' rest. Each time, they realized anew what a hard job their mother performed day after day—relentless, wearing, sit-down-and-stand-up work. Each day brought a numbing mixture of the Utah's alarms sounding intermittently, laboratory technicians coming to run new tests, people dropping in with requests for Bill to do something. In addition, it was a constant struggle to understand his speech, guess his needs and wants, boost his spirits, and meet all the little minute-to-minute needs of someone with a long illness.

Long before the day ended, the Schroeder kids were stunned to find themselves ready to collapse into the nearest chair, thoroughly exhausted. They could not imagine how their mother kept up that pace day in and day out. They were also keenly aware that if Mom was concentrating on Dad's health, she was going to neglect her own. Each time they saw her, her clothes seemed to fit a little more loosely; since coming to Audubon, she'd lost some twenty-five to thirty pounds. Because they couldn't be there to remind her, Cheryl hand-lettered a big sign and taped it to the wall in Margaret's room: TAKE YOUR MEDICINE, MOM! Margaret knew exactly what they meant, but she didn't want them to be concerned. She already felt bad that the kids now had, in effect, two parents in the hospital to worry about. The kids also began to realize that there was definitely another heart keeping their father alive—one that could never be removed or replaced, a heart more wondrous than any scientist could ever design. Bill himself had said on TV that he had a big purpose for living—and she was at his side each day, as together they made the longest and most difficult journey of their lives.

When visiting hours ended about 8:00 P.M., Margaret would carefully clean apould Bill's drive lines. She'd put on surgical gloves and remove the bandages covering the areas where the lines entered his body. By now the skin around them was healing so that each site looked something like a navel with a tube coming out of it. Margaret swabbed each area with gauze soaked in a mixture of peroxide and water, and used a hypodermic syringe to squirt the solution into hard-to-reach places. Then she applied new dressings, covered them with bandages and tape, and marked her initials and the date on the tape to show when the cleaning had been done. Such sterile procedure was vital for preventing infections, which would cause serious complications, so Margaret and the nurse performed the task scrupulously every evening.

Bill's day usually ended about 8:30 or 9:00 P.M., when he went to sleep for the night—unless some other complication kept him awake. The night nurse came on duty at eleven. The day nurse returned at seven the next morning, and it would start all over; business as usual.

As time went on, shift changes sometimes brought new tension into Bill's hospital room. Bill and Margaret didn't exactly welcome new faces among the nurses—at least not until they'd all worked together awhile. About ten nurses worked regularly with Bill, but substitutes were drawn from an even larger pool. When a new nurse came on Bill's case, it would be his or her first real experience with such a patient, and there was lots to learn: how the Utah and Heimes drives functioned in actual practice, which emergency numbers to call for various problems, what special data had to be collected, what supplies were to be used and where they were kept, and how Bill was doing physically and mentally on a given day.

The Schroeders came to feel that the most important component of a hospital stay isn't fancy medicine or sophisticated devices. It's nursing care. The doctors and the space-age technology may have been featured on magazine covers and in TV reports, but the nurses were the real backbone of the medical team, probably doing more work for less pay than anyone else. As if caring for a stroke patient with an artificial heart wasn't challenging enough, the nurses also had to deal diplomatically with a host of doctors and serve as go-betweens for a large, anxious family. They'd re-explain the doctors' explanations, spell out the options when the family faced decisions, and learn to communicate with eight family members who had their own individual ways of handling this ordeal.

As in any other profession, some nurses worked tirelessly, making it obvious that they really cared about Bill. Others weren't as efficient or enthusiastic. A nurse could set the tone for the whole day: If a good one was on duty, Margaret would breathe a little easier and go to bed earlier that evening; if a not-so-good one came on, Margaret usually stayed with Bill through the whole shift.

Because Margaret remained at his side every day, she observed individual nurses' ways, and had decided early on which methods were the most efficient and least troublesome for Bill. She'd helped change Bill's bandages, moved him in and out of bed, given him baths, and coaxed him into eating when no one else could. She'd held his hand to calm him when they came to draw blood or change an IV needle. She'd comforted him when he became weepy, and tried to cheer him when he was depressed. So she didn't take kindly to anyone making changes in their little routines. And she certainly didn't like someone telling her what Bill was trying to say or wanted to do. She'd lived with the man for thirty-three years and knew what he meant and felt, stroke or no stroke.

Margaret also pointed out all the physical changes in Bill that the staff might have overlooked. She found new bruises, skin irritations, eyesight and hearing problems, possible infections— all the tiny things you pick up when you're with someone every day and really care about him. Margaret made sure the nurses noticed these things, too, and they soon learned that her worries were often well founded. Then together they faced the challenge of calling attention to the problems she felt that the doctors had missed during their quick early-morning exams. "Gee," Margaret might say as the doctor was writing orders, "I wonder what this little red area is here . . ."

With similar attentiveness, Margaret would observe new

nurses, noting each mistake or variation in performing a task, such as getting Bill out of bed or finding a vein. The nurses sensed her tension, which added to their own. They were treading new ground just like everyone else. Not only were they unfamiliar with the experience of caring for a man with an artificial heart— they were cardiovascular nurses and for many of them, the long-term care of a stroke patient wasn't their area of expertise. They were also working in a fishbowl. Dr. DeVries had to document everything so carefully for the federal regulators that if a nurse made a mistake, the FDA would certainly scrutinize their work. If something went terribly wrong, it would be all over the news the next day. And the most unnerving part of all might well have been being accountable to their patient's own watchful wife, diary and pen in hand.

The stress of caring for the world's only living artificial heart patient took its toll. From time to time nurses asked to be removed from the case. The high turnover meant that Margaret and Bill continually had to get used to new nurses. No one under-stood why the hospital didn't just assign a core team of nurses to work with Bill from beginning to end. Polly Brown told them that such an arrangement would be ideal in theory, but she asked how, in real life, could you stretch that team over three shifts a day, seven days a week, and also accommodate sick days, vaca-tions, and emergencies? Still, the Schroeders felt that the nursing assignments could and should have been more consistent—but it would be months before the problem was resolved.

Just as Dr. Lansing had predicted in that first meeting to discuss the artificial heart, with all the daily comings and goings of staffers, quiet times for Bill and Margaret were few and far between. When they did manage to find a rare moment alone, it meant everything. Sometimes, amid the everyday hustle and bus-tle of the hospital, the couple simply created their own private moments. When Bill, for example, sensed that his wife was tired or worried, he'd take her hand, kiss it, grip it tightly, and pat it. Then he'd look steadily into her eyes for a long time, as if to reassure her that they were going to make it through this thing together, side by side, just as always.

Sunday, Jan. 6. The kids and I went out to breakfast. Came back and waited till after 12 o'clock for Bill to wake up. He seems so hard to wake up. I think it's the medicine he is taking.

We ate and then he went for a walk in the hallway. . . . He seems to have a hard time swallowing pills or capsules . . .

He can get up and get in bed by himself. He is getting stronger every day. Just wish he could talk to me. I need to ask so many things of him. His mind is still so confused. This medicine just makes him sleep . . .

Since the stroke he has been shy of the heart and the machine. I think he has to regain his knowledge of the machine and his trust of the people taking care of the machine.

Am going upstairs for the night, hoping things will go good tonight. I just feel like I must talk to someone. I miss having someone to share the day with. No one to talk to. The kids are so good, but to share your life with someone is another thing.

Goodnight.

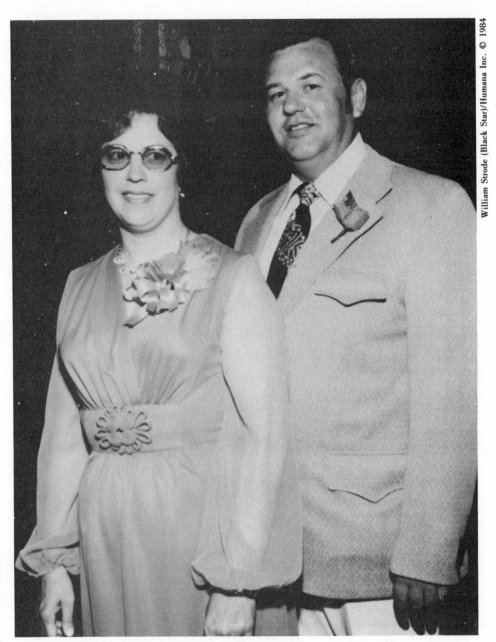

September 2, 1975. Margaret and Bill Schroeder on their twenty-fifth wedding anniversary.

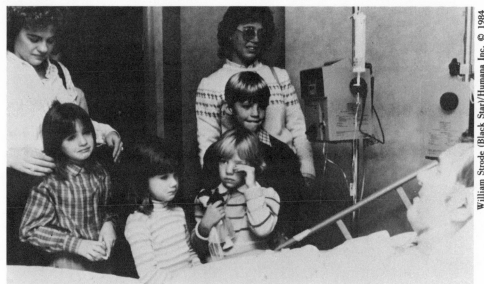

November 24, 1984. The day before Bill's historic operation at Louisville's Humana Hospital-Audubon, the family gathers at his bedside. (*Left to right:* Cheryl; Mel's daughters, Melanie and Abbie; Stan's daughter, Tracy; Moni's children, Vicki and Bobby)

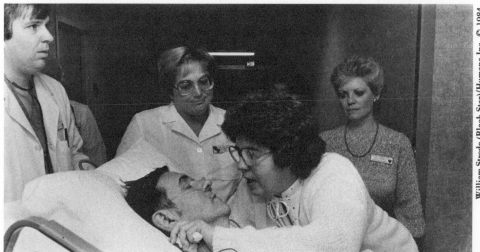

November 25, 1984. Just before 7:00 A.M., Margaret says a final good-bye to Bill as he is wheeled into surgery. (*Background, left to right:* Dr. William DeVries's surgical associate Dr. Ronald Barbie, director of the coronary intensive-care unit; Laura Wood, R.N.; patient coordinator Kevan Shaheen, R.N.)

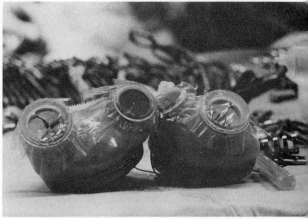

Still in sterilized wrappings, the two chambers of the Jarvik-7 heart lie alongside other surgical tools as Dr. DeVries opens Bill's chest.

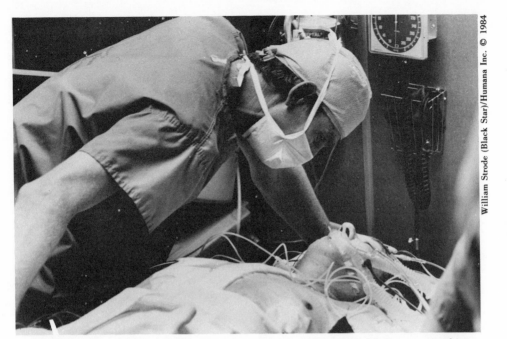

After the surgery, Bill is returned to intensive care with the artificial heart pumping his blood and the respirator forcing air into his lungs. Dr. DeVries leans close to tell his anesthetized patient: "Everything went perfect."

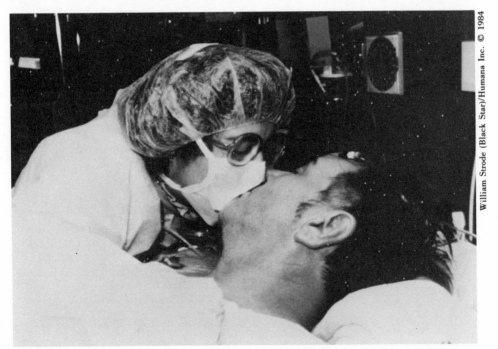

November 27, 1984. After the respirator tube has been removed from his mouth, Bill returns a kiss from Margaret, who is dressed in surgical garb to reduce the risk of infection.

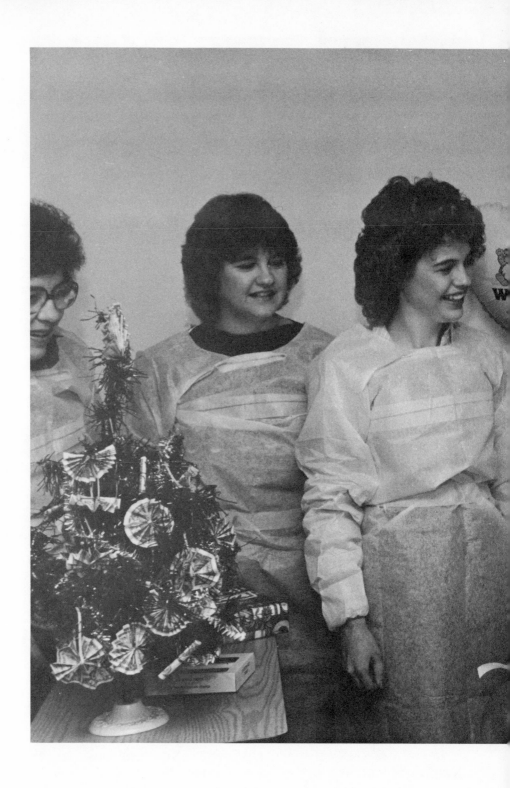

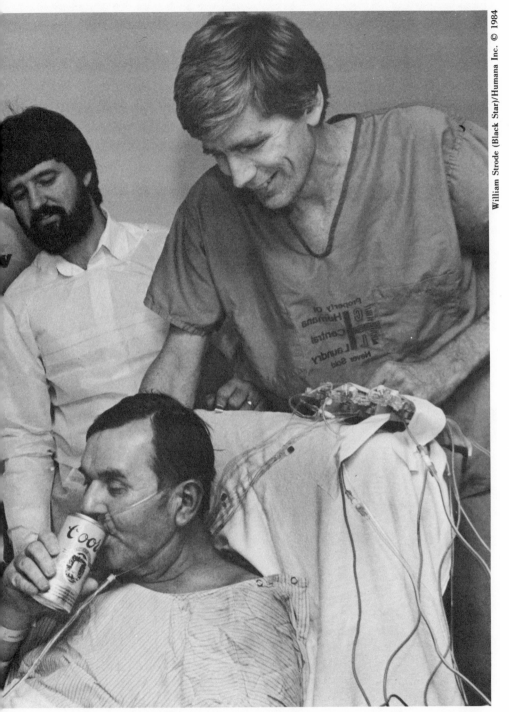

November 29, 1984. Bill gets the beer he asked for, and jokes about the "Coors Cure." (*Standing, left to right:* Margaret, Moni, Cheryl, Mel, Dr. DeVries)

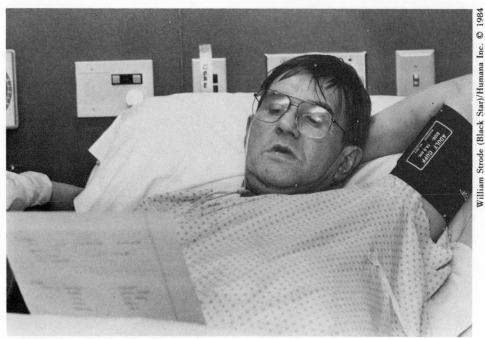

Early December 1984. Bill's miraculous recovery continues, and he looks like his old self again, reading over a handwritten list.

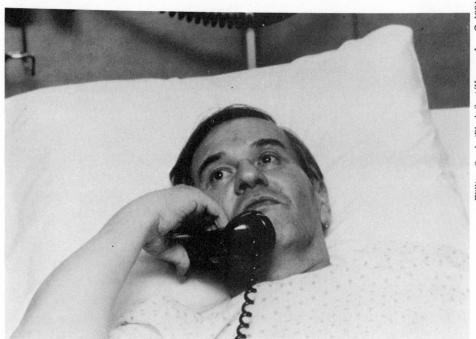

December 12, 1984. Bill upstages a congratulatory call from President Ronald Reagan by griping about a delay in getting his Social Security benefits.

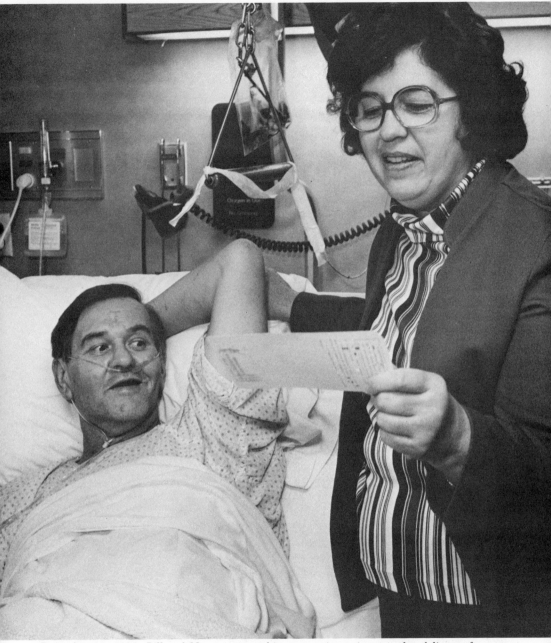

December 13, 1984. Bill and Margaret savor his success in getting next-day delivery of his Social Security check after just one phone call.

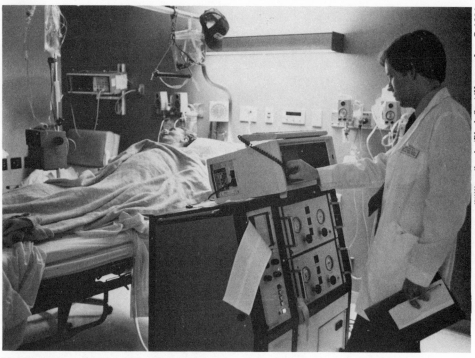

Mid-December, 1984. After the stroke, Bill sleeps a lot. Technician Brent Mays checks a readout on the computer atop the 300 + -pound Utahdrive.

December 23, 1984. Despite stroke complications, Bill begins to bounce back. (*Clockwise from left:* Moni, Stan, Rod, Terry, Margaret, Cheryl, Bill)

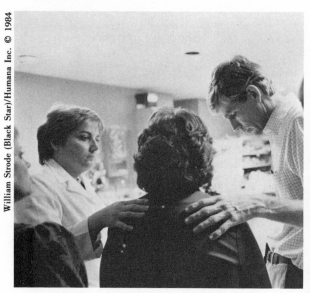

December 13, 1984. Within hours of receiving his Social Security check, Bill suffers a devastating stroke. Outside his intensive-care room, nurse Laura Wood and Dr. DeVries steady Margaret as DeVries explains.

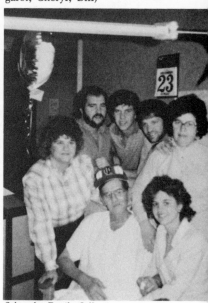

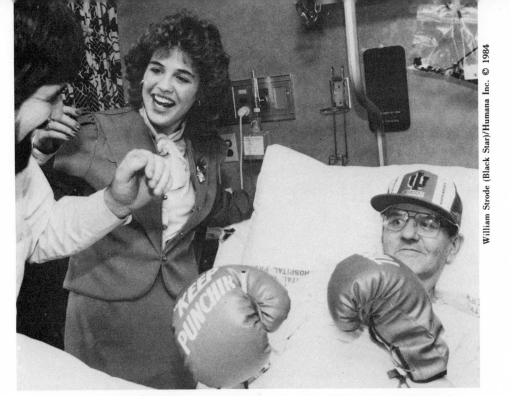

Christmas morning, 1984. Almost two weeks after the stroke, Bill is feeling well enough to kid around with Mel and Cheryl. He is sporting boxing gloves, compliments of a sporting goods company, and his favorite Indiana University cap.

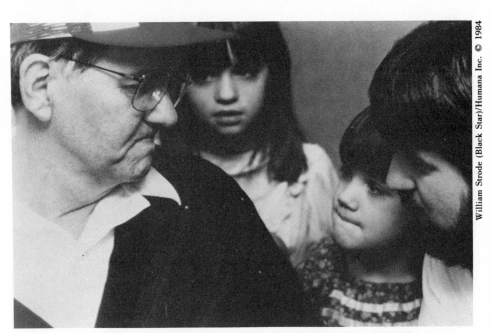

Christmas Day, 1984. As the whole family gathers at the hospital for Christmas dinner, Bill and granddaughter Abbie share a moment along with Melanie and Mel. It was a day that, without the artificial heart, Bill would never have lived to see.

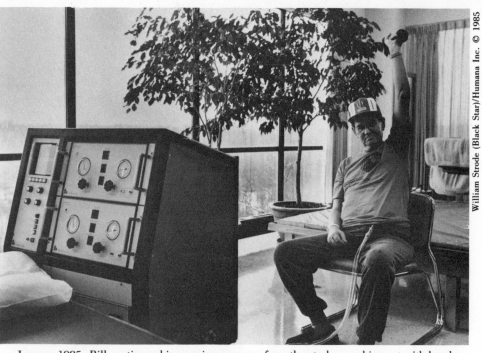

January 1985. Bill continues his amazing recovery from the stroke, working out with hand weights in grueling physical therapy sessions.

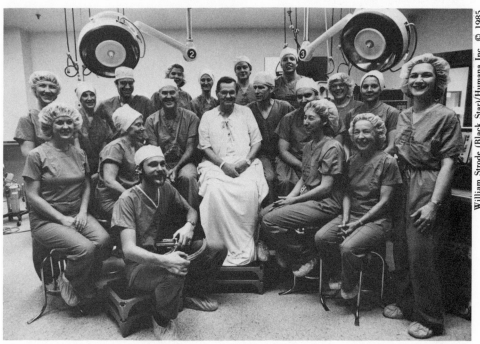

Bill poses in the operating room for a photo, flanked by Dr. Lansing, Dr. DeVries, and the rest of the surgical team. In the front, technician Larry Hastings cradles the Heimes portable drive.

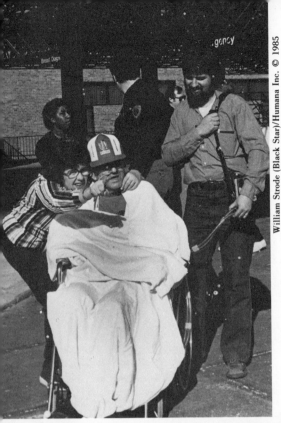

February 19, 1985. On Bill's first wheelchair ride outside the hospital—the first
one ever for an artificial heart patient—
Margaret points across the street to the apartment that will soon be their new home. Mel
shoulders the Heimes.

On the way back to Bill's room after his
first ride outdoors, the group stops by Murray Haydon's room, and for the first time,
two men with artificial hearts greet each
other.

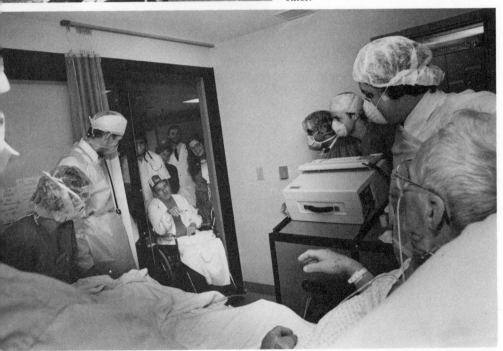

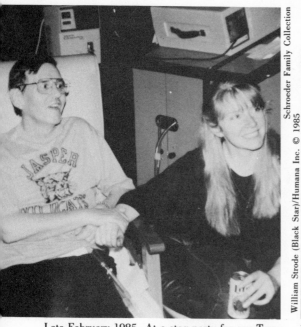
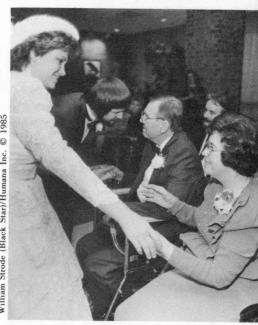

Late February 1985. At a stag party for son Terry in the doctors' lounge, Bill makes friends with technician Larry Hastings's wife, Vicky. Bill is enjoying the party immensely—at a time when critics of the artificial heart program are questioning his quality of life.

March 15, 1985. Julie and Terry offer Bill and Margaret the sign of peace at the wedding blessing. Bill acknowledges it tearfully. (*Background:* Peter Heimes, behind Bill, and Stan's wife, Terri)

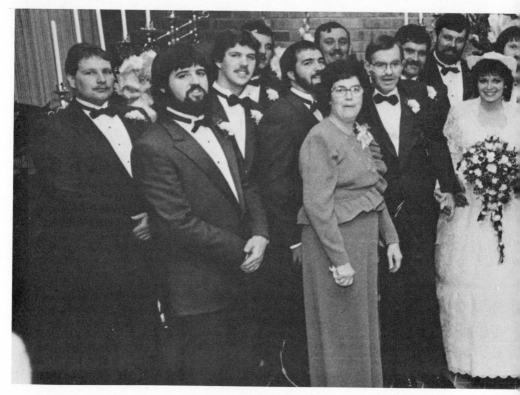

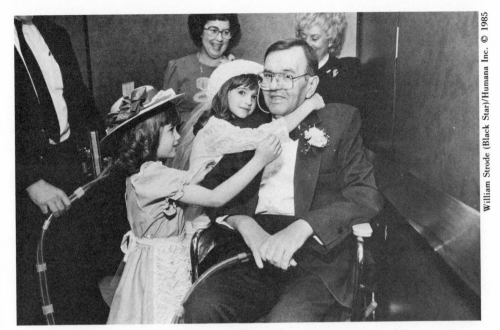

Bill and his granddaughters Abbie and Melanie ride an elevator to the wedding reception in the hospital auditorium. (*Background:* Margaret and Polly Brown)

After the wedding blessing in the hospital lobby, Bill stands with his family and holds the bride's hand as they all pose for pictures.

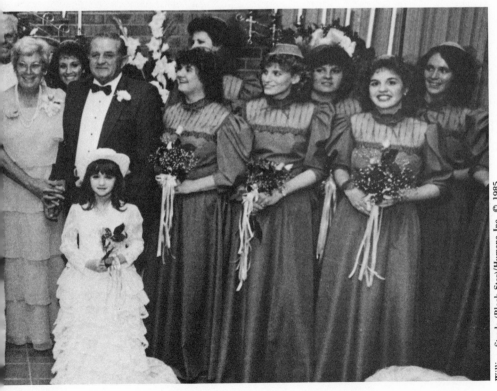

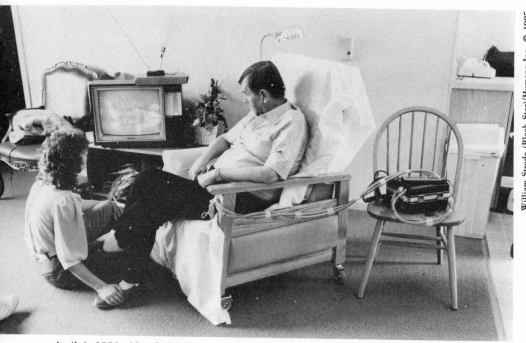

April 6, 1985. After Bill becomes the world's first artificial heart patient to be discharged from a hospital, he and Cheryl relax in the apartment living room as they watch bowling on TV. The Heimes drive rests on a nearby kitchen chair.

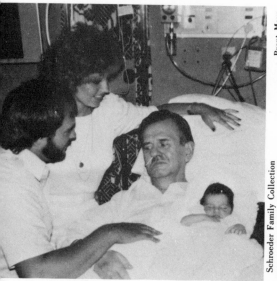

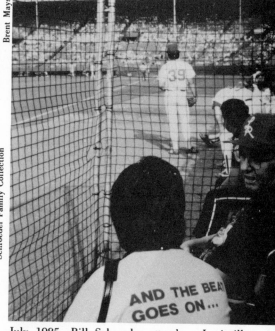

June 2, 1985. Almost a month after a brain hemorrhage sends him back to the hospital, Bill witnesses the christening of his brand-new grandson, achieving one of the cherished goals he cited as a reason for trying the artificial heart. Within days after this photo, he shows signs of yet another remarkable recovery. (*Left to right:* Stan and his wife, Terri, Bill, and grandson Lukas William Schroeder)

July 1985. Bill Schroeder attends a Louisville Redbirds minor-league baseball game with his four sons. Mel takes his turn sitting with his father and holds the portable Heimes.

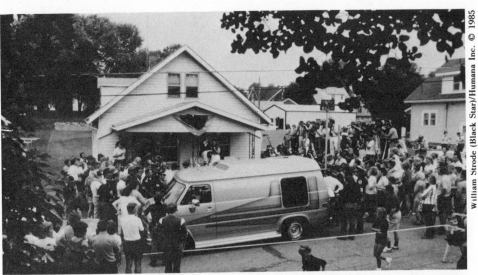

August 1985. Terry pulls the specially equipped van up to the curb at the Schroeder home on Mill Street, which is draped with banners for Jasper's annual Strassenfest. A crowd gathers to see Bill's triumphant return home.

Dr. DeVries and his wife, Karen, wait on the Schroeders' front porch as Bill's wheelchair is lifted from the van and he sees his beloved home for the first time in ten months.

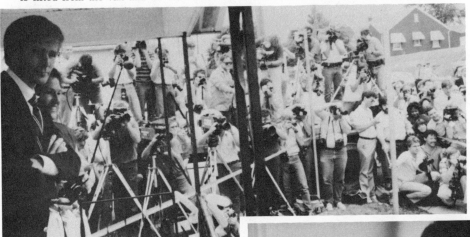

Late August 1985. After being discharged to the apartment a second time, Bill and Margaret have some family time with their grandchildren. (*Left to right:* Abbie, Tracy, Bill, Margaret, Lukas, Melanie)

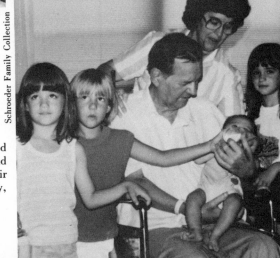

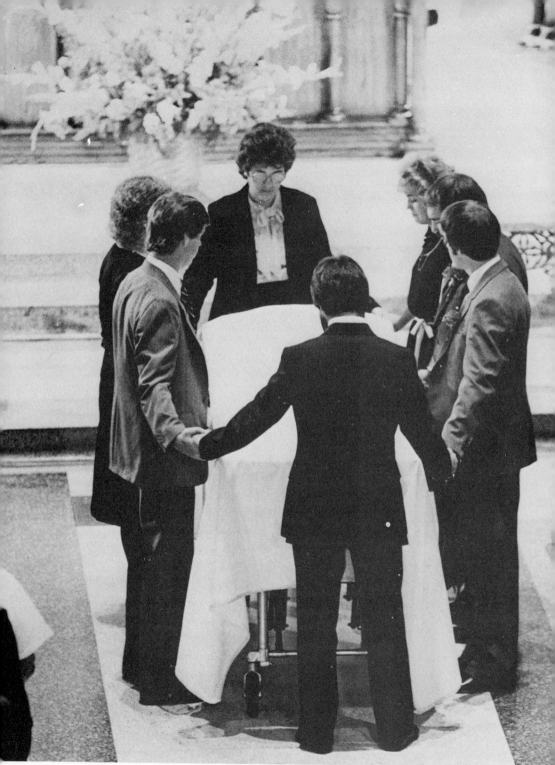

The Schroeder family, in a united gesture, hold hands
around Bill's casket during funeral proceedings.

Humana Inc.

CHAPTER ELEVEN

Throughout January, Bill's condition was as unpredictable as Louisville's weather. He might feel good and get stronger for a few days, only to have some complication send him sliding back down, leaving him weak and feeling lousy. It was like a roller-coaster ride. On good days he would stride the halls enthusiastically—covering the equivalent of four city blocks—and his entourage had to walk briskly to keep up. He'd be eager to get out of bed and brighten even more when family visited. On wheelchair rides Bill would point which direction he wanted to go, and he seldom wanted to return to his room. He was doing so well, in fact, that the medical team began planning to discharge him to the halfway house across the street.

However, each time Bill seemed to get better, complications developed. He began to have brief periods every few weeks during which he seemed to go into a trance, with his mouth drawn to one side. The episode would be over within minutes, and he'd appear fine afterward, but very drowsy. Doctors ordered an electroencephalogram, or EEG, in which several tiny electrodes were inserted in his scalp and earlobes to measure brain activity. The results suggested he'd had some kind of seizure, but the doctors weren't certain. They might also have been small strokes, caused by tiny clots that lodged in his brain but then dissolved without causing permanent damage. Lansing described those periods as "seizurelike episodes" or "periods of vacancy." There was no clear-cut explanation for them. Dr. Fox decided to try the anti-seizure drug Dilantin to see if prescribing it helped.

Bill was also continually weakened by anemia—in part a result of the Jarvik-7's action. His blood was being churned, in effect, by the harsh motion of the artificial heart's metal valves, which smashed oxygen-bearing red cells as they passed through. Such destruction of blood cells, or "hemolysis," wasn't as exten-

209

sive with the Heimes drive, which pumped more gently; Symbion researchers were working on a new Utahdrive that would pump more like the portable. But it would be months before the new Utah would be ready for Bill's use.

In the meantime, DeVries battled Bill's anemia by giving him transfusions every couple of weeks. Bill seemed to perk up after each transfusion, but would gradually become more tired and feeble over the next few days, as if his blood were being drained out of him, which in a sense it was. The number of transfusions had to be limited because whenever a needle pierced his skin, he ran a greater risk of infection.

Bill also developed stomach pains, which were so severe that the doctors gave him morphine. He endured more uncomfortable tests to find out what was wrong: A muscle near his stomach was hemorrhaging, due to excessive anticoagulation. The pain stopped after doctors adjusted the dosages of blood-thinners. About this time, Margaret pointed out to the doctors that Bill seemed to have trouble seeing with his right eye. An ophthalmologist confirmed her suspicion: Probably because of the stroke, vision in that eye was impaired. But because Bill couldn't converse well, it was difficult to determine the extent of the damage.

Like many stroke patients, Bill had a hard time concentrating. If several people in his room were all carrying on a conversation together, he might become confused or overwhelmed. Many times, Bill also seemed sad and listless, again typical for a stroke patient. He'd refuse to eat or get out of bed. He might refuse to take his medicine, or he'd hold the pill in his hand and hide it under the sheet when no one was looking. Sometimes he'd cry at the slightest thing. Dr. Mudd, the psychiatrist, prescribed antidepressants for Bill. Every few weeks or so, Bill appeared to have another seizurelike episode. It was often difficult to tell what was really happening, because at times he would pretend to be asleep and refuse to open his eyes. And who could really blame him? So many people were in and out of the room all the time; his eyes were the only doors he could shut. Bill had always been used to being in charge, and this was now one of his few means of exerting control on his surroundings.

A number of other nuisances occurred as the days and nights went on. Whenever anyone stuck Bill with a needle either for blood work or to monitor his diabetes, often several times a day, the blood-thinners he was given made him bleed more than normal. He was also having trouble swallowing, and had lost his ability to control certain other bodily functions.

In the beginning, it had all seemed simple: Replace Bill's bad heart with a good one, and get him well enough to go home. Now everything was so complicated. In a widely publicized article, Dr. Jarvik had written that the ultimate test of the artificial heart would be whether it was "forgettable." Yes, the machinery was pumping so flawlessly that it *was* sometimes forgettable—but only because there were too many other things to worry about.

The family had never dreamed that having an artificial heart could involve so many additional physical problems. When Bill had signed the consent form, he was like a drowning man going under for the last time. When somebody tosses you a lifeline, you don't think about what's at the other end. You just grab it, hold tight, and hope you're pulled to safety. Only then do you worry about what happens next.

Even though the list of Bill's complications grew longer and longer, he still showed flashes of the old spunk and spirit and sense of humor that had brought him this far.

One day that winter, when the kids visited him, he was feeling down. Stan stood by his bed and tried to give his father a pep talk, just as Bill had done for him during his high-school years.

"Come on, Dad! You got to get mad at this thing, if you're going to beat it. You just gotta hang in there and keep punching," Stan said.

Bill just stared glumly.

"You can do it, Dad. I know you can. You just got to get mad and *whip* this thing!"

Bill kept looking straight ahead, then whipped back his arm and socked his son with a roundhouse punch. Stan doubled over, groaning, and the others burst into laughter. Bill was laughing, too. So did Stan when he finally caught his breath. Bill had made it clear who would decide whether he needed a pep talk.

Another time, Bill's nurse, Sandy Chandler, brought in her morning cup of coffee, set it near Bill's bed, then left briefly. When she returned, her coffee cup was empty. Bill's eyes were closed as if he was asleep, but he had a huge grin on his face. Sandy couldn't believe it, and kept asking what happened. She'd been gone for only a minute—he must have gulped that whole thing in a hurry. Bill tried harder and harder to keep his eyes and mouth shut, but his body was shaking with laughter. Just as the stroke had dissolved some of his rough-and-tough exterior, it had also taken away his ability to keep a poker face when he played a trick on someone.

Despite all the special, irreplaceable moments the family shared with Bill, the stress was beginning to take its toll. Increasingly, the night-shift nurse would arrive to find Margaret still at Bill's side, taking care of him or dozing on the small couch. Dr. Richard Allen, a Louisville cardiologist, examined Margaret and recommended that she participate in Audubon's cardiac-rehab program. So she began going downstairs for periodic treadmill tests and to exercise on a rowing machine three times a week.

Back home, the kids still faced questions about their dad wherever they went. Cheryl's desk in the Kimball Company's main office was out front, and tour guides would walk by and point her out as Bill Schroeder's daughter. She was asked so often about his condition that finally she began answering, "Oh, he's doing okay." It always felt awkward. Was she really expected to go into a full-length explanation?

Whenever the family were out in public, they knew they were being watched. They heard the hushed whispers when they entered a bar, and in restaurants they would feel stares and glance up as someone was pointing them out. Sometimes, though, they couldn't be sure they'd been recognized—but even if they weren't being watched, it still felt that way.

And, of course, worries about both their parents were always with them. Anytime they left home, they'd wonder whether they would miss an important call from the hospital. It might have been easier if someone had told them what to expect or how long their dad's recovery would take. But nobody knew. In order to concentrate at their jobs, they learned to snap their emotions on and off like a light switch.

The kids had always dropped in at their folks' house once or twice a week. Now it was frustrating to have to plan and coordinate the long drives to the hospital. Since it was winter, they all paid much closer attention to weather and road conditions. Whoever planned to drive to Louisville would first stop by the Mill Street house to check for supplies or messages to take to Mom and Dad. If the kids went after work, they'd often arrive only an hour or so before evening visiting hours ended. They'd have to be ready for anything because Bill's condition was so unpredictable.

Before Cheryl left for Louisville, she'd gather her mom's clean laundry, mail, and phone messages, then pick up her prescriptions at a Jasper drugstore, and ride down with Glenn. Cheryl and Moni, more so than their brothers, would pitch in with Bill's nursing care and take over tasks to relieve Margaret and the nurses. Cheryl would bring snapshots of the latest family gathering to show her dad, and usually just talked with him for a long time. Sometimes she urged him to draw in a sketch pad using felt-tip pens. She'd have him trace her hand, and then his own. With her encouragement, Bill also traced other people's hands, sometimes drawing one over a picture of his own. He enjoyed seeing the results on paper, but got an even bigger kick when his subjects discovered that they had ink between their fingers.

For Moni the distance from the hospital was especially frustrating, now that her three-hour drive had stretched into five. She usually tried to arrange her work schedule so that she could stay two or three days at a time at Audubon because it was a relief for Margaret to have a family member there for more than just a few hours at a time.

Terry always brought his dad a new joke, and reported all the latest scores from the Jasper Wildcats games. While there, he'd balance the family checkbook, since Margaret had never done it before. Whenever he and Julie visited they also made sure that Margaret got out of the hospital for a while. Margaret didn't have a car with her; Bill had always insisted on doing the driving, even on long trips, to spare her arthritis and delicate heart. Back home, she occasionally drove The Boat when Bill was sick, but she wasn't about to get out on the streets of a city the size of Louisville. Besides, where would she want to go? Bill needed her, and his room was the only place she wanted to be.

Stan and his wife, Terri, visited as often as possible, although as time went on they grew busier with preparations for their new baby. But one evening they made a special trip to see Bill. As soon as Margaret went upstairs for a few minutes, Stan crouched in front of the chair where Bill was sitting and whispered to him.

"Dad, we've got a secret for you!"

Bill listened intently.

"We went for an ultrasound at Memorial today and guess what we found out? It's a *boy*! Terri's gonna have a baby boy!"

Stan took his father's hand and searched his face. "Do you

understand what I'm telling you, Dad? It's a boy! You're going to have yourself a *Schroeder Grandson!*"

Bill's eyes widened and he slowly smiled.

"Now, nobody's supposed to know, so we've got to keep it a secret, okay, Dad? Don't tell anybody. Not even Mom. Understand?"

Bill grinned and slowly shook his head. No, he wouldn't tell. When Margaret returned, Stan caught his dad's eye and each of them put a finger to his own lips. Even Margaret couldn't get Bill to tell her the secret.

Actually, Stan and Terri weren't supposed to learn the baby's sex. But an ultrasound technician at Memorial, who happened to be married to a Schroeder cousin, thought they'd want to know. Stan was grateful; like his siblings, he'd learned to savor each extra moment with his father, sharing time with him in the here and now without counting on tomorrow. So he and Terri had immediately decided to tell Bill but planned to let everyone else wait until the baby was born.

Rod also visited his parents whenever he could, but never for very long. Instead, he offered to do chores for them around the house in Jasper. He'd never lived on his own, and now he and Cheryl had to run the household themselves. Rod's girl friend, Lori, was away at IU in Bloomington, about two hours from Jasper, studying to be a nurse, so Rod had to carry on long-distance relationships in a couple of directions. He'd considered going away to study computer programming. But he decided that starting school would be too much to handle along with everything else, so he stayed with his wood-factory job. Margaret worried about all of them, but especially about her youngest, Rod.

Mel, as the eldest son, was stepping into his father's role, phoning his mom every day at lunchtime, coordinating the kids' visits, attending meetings with doctors, and bringing Patti and their daughters down for visits. When Margaret faced questions and decisions about Bill's medical treatment, Mel was usually the one she consulted first.

By late January, Margaret had been away from home for more than two months. The kids tried to persuade her to come to Jasper for Julie's bridal shower on January 25. At first, Margaret wouldn't hear of leaving Bill overnight. Just for the evening, the kids insisted, and they promised that someone would bring her back first thing in the morning. Margaret thought it over. No telling what the house looked like. Maybe she would go. Just overnight.

By this time, the hospital staff had decided that it was no longer necessary for a nurse to watch over Bill through the 11:00 P.M. to 7:00 A.M. shift. Nurses would look in on him a few times during the night, and pull the Utah up to the doorway. Then the security guard watched it from a chair in the hall, and if an alarm sounded or a light flashed, the guard called a nurse. Margaret wasn't entirely comfortable with that arrangement, so sometimes she stayed all night on the couch in Bill's room. That made her all the more reluctant to leave Bill for a trip to Jasper. But Mel insisted that if she came home, he'd sit up with Bill for the night.

The next afternoon, Mel arrived to take over, and a friend of Julie's from Louisville, Angie Beckman, came by to pick up Margaret for the trip home. But she still questioned whether she should leave.

"Mom," Mel assured her, "you just go on home. Have a good time, get some rest. Don't worry about a thing. I'll be right here. Nothing's going to happen. Go on. It'll do you good."

She finally consented, but only after carefully assuring Bill that Mel would be with him all night and that she'd return in just a few hours.

In her diary she described that day and the next:

Friday, Jan. 25. First time I went home since I left Nov. 11. I loved being home and seeing everything. But so much to do. I need to be home. Moni and Bobby and Vicki were there. The shower was very nice. Julie got lots of nice things. Did wash, picked up things. The kids were yelling for me to go to bed.

Saturday, Jan. 26. I woke up in my very own bed. First thing, I wondered how my husband was doing. I made a cup of coffee and forgot to drink it. Terri came and cut my hair. I got here in Louisville at 11:20 A.M.

As soon as Margaret returned Saturday morning, she hurried to Bill's room. He was glad to see her, and she was relieved to see he was doing fine.

"See, Mom?" Mel said proudly. "You didn't have a thing to worry about!" He didn't dare tell her that while she'd been away, Bill had given him the scare of his life.

After Margaret left Friday evening, Mel and his dad watched TV until Bill drifted off to sleep. Mel turned out the lights and drew the curtain between Bill's bed and the couch and watched some more television. Shortly after midnight, Mel was pretty sleepy himself, weary from a long week's work and the ninety-mile drive. He heard his father cough, so he pulled back the curtain to check on him.

In the dim light from the TV, Mel saw a big dark splotch covering Bill's right side.

"Dad?" Mel asked.

"Huh?"

"Did you throw up?"

Bill shook his head slowly. "No."

Mel turned on the light. "Well, what's—?"

Mel couldn't believe his eyes. The whole right side of Bill's body was stained with bright red blood.

"HEY! WE NEED A NURSE! QUICK! GET A NURSE IN HERE!" he yelled out the door. "Oh, geez, Dad! What in the—?"

Bill just looked at him blankly.

Oh, my God, Mel thought. *Something's leaking, that artificial heart is pumping away, all those blood-thinners—and here I am watching TV! Oh, God, Mom will* never *forgive me . . .*

The nurse who rushed in was just as surprised as Mel at first. Then she realized that the plastic casing for an IV needle had broken. Blood had backed up through the needle and was oozing out onto Bill's arm and pajamas, and the anticoagulants were making him bleed more than usual. She quickly got another IV going. It took about an hour to clean up Bill's blood-soaked bedclothes and linens and get him settled again.

Afterward, Mel kept wiping his face with his hand. Now he knew he wouldn't get to sleep for hours—if at all. Here he tells Mom he'd take care of everything, and *this* has to happen—the one night she goes home! What was more scary than anything was that no alarms had sounded, and Dad hadn't said a word. How long would he have kept bleeding like that in silence?

The next morning, Mel debated whether to tell his mom about the incident. Definitely *not*, he decided. She'd never leave the hospital again.

In the following weeks, there were more scares like that, mostly screw-ups due to "human error." Not long after the bleeding episode, Margaret went upstairs one afternoon for a brief rest. When she opened the door to Bill's room, ready to greet her husband and the nurse, the room was empty. No Bill, no nurse, not even his bed.

Bill!

Margaret put a hand to her own heart and ran down the hall, frantic, yelling for the nurses. One stopped her short, and told her that Bill had been taken upstairs for a sleep test. Margaret was furious—and she had every right to be. They could at least have told her that the test was going to be done. With so many doctors wanting to run so many tests on Bill, it was hard for *anyone* to keep track, but that was hardly an excuse for not warning her.

Another incident involved a small computer that was kept on top of the Utah to monitor the action of the heart and drive system. One afternoon the computer began emitting strange beeps. The technicians fiddled with the dials, but Margaret could tell from their puzzled faces that this problem was different from any they'd encountered. Bill was watching them, too. Margaret tried to reassure him, stroking his hand and talking to him. Ever since the stroke, Bill seemed wary if someone got near the machine or picked up his drive lines to move them. When strangers stood close to the Utah, Bill would watch them alertly, but he would relax if they moved to the other side of his bed.

The technicians finally surmised that phone lines might be causing the beeps. They'd rigged the computer to enable themselves and DeVries to dial in and monitor the Utah on home computers. After some tense moments, they figured out that someone from the outside was accidentally dialing in, which was making the computer beep.

Relieved, they assured Margaret and Bill that the heart and its machinery were actually working fine—it had been a wrong number. Just another little bug to be worked out of the program. *Some relief*, Margaret thought. What other little bugs were they going to find—or maybe *not* find in time?

CHAPTER TWELVE

Bill was still fighting to get well, and he made amazing progress. By late January—eight weeks after the implant—he was stronger than he'd been in months. His coordination had improved so much that often he could do many things such as eating or shaving with little or no assistance. It was still very difficult for him to talk. His long-term memory seemed intact, but his memory for events occurring after the stroke was lacking. Progress was coming in a series of tiny steps that were easier to observe from week to week than from day to day. By now the family began to accept that he might never again be the Bill Schroeder they once knew, but they were determined to help him be the very best he could be. He still had his enormous will to live, and the family had high hopes that he could still achieve some of his cherished goals: going to Terry's wedding and seeing the new grandbaby due in May and returning home to Jasper.

Then in early February, he began having high fevers. For no apparent reason, his temperature would peak at night—sometimes up to a dangerous 105 degrees—then it would fall as morning came. Bill would sweat right through his hospital gown, at times even through his bed linens. Margaret and the nurses tried to bring down the fever by placing him on a special "cooling blanket," a flat, thin plastic mat filled with cold water. Or they draped him with wet towels and sponged him with enough rubbing alcohol to take your breath away when you walked into the room. Strangely enough, when Bill was feverish, he could sometimes pronounce words more clearly and loudly than ever and speak in full sentences—although often they wouldn't make much sense.

Dr. DeVries, who still checked Bill every day, thought at first that Bill had merely caught a cold, or the flu bug that was making the rounds of the staff. When the fever dragged on all week, the whole medical team became puzzled. Of course, Bill had to endure more tests, and more tests meant drawing more blood—several times a day now. The lab technicians were coming so frequently that they'd walk in apologizing: "Hi, Bill, it's me again. Sorry, but I'm going to have to stick you one more time." Their job became increasingly tricky because veins had been stripped from one of Bill's arms for his coronary bypass, and those on his other arm were nearly collapsed from previous blood work.

Some technicians needed just one or two tries to get the blood going, but others had to stick him three or four times, leaving bruises up and down his arms. When Bill was first admitted to Audubon, he never flinched when blood was drawn. But now that they'd taken blood so often—and perhaps because the stroke had robbed Bill of some of his tough-guy bravado—every needle became painful. Margaret also found this increasingly difficult to watch. Sometimes when lab workers appeared at the door with their trays of tubes, all she could think was "Oh, no—here come the vampires again." But she'd have to set aside those feelings quickly, and keep talking to convince Bill and herself that the test was necessary, and hold his hand as the needle went in.

As usual, Margaret would query each doctor and collect all kinds of answers. Maybe the fever indicated the presence of infection, a constant worry. Or maybe it was a reaction to a combination of drugs. The doctors decided to try taking Bill off the antidepressants to see if that helped. While the doctors searched for answers, Bill continued to feel hot and miserable. When you have a fever, you don't feel like doing much of anything, and Bill grew so weak that he couldn't get out of bed to exercise anymore. He certainly didn't feel like eating, and had to take supplemental nutrition through a nasal tube. Day by day, Margaret could see the fever sapping the strength and spirit Bill had struggled so hard to recapture. Most of the time he just slept, and when he was awake, the look in his eyes made her ache to find a way to soothe him.

About that time, Dr. Jarvik dropped into town for a visit. He'd been back in Utah working on a new model of the heart that bore his name, and traveling around the world promoting its manufacturer, Symbion, of which he was president. The Schroeders had grown fond of the quirky thirty-eight-year-old inventor, partly because he could be so much of a kid himself, and partly because he'd said that Bill reminded him of his own dad, who suffered heart problems. To the family, Jarvik was a breath of fresh air because he came to see Bill not as a doctor, but as a friend. In fact, Jarvik had never treated a patient. He had gone to medical school in Italy, finished up at the University of Utah, then immediately had begun to work with artificial organs, making prototypes of the Jarvik-7.

When Jarvik came to visit in February, Bill recognized him right away and eagerly reached out to shake his hand. Jarvik had brought him some presents: crayons and a sketch pad to encourage him to draw, plus a black beret so Bill would really look the part of an artist. As Jarvik sat beside him, Bill selected a maroon crayon and used light, feathery strokes to draw a house with two big windows, way over on one side of the pad. On another page, Bill drew small rocket ships with red and yellow flames shooting out from the bottom. Jarvik talked with him for a long time, and promised to take Bill fishing when the weather grew warmer.

That evening Jarvik took Margaret out to a fancy restaurant, then to a downtown performing-arts center in the shadow of Humana's corporate headquarters, for a live ABC News broadcast on medicine and the media. ABC's *Viewpoint* producers selected Louisville as a backdrop for this program because of all the heart and hospital news generated there recently. Television anchor Ted Koppel moderated a panel discussion among several journalists and doctors, including DeVries. Afterward Jarvik took Margaret backstage to a surprise birthday party for Koppel, who asked DeVries to make the first incision in his birthday cake. But Margaret was anxious to return to the hospital and got a ride back with George Atkins.

The party reminded Margaret that Bill's own birthday was coming up soon—the fourteenth, to be exact. When she mentioned the date to hospital staffers, they thought she was kidding. February 14? The world's only man without a human heart was born on Valentine's Day? No one could believe it.

On the morning that Bill turned fifty-three, he woke up feeling sick and slightly feverish, and could barely hold up his head for snapshots of himself and the nurses. But he knew he'd reached another important milestone, and when all the kids came to help him celebrate, he perked up somewhat. When they turned out the lights and Cheryl brought in a cake with fifty-three candles on it from the Jasper City Bakery, Bill's eyes widened and he smiled broadly before blowing them out with the help from the grandkids.

The Schroeder clan crowded around Bill's chair to help him open presents. Stan and Rod added a T-shirt to Bill's collection: KISS ME—I'VE GOT A HEART ON. Any other time Bill would have modeled it and made sure all the nurses got the joke, but now he just smiled. Terry gave him gym shorts, teasing that he could give the staff a thrill by showing off his legs in the hall. Cheryl gave him a Yahtzee game to encourage him to exercise his hands. Margaret had slipped out to K mart and bought him a black sweat suit. Mel brought a tray of Indiana soil and lettuce seeds, reminding his dad of the saying around Jasper that you're supposed to plant your lettuce on Valentine's Day. It wouldn't be the same as running the tiller up at the forty acres, but at least Bill would have the distinction of being the hospital's only patient with his own garden.

Humana had put out news of Bill's birthday, so Audubon's mail room was soon flooded with cards, flowers, birthday cakes, and candy. Of course, the Schroeders' hospital family wanted to celebrate with them. Polly brought them champagne, Dr. Jarvik sent heart-shaped balloons, and the Audubon staff threw a little party in the auditorium with cake and punch. Bill was wheeled down to the party, but he didn't feel like staying long. As usual, there were plenty of leftovers, so the Schroeders wheeled a cartful up to the hall outside Margaret's room and invited the whole staff up for refreshments. As staffers drifted up to spend a few minutes with the family, the grandkids made sure they signed Bill's king-sized card, which the family had stored at the end of the hall. Meanwhile, the Schroeder family took turns visiting their dad. It wasn't like past birthday celebrations, of course, but it was still another precious day which would have been impossible without the artificial heart, another day for the Schroeders to be a family again.

Ever since Bill's surgery, the Schroeders had had inquiries from agents offering to sell their story. Everyone—hospital staff, friends, reporters, strangers—seemed to think that the family's story had the makings of a fantastic book or movie. They had no idea whether to pursue such an effort or, if they did, what this would entail. They did know that although their struggle was day by day, they also had to start planning for the future. The medical team was talking about discharging Bill to the apartment at the halfway house, and there was no way to know what expenses the family would face when he went home. The Schroeder kids knew for sure that they had to think about providing for Mom in case something happened to their father. Margaret, in turn, was concerned about the family's mounting travel expenses: Considering standard mileage costs for the 180-mile drive—and, usually, the purchase of a meal during the visit—each trip cost a total of thirty or forty dollars.

In a broader sense, the family had learned so much already about artificial hearts, doctors, hospitals, the media, and human experimentation—and learned it the hard way—that they felt obligated to help others who might face a similar ordeal. So, just as Bill had chosen to trust the advice of his doctors, Margaret and the kids decided to put themselves in the hands of professionals.

George Atkins from PR introduced them to Sheryl Snyder and Bill Hollander, lawyers, from the prestigious Louisville firm of Wyatt, Tarrant, and Combs. Atkins also arranged for a literary agent, Clyde Taylor from Curtis Brown Ltd. of New York, to fly down for a meeting.

After discussions with Taylor, the Schroeders were a little surprised to learn that again what had sounded so simple was becoming incredibly complicated. Taylor said that they could sell their story to a publishing house and let the publisher provide a writer, or they could hire their own writer, or perhaps they would be able to sell only an exclusive magazine article, or . . . The list went on and on. Nothing, it seemed, was standard.

The Schroeders couldn't help but think that if Bill hadn't suffered the stroke, he would have found out exactly what they should do, or whether they ought to forget the whole idea. Even if Bill wasn't well enough to attend meetings with the lawyers and agents, he'd be on the phone, asking all kinds of questions, making decisions, and ordering them to be carried out. It was difficult for the family to step into his place and guess what choices he would make.

Taylor checked around and returned a week later with an offer from *Life* magazine. *Life* would pay a flat price for exclusive interviews and photos, and since hopes were high that Bill could attend Terry's wedding in Jasper and move to the apartment soon, the magazine agreed to pay more for exclusive access to those events. Taylor would get 10 percent of the payment, and, after taxes, the Schroeders would wind up with a sum in the low five figures.

However, things became even more complicated. When the Schroeders had signed that release for the Black Star photo distribution agency—the day before Bill's surgery—Humana officials informed them that it was a standard form authorizing the hospital to use footage and photos of the family for educational purposes. Both Humana and the Schroeders had been under the impression that the hospital company and the family shared legal ownership of the photos. But after *Life* magazine requested previously unreleased photos of the family from Black Star, the Schroeders' lawyers discovered that, according to the document, the pictures were actually the property of Bill Strode and Black Star.

Humana had hoped that the arrangement would help avoid the appearance of the firm's profiting directly from the photos' distribution, since it was already being criticized for reaping free publicity from being involved with the artificial heart. Humana would pay Strode to take photos and Black Star would distribute them to all the media free of charge so no one could be accused of making money by selling pictures of the patient and his family. Of course, photos of the Schroeders brought Humana free advertising anyway, dramatically increasing the firm's name recognition worldwide.

Humana officials now realized their oversight concerning ownership of the photos. Because all parties agreed on the original intent of the contract, a new one was drawn up, stating that the family owned the rights to use any photos as they saw fit, and that Humana also had the right to use them for educational purposes. Working out this contract required lengthy sessions between Black Star representatives, Humana's lawyers, and Snyder and Hollander, the lawyers who had offered to donate their legal services to the family, unaware that the negotiations would drag on for months.

The Schroeders were confused about what to make of it all. They had never dealt with lawyers before, and now they had not only doctors, nurses, a PR staff, technicians, therapists, security guards, a photographer, and a social worker, but also a literary agent and a magazine contract to be concerned with. And there were new worries: Were they doing the right thing? Was it really what Bill would want? Did they need to get mixed up with agents and additional legal contracts? Could the *Life* article somehow cause problems for Bill? And if the family were entitled to make some money from their story, how could they be sure they weren't being taken advantage of?

The negotiations also revealed something amazing: If photos of the family had been sold instead of distributed free, overseas royalties alone would have netted several hundred thousand dollars for the pictures' owners. Although the Schroeders were more than willing that the photos be used for educational purposes, they were astounded that an outside party could have profited so much from the medical ordeal of their husband and father.

For the Schroeders, money wasn't the point and had never been. The family would have given anything to have Bill healthy and at home. They would have been perfectly happy never to have faced any of these decisions, and certainly wouldn't have minded if their knowledge of the artificial heart had never gone beyond what they saw on TV. But after Bill chose to get that artificial heart, it was as if a door had closed behind them forever. Now the only thing the family could do was keep on walking hand in hand through the doors ahead.

News travels around a hospital faster than running water—and gossip is even quicker. If you stick around long enough and keep your ears open, you can find out exactly who's doing what to whom. No wonder TV soap operas are so often set in hospitals.

By mid-February, even before Dr. DeVries told Margaret, she'd known for a couple of days that the screening committee had selected another artificial heart candidate, a fifty-eight-year-old retired barber from Louisville named Murray Haydon. Once again, the media descended on Louisville, and Humana reopened the downtown briefing center.

In her diary the next day, Margaret wrote:

> Went to get my hair done. Had to wait on a cab, then wait to get back. Ran into the camera crew for the new heart transplant. They took some pictures of us. I felt real silly, like I was in the way walking down the hallway.

Back home, the kids' phones were ringing off the hook with reporters calling to ask how the family felt about the new implant. They could only say that the family wished the Haydons well and hoped they could be of help.

Privately, the Schroeders had mixed emotions. Sure, it would be great not to feel so alone, and finally talk with another family going through an ordeal that couldn't be understood by someone who hadn't been there. But at the same time, it was scary. When they thought about how much attention the doctors gave Bill at the beginning, they had to wonder: Would another patient divert this attention from Bill? DeVries had told Bill at that first meeting that he wasn't sure that the medical team could take care of more than one artificial heart recipient. What made him so sure they could handle another one now? And since the doctors could start over with a patient who hadn't had a stroke, would they subconsciously try harder to help that new patient get better?

Those were selfish feelings, but they seemed normal under the circumstances. The Schroeders certainly didn't begrudge anyone the same care Bill received. When a loved one is sick, however, you want the very best for that person, no matter what. DeVries himself had said on the ABC *Viewpoint* panel that, as a father of seven, he fully sympathized with desperate parents who use the media to seek organs for dying children. "I would bite, scream, scratch—anything—to get that liver to my child," DeVries had said. The Schroeders felt the same way about Bill.

So it was somewhat painful to hear Dr. Lansing say on TV that the new patient was the "ideal candidate" because, unlike Bill, he didn't have coronary-artery disease, diabetes, or other recent surgeries. Unlike Bill and Barney Clark, who were close to death at the time of their implants, Murray Haydon was healthy enough to live another two or three weeks, making him "a much more adequate test or evaluation of the mechanical heart and its function itself than anyone before," Lansing said. And thanks to what they'd learned from their work with Bill, he said, the doctors would start administering anticoagulation drugs earlier for Haydon, in hopes of preventing a stroke.

There would be another change based on the lessons learned from Bill's experience: Lansing now planned to meet regularly with other members of the medical team to compare notes before press briefings, to avoid conflicting reports that might upset the Haydons. It was becoming increasingly apparent that almost every aspect of the experiment was a learn-as-you-go, trial-and-error process. The Schroeders' only hope was that the knowledge that came at the price of their own pain might spare future recipients' families some grief.

On Saturday hospital officials introduced Haydon's wife, Juanita, to Margaret. They spoke briefly; it was hard to know what to say. The news of Haydon's impending operation had brought memories rushing back to the whole Schroeder family—those fearful early days, the worries and the what-ifs, the sense of being the only ones going through such an experience. The Schroeder kids couldn't understand why the heart institute hadn't arranged a meeting for them with the Haydons' three grown children. Why not provide the new recipient's family with all the information available? You can get only so much from reading pamphlets, talking to doctors, and watching videotapes. Back in November, the Schroeders would have given anything to talk with another family of an artificial heart patient. Even if the other family didn't have all the answers, it would have been easier to know what to expect. Most of the time, it seemed that the complications themselves weren't nearly so hard to handle as simply having no idea what would hit next.

So when the kids visited the hospital that weekend, they tracked down the Haydons, who had gathered in a waiting room for the operation. The Schroeders introduced themselves and wished them good luck, promising to be available if the Haydon family ever wanted to talk. "You're in our family now," Terry told them. "Just make sure you all stick together through this. Then you can handle whatever comes along." The Haydons were grateful, but the Schroeders were a little surprised to find that the mood in the waiting room was more casual than theirs had been on the day of Bill's surgery. Maybe it was just the way the Haydons handled such things, but, on the other hand, maybe artificial heart surgery was already beginning to seem almost routine. In fact, Haydon's operation went so smoothly that one nurse called it "dull."

That night Margaret wrote:

Today was the day our family grew larger, as a Mr. Haydon had an artificial heart put in. He is fine and did real well in surgery. Now there are two families with the same problem.

Bill is a little stronger today, I believe. His temperature is down to 99 degrees tonight. Mel, Patti, the two kids and Terry and Julie all come to see Bill. Then [Stan's in-laws] Buck and Mary, Stan and Terri come to see us.

They all left and it's so lonesome. But I have Bill and he has me, too.

Margaret tried several times to explain to Bill that Dr. De-Vries was putting an artificial heart in another man. She wasn't sure that he understood, but maybe he did because he smiled weakly and nodded when she talked to him about it. The next morning, Margaret turned on the television set in Bill's room so he could watch Dr. Lansing brief the press on Haydon's progress. However, reporters kept turning the line of questioning back to Bill's condition.

There wasn't that much to say about Haydon, for a couple of reasons. First, as the Schroeders knew, very little was expected to occur during the hours immediately after surgery. Second, Haydon was a very reticent, private man. He had even told De-Vries that he didn't want an artificial heart if it meant enduring the kind of attention that Bill received, so DeVries had assured him that Humana would try to release a minimum of information about his case.

When reporters kept pressing to learn how Bill was, Lansing told them exactly what he thought—and he wasn't encouraging:

"If he does not get stronger, if he does not get over the fever, he will remain discouraged and that will be a threat to his life," Lansing said. "I agree absolutely that an individual's spirit is a very important determinant of his survival."

What?! One of the doctors was worrying aloud on national TV that his patient might lose the will to live? Margaret couldn't tell if Bill had heard it, but she turned off the TV right away so he certainly couldn't hear any more.

Lansing's comments didn't make any sense. Why, Bill was doing better that morning than he had in a couple of weeks! When was the last time Lansing had really spent some time with Bill? She often saw him more on TV than she did in Bill's room. When DeVries came by that morning, she told him how upset Lansing's statements had made her. DeVries assured her that Bill was indeed doing better, and advised her to just stop watching the televised briefings because they couldn't possibly describe Bill's condition completely. When Mel called that day at lunchtime,

Margaret warned him about the TV reports and told him to pass on DeVries's suggestion to the other kids. But the rest of the family had already stopped reading the papers or watching TV reports about their dad because the stories always seemed to be conflicting or inconclusive.

Apparently, words were exchanged among the medical team, and that afternoon Lansing gave a much more optimistic assessment of Bill's condition, acknowledging that the Schroeders had been "very upset" over his earlier comments. He'd checked Bill late that morning, and he did indeed seem better. He added that Bill still seemed depressed, but speculated that it was probably just because he felt sick. He would probably feel a lot better if he could get out of the hospital soon, either when he was discharged or just for a brief wheelchair ride outdoors, Lansing said.

That evening Bill's fever seemed to abate a bit, but at night he coughed a lot and had occasional trouble swallowing. The next morning, Bill was well enough to sit in his wheelchair, so Margaret got him ready for another ride around the hospital. She gave him his favorite IU cap to wear, and draped a hospital blanket over him because the blood-thinners made him feel chilly. They were joined by Larry Hastings, nurse John Lammers, a security guard, Bill Strode—who was there to take pictures of Haydon—and Mel, who'd stopped by for a visit. Mel mentioned that it was surprisingly warm outside for February.

He turned to Larry. "Hey, why don't we take Dad outside? Any reason why we can't?"

Larry, easygoing as ever, smiled and shrugged. "I don't see why not!"

"Dad," Mel asked, "you want to go outside?"

Bill's eyes widened. *"Yeah!"*

On the way downstairs, they were joined by Polly and Donna Hazle from PR. As they went out the hospital's heavy glass doors, they all felt a little thrill. If they'd gone through channels to get the excursion approved, there might have been all kinds of meetings, discussions, assessments, precautionary measures, and public-relations groundwork—and by the time everything was finished, the weather would probably have turned cold again. Mel and Margaret felt great about finally doing something spontaneous.

They cautiously wheeled Bill out onto the sidewalk. Even though it was still February, the weather felt like spring. For the first time in months, Bill could feel the sun's warmth on his face and breathe fresh air. Those were such small things, so simple, and yet at that moment they meant everything. Bill squinted and smiled. The group came to a stop, and as Mel stood by with the Heimes over his shoulder, Margaret put her arms around Bill from behind, kissed him, and turned his attention to the apartment building across the street.

"See, honey, that's going to be our new home! You get better and we'll move out of the hospital, and you and I can have a place to ourselves. Okay?"

Bill looked across at the apartment, smiled, and nodded. Margaret knew that Bill always needed a goal to strive for, and she seized the chance to point out another one.

Bill looked delighted to be outside. Several times Larry, John, or Margaret asked if he was ready to go back in, but Bill would shake his head. Strode took some pictures. Two little girls recognized Bill as they walked by, and came up to ask permission to meet him. Because it was the first time he had been outside the hospital, no one knew what to expect, but the girls were polite and respectful, and Bill seemed to enjoy shaking their hands as they wished him good luck.

After fifteen minutes or so, the group went back in. The brief trip really did boost Bill's spirits. He seemed perkier the rest of the day, and even had a good appetite at supper. Finally, after two and a half weeks, his fever had started to drop. Humana proudly released this upbeat news to the reporters who were in town to cover Haydon's implant. That night Margaret wrote:

Tuesday, Feb. 19. Today we made history. Bill went outside for the first time. He was so happy. He didn't want to come back inside . . .

The next day was also warm and sunny, so Margaret gave Bill pep talks all morning about how they'd go outside again. DeVries was disappointed to learn that he had missed the first trip, so he planned to go along this time. Meanwhile, PR was catching hell from the press for not giving them prior notice that news was about to be made. Now there was a bigger problem: A mob of TV camera crews, reporters, and photographers had camped just outside the hospital door, hoping to capture Bill's second trip for the evening news—the very thing everyone had hoped to avoid.

Margaret was happily preparing Bill for his second ride outdoors when Dr. DeVries came in. "Margaret, the media's all over the place," he said. "You can't take him out there today."

Oh, come on. Bill had been looking forward to this all morning—she'd already told him they were going. "Well," Margaret said incredulously, "go out there and tell them to let us alone!"

DeVries laughed softly and shook his head. "It's not that easy, Margaret. Those people just won't take no for an answer. Come here, look . . ."

DeVries led her to a window over the parking lot, and pointed to the cluster of cameras aimed at the hospital entrance.

Margaret looked up at the doctor in disbelief. "Well, we seem to be prisoners! Are we going to be prisoners all our lives?"

DeVries looked out at the crowd. Margaret still couldn't believe it. "Haven't they gotten enough of him yet?" she asked. "When are they going to get enough and leave us alone? Is it going to be like this when we get home, too? Are we going to have to stay inside our house and be afraid to go out because of all the people we don't want to meet?"

Once again, DeVries had to admit that he didn't have the answers to her questions. All he knew was that they couldn't make Bill face all those cameras and strangers shouting questions at him. "It'd be a zoo, Margaret. No telling what would happen," DeVries said. "We just can't go out there today. I don't know what we'll do, but we'll have to do something. This can't go on."

So that day Bill had to settle for a ride through the hospital corridors and looking out the big picture windows at the end of the hall. As the group passed coronary intensive care, someone suggested that Bill might enjoy seeing Mr. Haydon. It didn't sound like a bad idea, and they detoured into the unit.

Haydon still wasn't receiving visitors, so the group stayed outside the sliding glass door to his room. Margaret wheeled Bill up to the door so that he could look in.

"See, Bill?" Margaret said. "That's Mr. Haydon. He's another member of our 'family'!"

Bill's mouth slowly dropped open and his eyes widened. He looked astonished to see another Utahdrive hooked to someone. He stared first at the other man's Utah, then at his portable drive strapped over the technician's shoulder, then back at the other man's Utah. Bill pointed at Haydon's machine and gave Margaret a questioning look.

"Yes, honey. That's his Utah. Yours is in your room. It's all right, sweetie. There's two people with Utahs now. You still have yours. It's okay." Margaret hoped he understood.

They wheeled Bill back to his room, switched him back to the Utah, and put him to bed for a nap. In the evening Bill felt well enough to take a few steps with some assistance. Now that his appetite was coming back, the feeding tube was removed, and a dentist came to fit him with dentures for the first time since his teeth were removed in November. Now Bill really looked like his old self again.

DeVries's associate, Dr. Sam Yared, strolled in waving a twenty-dollar bill and asked if anyone wanted to send out for dinner. Nurse Sandy Chandler grabbed the bill and spent it all on pizza for everybody. The nurses gave Bill a slice, and even though he wasn't particularly fond of pizza, he dug in as Strode took pictures. After three months of hospital food, any kind of fast food had to be a treat. The media didn't get photos of Bill going outside that day, but they did pick up on the news that Humana released. SCHROEDER WALKING, EATING PIZZA; HAYDON SITS UP, proclaimed the *Louisville Times*. Sometimes it seemed Humana was eager to put a line in the water, and the press was anxious to bite.

Meanwhile, DeVries told the PR staff that they had to do something about the media stakeout. A pool of reporters and photographers was set up to cover Bill's next trip outdoors. Sometimes you just had to give the media something—anything—to make them leave you alone for a while.

The next day was cool and sunny. A little before 2:00 P.M., Margaret and the nurses got Bill out of bed and technician Larry Hastings switched him to the Heimes. To make sure that Bill would be warm enough Margaret saw he was dressed in a windbreaker and the beret Dr. Jarvik had given him. Then she and nurse Sandy Chandler wheeled Bill down to a side door of the hospital, along with a security guard, Laura Wood, Polly Brown, and Larry Hastings, who carried the portable drive. Through the door, Margaret could see reporters and photographers, but there weren't nearly as many as the time before, and they were in a special roped-off area. Strode and some people from PR were also there.

"Everybody ready?" Polly asked. "Bill, you ready? Here we go!"

Sandy wheeled Bill toward the press, with Margaret and the others walking alongside. Again, Bill's big smile showed that he was happy to be outside. He smiled and waved at the people up ahead, but so many strangers being there became confusing, and he began to look puzzled. Then Bill spotted Strode's familiar face, and slowly pointed at him with a little grin.

The group came to a halt a few feet in front of the reporters. Robert Bazell, NBC's medical correspondent, crouched in front of Bill's wheelchair and held out his hand. Bill slowly smiled and held out his own.

"How are you feeling, Mr. Schroeder?" Bazell asked. "How do you feel?"

Bill leaned toward him and looked into his eyes. He struggled with a couple of syllables, then said in a soft, pinched voice, "I feel real fine." Margaret repeated his words a little louder: "He said he feels real fine."

Did Bill want to say anything to his friends and well-wishers? the reporter asked.

"Tell them something good," Polly kidded Bill. "Better tell them something good."

Bill slowly looked down at his hands. This was all getting so complicated. All these people . . .

He looked up again and tried to say something else, but he was tired and overwhelmed. Sandy turned his wheelchair around, and the group headed back toward the hospital. The reporters pulled Margaret aside for a few quick on-camera questions. She wasn't eager to be interviewed, but figured it was better that they talk to her than bother Bill just now. With all the suffering he had been through lately—the tests, the complications, the fevers—it was going to be hard to sound real optimistic. But now she *had* to say something. *Just be honest,* she thought. *Just say the kinds of things Bill would say if he could.*

How did she feel? a reporter asked.

"Oh," Margaret said, working at a smile, "it feels good just to have him come out. That's the main thing. He did just great. He always did love people . . ."

And how was her husband doing?

"He's really on the way to recovery," she said, knowing that Bill might see this interview on TV. "I don't want him to be frightened of everybody when he comes out the door. He feels like everybody's going to look at him or something. When he gets more around to talking to everybody, he'd be glad to come out and talk to you."

How did she feel about recent pessimistic news reports about her husband?

"Well." Margaret's smile was even bigger now. "The TV is real close and I can turn it off!" The reporter thanked her for her time, and she hurried off to catch up with Bill.

Bill napped until about 7:30 that evening. When he woke up, it was obvious that the excursion had done him good. When some folks from Jasper visited that night, Bill was wide awake and smiling. And when University of Louisville basketball coach Denny Crum came by later, Bill recognized him instantly and eagerly shook the hand of the man he'd seen so often on TV ball games.

However, Bill's recovery continued to be a roller-coaster ride—a promising couple of days followed by a depressing one. For example, the next morning, Bill vomited and appeared to have another brief seizurelike episode, which meant he had to have another EEG. The doctors also started giving him vitamins intravenously. That afternoon DeVries appeared at a press briefing where he announced that he was going to stop releasing so much information about his patients. He maintained angrily that so much news coverage had repeatedly hurt his patients and their families—the bleak headlines based on Lansing's comments, the canceled wheelchair ride, the contrived trip outside for the media pool. The public simply no longer needed to know what Bill Schroeder had for breakfast or the latest results of tests on his kidneys, he said. Except for major changes in his patients' condition, such as a stroke or being discharged, he would publish this information months later in scientific journals.

"You can't tell what the quality of life of the patient is by reading about it in the newspaper. I can tell you that for sure. You just have to be there," DeVries said. "I think there are people who would see Mr. Schroeder and not want to go through that. But I think there are people who would see Mr. Schroeder and would just jump at the opportunity to have that quality of life. How do you compare my quality of life to your quality of life? What measures, what yardsticks do you use?"

The media reacted with complaints that Humana and DeVries wanted to release only the good news and hide the bad. But

DeVries's new stance was fine with the Schroeders. By now they were ignoring the press anyway, and they hoped that this announcement would make reporters lay off for a while. On the other hand, they wondered, would a news cutback lead to the problems Humana had set out to avoid, such as patients and their families getting harassed? Once again, they'd just have to play wait-and-see.

DeVries was definitely right about one thing: No one on the outside could judge Bill's quality of life by what was reported in the news. Here he was, not just lying in bed, but trying his damnedest to recover from complications of a stroke that might well have killed him if he hadn't had an artificial heart. You only had to spend a little while with him to see how hard he was fighting. Or see the look on his face when Mel's wife, Patti, a seamstress, came up that week to measure him for the tux he was to wear at Terry's wedding. You only had to watch him perk up and try harder in physical-therapy sessions when Margaret mentioned that grandbaby due in May.

Then there was Terry's stag party. By this time Bill was recovering well enough that everyone hoped he could attend Terry's wedding in three weeks. Some of the Schroeders and the hospital staff planned a little get-together in late February for Terry, his dad, and the male hospital workers. For days the staff and the Schroeder boys kept pumping up Bill's spirits by reminding him of Terry's stag party, and made a big deal of keeping it a secret from Margaret, assuring Bill it would be "just guys." Bill was delighted. They also told him they might even bring a stripper to the party, which was to be held downstairs in the doctors' lounge.

But the evening of the party, everybody had been talking it up for hours, and Bill couldn't wait to go downstairs. Margaret and the nurses couldn't make him stay in bed to rest. He still didn't feel up to taking more than a couple of steps at a time, but when Terry and Stan got Bill into the wheelchair, they had to put the chair's brakes on because he kept trying to push himself out the door. Margaret didn't know exactly what they'd planned, but every time she asked if she could come along, Bill would shake his head vigorously and say, "NO!" This was definitely going to be just guys. At the last minute, though, DeVries canceled the stripper, saying that they'd be sunk if the media ever got hold of *that* story.

Terry and Stan took Bill downstairs, along with Brent Mays, the technician, and nurse John Lammers. In the lounge, some guys from Jasper and some male staffers played poker, smoked cigars, and drank some brews. DeVries and a few other doctors came by and shot pool. Guys would come over to talk to Bill, shake his hand, and get him to laugh at an off-color joke or two. Bill watched a couple of Stan's pals playing checkers, and couldn't help smiling and shaking his head when they razzed each other about bad moves. Then technician Larry Hastings, who had the night off, dropped in to say hello. Because Larry was going out that evening with his wife, Vicki, an attractive woman with long, strawberry-blond hair, he brought her along. At the sight of Larry's wife, Bill's eyes widened and he nudged Terry expectantly.

Oops. Nobody had thought to tell Bill that the stripper had been canceled at the last minute. Terry debated whether to explain this now. Vicki sat down beside Bill and talked with him for quite a while. Bill just kept grinning and holding her hand. He was doing so well that no one was really paying much attention when Larry and Vicki said their good-byes and stood up to leave. The next thing anyone knew, Bill was out of the wheelchair and on his feet, following her to the door, stretching out his drive lines as far as they would go. Brent dove for the Utahdrive, as John scrambled to catch up with Bill. No one knew that Bill was strong enough to get up and walk like that. The "experts" on the outside could debate quality of life all they wanted, but one thing was certain: Bill enjoyed the hell out of that party.

CHAPTER THIRTEEN

Ever since Bill had said on TV that he wanted a customized van, a number of people began working behind the scenes to make his dream come true. Paul Uebelhor, the automobile dealer, and another Jasper businessman, Arnold Habig, founder of Kimball International, donated a gleaming 1985 Chevy van in the shades of blue and silver that Bill had chosen when Paul visited two days before the stroke. A Louisville firm, Komfort Koach, agreed to customize the van for free. Again, everyone was treading new ground: No one had any idea what was required to outfit a vehicle for a person with an artificial heart. It took DeVries and the technicians, Margaret, Uebelhor, and the Komfort Koach people several meetings to determine what modifications the van would need.

The final list of options kept the Komfort Koach people busy for a couple of months. They added a wheelchair lift strong enough to raise the heavy Utahdrive, and fastened a mount behind the driver's seat to hold the machine in place. They put in another mount to secure Bill's wheelchair so that it faced a large tinted side window. An electrical outlet was added so the Utah could be plugged in. In the rear of the van, they added an extra seat with a rack underneath for storing the Utah's spare air tanks.

Komfort Koach installed devices for every emergency imaginable: a cellular phone, a CB radio, a public-address microphone and loudspeaker, a siren, emergency flashing lights under the grille, bright headlights that flashed alternately like those of a police car. Only later would they learn that the van had to be licensed to use the siren and emergency lights.

As the list of options grew, the Schroeders began to realize that without such a vehicle, Bill's mobility outside the hospital would have been extremely limited. It was another jarring discovery that simply confirmed that so much of the artificial heart experiment involved deciding how to cross bridges only after the family and medical team had come to them. No one even knew where the next bridge would be.

The van was also equipped with a panel over the driver's seat that controlled an elaborate system for lighting various parts of the interior, and an alarm system that would set off a siren during a break-in. A five-inch color TV was mounted overhead behind the driver's seat for viewing by passengers in back.

There were also the usual standard options plus power brakes, power steering with a tilting wheel, cruise control, and an AM/FM cassette deck. The whole interior was lined with plush blue carpeting. In honor of Bill, the van's rear window was engraved with fancy frosted letters proclaiming: THE HEART AND SPIRIT OF JASPER. In short, Uebelhor & Son Chevrolet and Komfort Koach did a wonderful job—wonderful to the tune of $45,000.

For tax purposes, the van was not given to the family, but to a nonprofit foundation of Humana Heart Institute International. So, although Bill had been instrumental in obtaining the vehicle, and although the family had worked out the particulars with Uebelhor, the Schroeders had to make arrangements with the hospital anytime they wanted to take Bill out for a ride.

Even though the keys were ceremonially presented to Margaret at a technical briefing for the media at Komfort Koach headquarters, there were still many unresolved questions about the van's intended use and how that would work out in actual practice: Would the Schroeders be allowed to take it to Jasper if Bill moved back home? What if several more implants were performed and all the artificial heart patients had to take turns using it? Could the family ever just take Bill for a spur-of-the-moment trip without having to round up nurses, technicians, and a security guard?

On March 9, about a week after the van was delivered to Audubon, the family decided to take Bill out for a ride in the van. Once again, Margaret first made sure that Bill was presentable, helping him put on his black sweat suit. She'd been preparing him for his first real trip in the van for quite some time now. The weekend before, Terry, Stan, and Larry Hastings had wheeled Bill downstairs to show him the vehicle, and they decided that as long as Bill was on the Heimes, they might as well take a test drive. So they put him in, climbed aboard, and took an impromptu spin around the parking lot. Everything had gone fine.

This time, for Bill's first official trip away from the hospital, technician Brent Mays again switched Bill to the Heimes. The medical team had decided to use the portable drive whenever Bill rode in the van, and brought along both a spare portable and the Utah, in case something went wrong or their return to the hospital was delayed.

As the usual group gathered in Bill's room for the outing, DeVries joined them. He seemed as eager as the others that this test drive would be a step toward many excursions not only for Bill, but for future artificial heart patients, too.

"Okay, Bill," Margaret said. "Ready to go?"

Bill's eyes widened with excitement. "Yeah! I'm ready!" he answered. Cheryl lifted the Heimes onto her shoulder, and they were off.

As Margaret wheeled Bill out into the hall, and Brent pushed the spare Utah behind them, the whole staff knew exactly where they were going. Everyone reached out for a handshake from Bill and wished him the best. Bill took their hands and patted them, getting a little teary-eyed. The security guard hurried ahead to hold an elevator.

Downstairs the group waited by a rear door to the hospital while Mel brought the van from the doctors' underground parking lot, and eased the passenger side up to the curb. Several people helped roll the spare Utah onto the lift, which was activated by pressing a button. When the heavy machine was level with the van's floor, Mel and Brent pushed it inside and secured it.

"Dad, ready to get in?" Mel asked.

Bill smiled. "Yeah!" Bill was checking out the van as if he still couldn't believe it. Mel and Brent pushed his wheelchair onto the lift. While Bill sat there, DeVries leaned over and asked him how he liked the van.

Bill didn't answer, but he grabbed the doctor's big hand, squeezed it tightly, and patted it hard. Misty-eyed again, he held DeVries's hand for a long time. Finally, he let go of it and began waving to each of the hospital staffers.

Suddenly it hit everyone: Did Bill think he was going home and leaving the hospital for good? Margaret put her arms around his shoulders and tried to explain: "No, honey, we're not going home yet. Right now we're just going to sit inside for a while. We've got to take it one step at a time, sweetie, remember? We'll go home another day." Bill looked puzzled.

When the wheelchair had been raised level with the van's

floor, they realized for the first time that Bill would always have to duck his head to be wheeled inside. Another bug to be worked out. After Bill's wheelchair and the spare Utah were safely locked in place, there was little room for anyone else. Margaret and Cheryl crawled in next to Bill, and DeVries bent his lanky frame to get in the very back.

Mel climbed into the driver's seat, and the security guard got in on the passenger's side. Brent squeezed in beside the Heimes. A nurse sat on the floor in front of Bill and DeVries and closed the door. Now the van was packed—so packed, in fact, that Patti and the two girls, who'd come along, couldn't fit in and had to stay behind.

Bill just kept looking around as if to say, "WOW!" Mel couldn't resist revving the engine. "Everyone ready?" he asked, looking in the rear-view mirror.

"YEAH!" Bill answered. "READY!"

As they pulled out of the parking lot, Margaret called to Mel, "Are you sure you can drive this thing?" The Utah blocked her view out the front window, and as she and Bill looked out the side window, they could see only what whizzed past, as if they were on a train. They couldn't see where they were headed at all. Margaret had always been a backseat driver, but now she was having a really hard time.

"Melvin!" she called up to the front. "You be careful now!" Mel just grinned and kept trying out all the accessories— the siren, the cellular phone, and the flashing lights. Since none of them had any idea of where to go, they just cruised around some quiet streets in a nearby neighborhood.

DeVries kept patting Bill's arm, asking, "Isn't this a great van?" Bill would smile and nod as he looked out the window.

After about twenty minutes, Bill began to get weary. The security guard used his two-way radio to notify his base: "We're coming in!" After they returned, the slow process of loading everything onto the van was reversed. Bill must have realized that he wasn't going home, but it must have been confusing for him. Mostly, he was just tired and ready for bed. The others felt terrific. After many weeks of watching the medical team do all kinds of things supposedly in Bill's best interest, the family could finally do something for Bill that he clearly enjoyed.

Everyone who went on the ride had a great time, but the PR staff caught hell for it from the press. Bill's first trip off the

hospital grounds—the only one ever for an artificial heart patient—was supposed to be another carefully orchestrated media
event, with fair and equal access to all the press. By now everyone involved in the artificial heart program had learned that the
media would come down on them hard if they weren't provided
with some information on these occasions. This ride had been a
definite no-no. But the Schroeders had to chuckle a little at the
belated news reports of Bill's first trip. They'd gotten away with
something for a change!

Now that they knew the van would work out, the family
began dreaming of all the other trips Bill could take. But like
everything else, it all got much more complicated than they'd
imagined. The medical team insisted that a security guard go
along, just in case of trouble. A doctor's order was required for
each van ride, and the technicians would need at least a day's
notice to prepare for it. The Schroeders had hoped that the rides
would be as simple as loading Bill into the van when he felt good,
just taking off together on a fishing trip or picnic, like old times.
It soon became evident that such outings would never again be
"just family."

CHAPTER FOURTEEN

The first week of March 1985 was full of news about artificial hearts. Murray Haydon was returned to surgery about two weeks after receiving his implant. As with Bill, De-Vries had to reopen Haydon's chest to stop bleeding aggravated by the blood-thinners used to prevent strokes.

And in Tucson surgeons at the University of Arizona used a mechanical heart as an emergency "bridge" on a thirty-three-year-old man after he received a transplanted human heart that failed. The "Phoenix heart" model, which had been designed by an Arizona dentist, didn't have FDA approval yet, but it kept the man alive for eleven hours until he received a second human heart. However, the patient died two days later because of other complications.

A year ago, the Schroeders wouldn't have paid much attention to such reports. Now they followed them all, their ears perking up at foreign-sounding medical terms that had become familiar, comparing symptoms and treatments, and wondering about the possible implications for Bill. They realized how those cases confirmed what they were learning on their own—that so much of modern medicine was still just trial-and-error guesswork.

They were also increasingly amazed at the number of people hospitalized with some kind of heart disease or disorder. Audubon, a relatively large 484-bed hospital, had a whole floor reserved for heart patients; every room was occupied and more patients were on a waiting list. Until Bill's lengthy hospital stay, the Schroeders hadn't realized how pervasive heart disease really was.

Each time artificial hearts were in the headlines, the Schroeders received calls from reporters asking how they felt and what advice they'd give to people in similar situations. The family had learned by now that when the media started asking questions, they wouldn't let up until they got something. The family found it easier just to cooperate and give reporters a little comment or anecdote to keep them away for a while. In general, the Schroeders didn't dislike reporters. They could see that they had a job to do, but the news coverage often got in the way of sharing happy times with Bill. It was like having a party where somebody shows up uninvited.

By early March, the family were not only preoccupied with Bill, but were making plans to get him to Terry's wedding on the sixteenth, now just days away. After Bill's fever began to subside in late February, he slowly regained his strength. Every few weeks he'd have a seizurelike episode, staring for a few minutes and then appearing very drowsy. But he always seemed fine within hours, and the doctors were at a loss to explain it.

Nevertheless, Bill still worked so hard at rebuilding his strength that the Humana staff and the family began preparing to get him to that wedding. It had been touch-and-go during the fever, but now it could well be a "go." DeVries kept saying they'd all have to wait and see, but he was clearly hoping that his patient could make the trip, and agreed with the family that since the fever had begun to abate, Bill indeed looked stronger.

The whole town of Jasper was hopping with the news that Bill would attend the wedding. Brides usually have last-minute checklists a mile long, and here was Julie trying to tie up the usual loose ends in addition to planning around a major media event. There'd be no keeping this a secret—the first and only trip home for someone with an artificial heart. Reporters were already calling the kids to find out the arrangements. The Humana PR team was working feverishly to satisfy the press and also give the family some privacy. ABC News had already scouted out the town and the church, and at least seven other camera crews had expressed their interest. Meanwhile, the family were trying to accommodate the *Life* contract by giving the magazine the inside story while providing enough leftovers for the rest of the media.

Working out the logistics of taking Bill to the wedding was another problem. One idea called for flying him to Jasper in a helicopter, but no one knew how the Heimes drive would function at high altitudes. A more likely scenario would be for Bill to ride up in the van, rest in a room at Jasper Memorial Hospital, attend the wedding, rest awhile after the ceremony, then return to Louisville that night. The medical team also decided it would have to find a hospital along the route between Louisville and Jasper prepared to admit Bill in an emergency. They had to decide also how to transport all the medical equipment, such as spare parts for the drive systems and IVs. The team would have to plot a route in and out of the church for Bill's wheelchair. And the family made sure Bill's uncle, Father Sylvester Schroeder, would limit the ceremony to twenty minutes or less so Bill wouldn't get worn out.

Since this would be the public's first chance to glimpse someone with an artificial heart, the Jasper police department were nervous about the responsibility of protecting the family, not to mention Bill. The Jasper cops were used to writing traffic tickets, investigating fender-benders, and escorting victorious high-school teams through town. Now they would have to devise contingency plans for crowd control and an escape route for Bill's van in case he had a medical emergency. Maybe they should·rope off the church parking lot and station members from each side of the family at the entrance to screen guests. Or maybe they should require everyone to bring their wedding invitations and flash them at the door to be admitted. Nobody knew what to do, and there was really no one to consult. The police had no idea how many reporters, photographers—or crackpots—to expect. But considering that Bill had become so famous, they had to expect that the scene could get even crazier than the night Bill's surgery was announced.

In addition, the family were getting Bill ready for the big day. When he became discouraged, they and the staff could usually get him to try once more by reminding him that he had to get stronger to go home for Terry's wedding. Bill still seemed confused at times. He'd answer some questions with a "no" when he meant "yes," but whenever he was asked if he wanted to attend the wedding, he made his wishes perfectly clear. He wouldn't say just yes or no. He'd smile, nod his head vigorously, and say, "Surrrre!"

But Bill was coughing more frequently now and occasionally choking on his food. Margaret and the nurses had told the doctors about the problem for some time, so a test was ordered in which he had to drink a liquid containing barium, which would show up on X-ray films. The test showed that the stroke had damaged some of the nerves in Bill's throat that were responsible for swallowing.

Concentrate for a moment on not swallowing, even for a minute, and you'll get a sense of how awful that must have felt—like keeping your mouth open for the dentist. Secretions would collect in Bill's mouth and the back of his throat and choke him until they were removed with a suction tube. Sometimes suctioning was done through his mouth, but other times a longer suction tube had to be inserted through the nasal passages. Bill hated suctioning more than anything. It must have felt like the breath was being sucked right out of his throat—that same helpless, drowning feeling he'd suffered when he was in severe congestive heart failure. Sometimes during that week before the wedding, Bill had to be suctioned every couple of hours, usually during the afternoon and night, and Margaret stayed with him the whole time so he could grip her hand whenever the nurse had to do it.

Still, the family had high hopes of bringing Bill home on Saturday. They were scheduled to meet with Dr. DeVries on the Wednesday night before the wedding to firm up their final plans. On Monday several Humana staffers, including Kevan, Brent Mays, and Donna Hazle, went to Jasper to scout out the church and the town. They reported to DeVries that the excursion would be very difficult and complicated. But the family figured that if the staff had gone this far to check things out, Humana certainly was committed to finding solutions to any logistical problems.

On Monday Bill developed a fever of about 100 degrees, but aspirin seemed to help. That afternoon DeVries sent Strode to take pictures of Bill. Strode hadn't been around much lately, but it soon became clear what DeVries was up to. The hospital's other artificial heart patient, Murray Haydon, was going on a wheelchair ride, and DeVries wanted him to meet Bill. DeVries and some other staffers came into Bill's room, followed by Juanita Haydon, pushing her husband's wheelchair. She wheeled Murray up to face Bill, who was sitting in his cardiac chair. DeVries perched on the bed between them as he introduced his patients.

"Look, Bill," Margaret said, "there's another member of 'the club'!" What was she supposed to say? As usual, Bill smiled at meeting someone new, and reached out to Mr. Haydon. For the first time in history, two men without human hearts shook hands. Strode took a picture.

In the morning on Wednesday—hours before the Schroeder kids were to meet with DeVries—their phones began ringing nonstop. This time, reporters were calling to ask if it was true that Bill wasn't going to the wedding after all. The only thing the kids could say was that no one from Humana had told them anything like that. Somehow word had gotten out to the press, even if it hadn't reached the family. The reporters also wanted to know how they felt about the fact that Terry's wedding day would also be the day that Bill tied Barney Clark's 112-day record for having an artificial heart. With everything else they had to worry about now, the kids hadn't given it any thought. Besides, the question implied that they were somehow keeping score, which was ridiculous.

By the time the family members got together for the ride to Louisville that night, they'd all heard that DeVries and the other doctors had unanimously decided Bill was too sick to make the trip. They didn't believe it because several members of the medical team had told them that if it was at *all* possible for Bill to go, Humana would do everything in its power to see that he got there. Besides, they figured, if Dad was well enough to sit up in a chair for a few hours a day, he was well enough to sit in a wheelchair for a three-hour round trip and twenty-minute ceremony. By the time the kids neared the hospital, they were ready for a fight.

Moni, who'd been down to visit the weekend before, couldn't attend the meeting with DeVries, but when Margaret phoned that afternoon to ask her what she thought about the rumors that Bill couldn't go, Moni was furious, too. "Don't ASK the staff, Mother!" she said. "Just TELL them what you're going to do. They don't have any right to keep Dad from going home."

When the caravan of cars arrived, the kids first went to see their dad. He looked pretty good, recognized them all, and reached out to hold their hands, but he was coughing a bit and still having a hard time swallowing. Mel's wife, Patti, Cheryl's boyfriend, Glenn, and Julie, all had come down with the Schroeders and stayed with Bill while the others went to the conference room down the hall to wait for Dr. DeVries. Finally, he came in with Kevan Shaheen and Gary Rhine, the social worker. DeVries sat down and took a deep breath. It was clear he knew he was in for a fight and he didn't really know how to begin.

"Well," DeVries said, "I take it you've already heard about my decision. I'm not going to let Bill go to the wedding—"

The kids all groaned and started to protest. DeVries held up a hand. "Now, let me tell you why I made that decision."

He explained that a couple of days earlier, Bill had had

another slight fever. Then there was Bill's swallowing problem, which would require taking along enough equipment and personnel to suction him at a moment's notice. And, as they all knew, he still hadn't regained all of the strength he lost in February.

"I've consulted with every one of your dad's doctors, the technicians, and social-work people," DeVries said. "I've asked everybody involved and they've all told me the same thing: It is just not in Bill's best medical interest to go to that wedding."

He paused, then added reluctantly, "And I have to agree with them.

"Now, one thing we've learned from this experiment is that when it comes to making medical decisions, we've got to treat a patient with an artificial heart just the way we treat any other patient. And in my judgment, a patient in Bill's condition should not be allowed to make a one-hundred-eighty-mile round trip. Not for anything."

The kids shook their heads, waiting for him to finish.

"Now, on the other hand," DeVries continued, "if you all wanted maybe to have some kind of activity for him here at the hospital, then we'd certainly do everything we could to—"

"Wait a minute!" Terry interrupted, holding out his hands as if protesting an umpire's call. "THAT'S IT??? Hey, can't we even discuss this a little more?"

DeVries shrugged. "There's nothing to discuss. I've made my decision and no amount of arguing is going to change it."

"But you don't understand—!" Cheryl began.

"Look, Dr. DeVries," Mel began. "You know as well as we do that Dad's been *living* for this wedding. He's been talking about it ever since he got here. I remember him telling you in that very first meeting right here, with Mom and me and all the doctors, that he definitely did not want to miss Terry's wedding!"

"I know," DeVries said evenly, "and I told him we'd do our best to get him there. And I really thought he was going to be able to go. Back when he was so sick with that fever, I would have said definitely not, and I think all of you would have agreed."

The family nodded.

"And then he was looking better, and I really thought he could make it," DeVries continued. "But it's a whole different ball game now—especially because of his swallowing problems. Sometimes this week he's had to be suctioned two or three times an hour. If he starts having trouble during the ceremony, there'd be all kinds of commotion and we'd have to rush him out of there to suction him. Plus there's the fact that he's never traveled outside the hospital for that length of time, so we don't know how he'd tolerate it. There's just a whole slew of logistical problems. I can tell you for sure that the Jasper police chief is beside himself at the thought of having Bill come up there."

Those were just excuses and the kids weren't buying them.

"But Dr. DeVries," Cheryl said, "you don't understand what this wedding means to Dad. We've been talking to him about it all the time, and he's been looking forward to it. If anything, it'll help him."

DeVries shook his head. "The risks would far outweigh the benefits."

"You can't know that for sure," Cheryl said.

"She's right!" Stan said. "You can't be *sure* that something bad would happen to him. But on the other hand, there's no question that he'd really get a boost out of going home and seeing everybody. He'll get up for it the same way he has for everything else: Christmas, the stag party, his birthday—you know he didn't feel great on his birthday, but he got psyched for that, too. I *know* he'll do it for the wedding!"

"I know how important this wedding is to you," DeVries said. "And I know how important it is to Bill. But we also have to look at the long run. If we're cautious now, and we wait for Bill to get stronger, and his physical condition improves, maybe he could take a trip home later—maybe even several trips, I don't know."

"But you said yourself you don't even know how much longer he's going to live, right?" Terry said. "RIGHT?"

"That's right," the doctor acknowledged.

"So maybe this is Dad's only chance to get back home," Terry said. "If there's no guarantee he's going to live one more day, why don't you just let him do what he's been trying so hard for all this time?"

"That would be real nice," DeVries said, "but it's not that simple. A trip to Jasper could be very dangerous for him. Besides, you know that your dad has very little short-term memory—he might not even remember the wedding the next day. Would it really be worth taking all those risks? What if he starts choking in the middle of the ceremony and we have to suction

249

him right there? What if he has a seizure? Is that really the way you want your friends back in Jasper to remember him?"

Margaret couldn't believe he was giving such excuses.

"Okay," Mel said, "maybe it isn't the best thing for him *medically*. Maybe going to Jasper might make him weaker, maybe it might even cause some other complication—but then again, maybe not. Nobody knows. What we do know for sure is that this is something that he said he *really* wanted. And it's also a chance for us, the family, to do something special for him. After all that Dad's done for you, as hard as he's tried for you, after everything you people have learned from all those tests—don't you think you at least owe him the *chance* to try to get home?"

DeVries shook his head. "I understand—"

"Obviously, you *don't*," Terry said, folding his arms in disgust.

DeVries took a deep breath and tried again. "I think I do understand. And I want him to go home just as much as you do, but it's a lot more complicated than that." He began counting on his fingers. It was a whole combination of things: not only Bill's physical problems, but how worried the Jasper police were, and the fact that the nurses who usually cared for Bill were licensed to practice in Kentucky but not Indiana, so malpractice insurance wouldn't cover them if something went wrong. They'd have to get nurses with Indiana licenses and train them to care for an artificial heart patient.

"Oh, geez, what a copout!" Stan said, rolling his eyes. "Man, you know that if you really wanted to work something out, you would. Even if you couldn't, I'm sure Humana could find a way."

"Wait a minute," Mel said. "In other words, what you're telling us is that before you didn't know any of this about security and nurses' licenses and all that kind of stuff. What you're saying is that all along you've been letting Dad hope that he could go to Terry's wedding, but you didn't even have any idea how you were going to do it! Is that right? You never even had any idea?"

"Of course I didn't!" DeVries answered. "None of us did— nobody'd ever done it before! You can't know what the problems are going to be, or what questions are going to come up, until after you've already gotten into something like this. That's what the experimental process is all about: Every answer you find raises ten new questions, every mistake you make teaches you something that will help somebody else. And I can tell you right now that we've learned that having a patient with an artificial heart gets very, very complicated. Much more complicated than I ever would have imagined."

Great. The family weren't talking about human experimentation. They were talking about something their husband and father had worked so hard for, about yanking his dreams right out from under him, about tearing up his will to live . . .

"You have to think about this question," DeVries was saying. "Could this family live with the fact that if Bill does go to the wedding, something horrible might happen to him?"

"Of COURSE!" Terry said. "We live with that possibility every day!"

"Yeah!" the other kids said, backing him up. Since Bill was unable to speak for himself, they were going to hold their ground the way he would have.

"What I mean is," DeVries said, "could you live with yourselves, knowing that you'd be taking Bill on a trip that could *kill* him?"

The family looked at each other, then nodded at the doctor. They knew Bill had never hesitated to take a risk if it involved something that was important to him.

"Okay," DeVries said. "Let me get this straight. In other words, what you're telling me is that you wouldn't mind if Terry had to remember his wedding day as the day his father died because this family decided it was in his best interest to take him on a one-hundred-eighty-mile round trip?"

Margaret hadn't heard him put it that way before. She looked at her kids.

"Hell, yeah, we can live with that!" Terry said stubbornly.

DeVries shifted in his chair. "Well, *I* can't," he said.

"Look, Dr. DeVries," Terry said, "ever since November, we've had to take this whole damn thing day by day. If there's a possibility that Dad might die next week or next month, why can't we spend a few hours this weekend doing something that he's wanted to do all this time? Why do you think he said he wanted to go through the operation in the first place? I'll tell you right now, my wedding was a hell of a lot more important to Dad than trying to set some stupid record for living with an artificial heart."

DeVries was running out of reasons. "Do you understand

what I'm telling you? That there's a possibility that your father could *die* if he goes to that wedding—?"

Terry shouted back: "Maybe there's WORSE things than dying!"

DeVries studied the table for a long time, then said quietly, "All I can say is that I am legally bound to protect my patient."

Margaret just kept quiet, listening to both sides.

"Doesn't his family have any say-so at all?" Cheryl asked. "I mean, what *do* we have the right to decide?"

"Well," DeVries said, "I don't know if you want to get a lawyer involved, but I guess you could get one to take it before a judge and have me overruled."

"Yeah, right, with the wedding three days away," Stan said. "This is a waste of time. We're just letting him down." He got up, slammed his chair into its place, and stalked out the door.

"Well," Margaret finally said to the kids, "there's no use arguing anymore. He just isn't going to let him go, and there's nothing we can do about it."

"Margaret, I'm sorry. I really am," DeVries said. "But that's my decision, and the whole staff backs me up. I'm still willing to do something here at the hospital if you decide you want to, maybe have a little ceremony or a rehearsal or something."

"Oh, *great*," Terry muttered. "An artificial wedding."

DeVries stood up. "I'll let you all think about it for a while," he said and walked out of the room. Kevan and Gary tried to pursue the idea of having some kind of "mock wedding" at the hospital, but the family wouldn't hear of it. After a few minutes, Kevan and Gary left to give the family some time alone.

It didn't seem fair at all. Who was supposed to make these decisions anyway—the doctor or the family? Bill had clearly indicated his own wishes, and the family members were trying their best to carry them out. Did the hospital only want to keep Bill around to do more experiments on him? Now the Schroeders were not only angry but hurt. They'd thought Dr. DeVries was on their side.

The family hashed it out again and again. They were united in their belief that Bill should go, no matter what. Mel got up and walked around the room, restless. On the conference-room blackboard, he wrote in big letters: JASPER OR BUST. Margaret wondered if she should call Dr. Salb—*he'd* know how important the wedding was. DeVries obviously didn't understand what it meant to Bill.

The kids wouldn't budge, but Margaret knew that DeVries wouldn't either. Finally, she calmed them down. "There's no use arguing. You heard him—he's not going to listen to reason," she said. "We'll just have to make do with what we've got." Her kids could see she was as heartbroken as they were. She didn't need a doctor to tell her how disappointed Bill was going to be. She couldn't stand the thought of the look on his face when he heard the news.

Mel seemed to read her mind. "Well, if it's DeVries's decision, I think *he* should tell Dad."

The rest agreed, but Terry just kept shaking his head. He'd really thought he could win this argument. "This is going to ruin the wedding," he said again and again. "It'll kill Julie when we tell her."

When Dr. DeVries returned, the family informed him that they'd abide by his decision, provided that he broke the news to Bill.

The doctor's jaw tightened. DeVries hated this just as much as they did. But it was his decision, his responsibility, and if anybody was going to be the bad guy, he was.

"Okay," he said. "I'll tell him. But I'm warning you right now that he might not even understand what I'm saying."

Just then, the doctor's pager beeped. "I've got to answer that," he said. "I'll meet you down in Bill's room in a few minutes."

The family filed back into Bill's room, looking woefully at Bill, who was sitting up in a chair while Stan and the others kept him company. Terry just shook his head sullenly at Julie. Some of the kids were on the verge of tears, but they tried not to let Bill see. After a few minutes, DeVries came in. Bill greeted the somber surgeon as he usually did, with an eager smile. Margaret put her arms around Bill from behind as DeVries sat on the bed in front of him, face to face.

Okay, Dr. DeVries. Let's see you do it.

The surgeon patted Bill's hand and said they had to talk very seriously for a moment. The family could see that this was going to be hard for him.

"Bill," DeVries finally began, "I know I promised you that

you could go to Jasper for Terry's wedding. And you've been doing pretty well lately. You've been trying real hard, and I appreciate that. But you've still got some complications that we need to work on before you can leave the hospital. So I've decided that medically it's not in your best interest to go . . ."

Bill looked like he was carefully thinking over each of the doctor's words. Then slowly an expression of disbelief crept over his face as he began looking around the room, from one family member to another.

"Now, Bill," DeVries said, trying to catch Bill's eye again. "I don't want you to blame your family. Believe me, they all want you there at the wedding. So if you're going to blame anybody, blame me. I'm your doctor, and I'm the one who made the decision, based on what I think is best for you. And I'm going to stick by it. You can blame me if you want. But I'm not letting you go to Terry's wedding."

Bill just stared at DeVries for a moment, and began to cry. Margaret held him and stroked his arm, saying, "It's okay, honey. We'll go back to Jasper someday."

Bill was crying loudly now, in big, shuddering sobs. The kids stopped fighting their own tears. Ever since the stroke, it had never stopped being painful to watch their dad weeping.

DeVries sat looking at the floor, arms folded across his chest. Bill was still sobbing, but now he couldn't swallow and began to gag and choke. DeVries looked up. Bill's face was turning red. DeVries quickly grabbed the small suction tube.

"Here, Bill, let me get some of that for you . . ." DeVries held the tube up to Bill's mouth, but Bill turned his head away, still crying and choking.

"Here, Bill." DeVries tried it again. Margaret grabbed the suction tube from him and pushed away the doctor's hand.

"YOU have done enough!" she said, and started to suction Bill herself.

Mel looked at DeVries. "I think you'd better leave."

"All right," the doctor said. All eyes followed him as he got up and walked around the bed.

When DeVries reached the door, Terry asked bitterly, "Do you think he understood what you said?"

DeVries left without another word.

Margaret finished suctioning Bill's mouth. Now he was whimpering. Terry went over to him. "It's okay Dad—" he began.

Bill looked at him for a long time. Terry could see so much going on in his father's watery eyes. All of a sudden, Bill took Terry's hand, slowly pulled it to his lips, and kissed it.

Terry wasn't ready for that at all. Not from Dad. His father's arm around his shoulders maybe, or a firm handshake. But not *this*. His own eyes stung with tears.

Margaret kept assuring Bill that she wouldn't leave him, that if he had to miss the wedding, she would miss it with him. *Oh, terrific,* Terry thought, *now I won't have either one of my parents at my own wedding!*

Since the family hadn't been able to get DeVries to hear them out, they kept going over it with each other, again and again. They were feeling not only the pain and anger of betrayal, but the shock. They'd thought DeVries was Bill's good friend, that he shared Bill's values, and understood what he'd been working so hard for all this time.

DeVries and Lansing had gone on and on to the media about the importance of the patient's will to live and having a close-knit family. But the doctors obviously didn't understand how all those things fit together. DeVries had just yanked away something Bill had been holding on to for support through all these difficult, frustrating times.

No doctor would have ever given Bill an okay to attend that wedding reception back in November, the day before he was admitted to Audubon. But no doctor could have kept him from going, either. As weak and breathless as Bill had been, he'd managed to walk into that gathering because family occasions were so important to him. Because they were his life.

The kids had to be back at work the next morning, so they reluctantly left their parents. They were still seething, but also knew that now, as so often in recent months, they'd have to accept the situation and make the best of it. They all agreed that DeVries's decision would cast a shadow over the whole wedding—and that their relationship with him would never be the same.

CHAPTER FIFTEEN

When Dr. DeVries made his early-morning rounds the next day, it was as if a gust of cold air followed him into Bill's room. Margaret didn't speak to him, and he stayed just long enough to make a routine check of Bill's chart.

Then Polly, who'd been out of town the day before, hurried in and took Margaret down to her office. "Sit down, Margaret," Polly said, settling in at her desk and kicking off her shoes. "I've got work to do."

Polly always seemed to find a way to get things done, no matter what it took—that's how she'd managed Lansing's practice all those years. She'd seen experimentation firsthand many times before, had worked with the state's first kidney-dialysis patients and first kidney-transplant team. So she already had a sense of the soaring highs and discouraging lows in store for artificial heart patients' families, as well as their nurses.

Now once more Polly was determined to get results. "Margaret," she announced, "we are NOT going to have a bunch of long faces at that wedding. We've got to do something. First, we need to get the children feeling good about whatever we all decide."

Margaret wasn't sure about that. She knew the kids were awfully disappointed and angry. "Well, what do we do?" Margaret asked.

"I don't know yet," Polly said. But in a minute, she was in her usual mode—a human whirlwind, chain-smoking, making one phone call after another, with still more callers on hold. She phoned around to investigate the possibility of a live remote TV broadcast of the wedding or making a videotape for Bill. Those, however, didn't seem to be enough. By 9:00 A.M., she was calling Mel at his office.

All the Schroeders were still seething over DeVries's deci-

257

sion. As soon as Mel arrived at work that morning, his phone began ringing. Reporters wanted to know why Bill wasn't going to Terry's wedding and—of course—how did the family feel about it? This was one time Mel was careful not to go into detail. First of all, they'd have to edit out a lot of expletives before they could print his comments. More important, the family felt bound to keep up at least some kind of friendly relationship with the doctors. They couldn't just check Bill out of the hospital against medical advice and make off with the expensive equipment that was keeping him alive. Bill had become a kind of hostage to the hospital, and the family didn't want to alienate the medical team.

And now here was Polly.

"Mel," she said, "I want to do something at the hospital so we can include Bill in the wedding—maybe a mock wedding or rehearsal or something."

Oh, brother. "I don't think you understand, Polly," Mel said. "The kids already talked it over last night and we all agreed that if Dad can't come to the wedding, then we didn't want to settle for anything less. We don't want anything to do with a mock wedding, or whatever you want to call it."

Polly wasn't about to be put off that easily.

"Well, I've talked to Margaret," Polly said, "and she thinks that maybe it would be a good idea."

I do? Margaret thought.

"Well, let me talk to Mom," Mel said. Margaret picked up the other line.

"Hi, Mom, what's going on there?"

"Well . . ." Margaret said, "I don't really know, hon. Polly's talking like maybe we could do something here for Bill."

"Is that what you want, Mother?"

"Well . . ." How was she supposed to decide?

Polly cut in and told Mel that their first step would be to get all the kids feeling good about some substitute for the real thing.

Mel was still skeptical. "That won't be easy, Polly. I have to tell you, everybody is *really* ticked off."

"Let me take care of that," Polly said.

"Well," Mel said finally, "if it's what Mom wants, I'll see what I can do." Mel called Terry and Julie and presented Polly's suggestion.

Terry thought it was the stupidest idea he'd ever heard. It

would take away from the wedding, he said. If the people at the hospital really wanted to do something for Dad, they should let him come home—there was no substitute for that. Besides, even if they did try something, there was no way to get it together in just two days. Terry and Julie already had more than enough to keep them busy right up until the wedding at one o'clock Saturday afternoon.

Mel polled the other kids by phone. Nobody was very enthusiastic about the idea. But, they all added, if it would make Mom and Dad happy, they'd go along.

After another quick round of calls between Polly and the kids, the family agreed that maybe it wouldn't be so bad to have some kind of wedding "blessing" at the hospital. Terry still thought the whole idea was stupid, and didn't want to help with it.

However, that was enough so Polly could proceed full steam ahead. She phoned Mel again to work out the logistics. He told her there was no way to round everybody up to get to the hospital by that evening. That left only Friday night, and that was when the wedding rehearsal was scheduled, which would be followed by a rehearsal party, and then the wedding on Saturday.

"Well?" Polly asked.

Mel figured that the only option was to hope that both the church and the priest would be available to reschedule a rehearsal for early Friday afternoon. If that could be worked out, then they'd have to call everyone to see if they could all leave work early that day to go to the rehearsal, then travel to Louisville for the blessing. And *that* would mean rounding up the seven other couples in the wedding party, plus the parents, plus Father Sylvester, plus the bride and groom, and God knows who else. Maybe they'd just better forget it.

"Mel," Polly said, "what's it going to take to get everybody down to this hospital?"

Mel just shook his head and laughed. "Well, Polly, I don't know. I guess you're just going to have to charter a bus."

"Okay, leave that to me," Polly said, and hung up.

Mel smiled. That should keep her busy for a while. In the meantime, his phone wouldn't stop ringing. His brothers and sisters at first agreed that if they did go to Louisville, they'd just wear casual clothes, but then they decided that if they were *really* going to do this, then, hell, they might as well go all the way. This meant more calls to and from the tuxedo-rental firm, and from confused members of the wedding party, Father Sylvester, and in the meantime, of course, from reporters. Mel was also struggling to work out a time when the whole family could sit down for a couple of hours with the reporter from *Life* magazine, who planned to be in Jasper for the wedding.

It was getting crazier by the minute. Every time Mel got up to take care of some of his own work at the office, the phone would ring. Finally, he just gave up, slid the phone to the center of his desk, pulled up his chair in front of it, and waited for the next call.

Rrrring!

It was Polly again. "Mel, I've got you a bus. It'll pick everyone up at Saint Joe's tomorrow afternoon at three o'clock sharp."

Mel pulled the receiver from his ear and looked at it. "What?" Damned if she hadn't done it.

"Well," he said, "okay . . ." He thought a moment. As long as she was granting wishes, he asked, "Hey, could you put a couple of iced-down cases of beer on that bus?"

"Mel, don't be ridiculous."

The other members of the wedding party now ran around trying to get everything squared away. Everything was happening so fast. There were still so many what-ifs, and they knew that all these loosely thrown-together plans could fall through at any time.

Terry was still steamed up, and refused to have anything to do with the preparations. Julie was frantically calling all the folks on her side of the family, trying to explain what Humana and the Schroeders were up to—although she wasn't exactly sure herself. And somehow, everyone managed to get free Friday afternoon.

Meanwhile, Polly had sent the hospital into a frenzy of preparations. Staffers were already transforming the briefing room into a reception hall. Polly even had a band lined up, but then Margaret remembered that the Stonemill Band, a local country-western group, had offered their services if the Schroeders ever needed some kind of fund raiser.

Fine, Polly said. Despite the short notice, the band agreed to come in the following night to play at the reception. Polly and Donna Hazle from PR arranged to get donations of floral arrangements, and a big wedding cake. A work crew labored most of Thursday night to convert the hospital lobby into a chapel, complete with a sound system, royal blue drapes to separate it from the rest of the hospital, candelabra, potted plants, and a set of fifty chairs with an aisle.

At 2:00 p.m. the next day, Friday, the wedding party went through a quick rehearsal at St. Joe's. Afterward, the forty or so family members and friends and the priest waited in the parking lot, tuxes and bridesmaids' dresses in plastic bags draped over their shoulders, coolers packed with beer and wine at their feet. Everyone was still a little skeptical about whether this was all going to come off—until a spanking-new bus turned the corner and pulled into the parking lot. The doors opened, and social worker Gary Rhine bounded down the steps, yelling, "We found you guys!"

The folks from Jasper were amazed. They'd expected some old school bus or broken-down crate, but Polly had sent them a spacious, air-conditioned cruiser with comfy reclining seats. It even had a clean bathroom. Everyone piled on, hanging their wedding finery from the overhead racks, giving the bridesmaids' hats a seat to themselves, setting coolers in the aisles. As the wedding party rode through Hoosier National Forest and past the turn-offs for the towns of Birdseye, Paoli, Palmyra, and Marengo, the group played cards, popped brews, passed around wine bottles, and took snapshots of each other. Even Terry was grudgingly warming up to the idea; after all, this *was* a party. He began teasing Julie that they'd have to celebrate two wedding anniversaries each year.

Polly had left orders for Gary to phone the hospital from the Georgetown exit, about twenty minutes out of Louisville, to alert the hospital security guards that they were on their way. When the bus stopped so he could make the call, everyone hurried over to a nearby liquor store to replenish their supplies, then piled back on the bus.

After the bus pulled into the parking lot at Audubon, Polly directed the guys to one unused hospital room and the girls to another so they could change into their wedding clothes. Terry and Julie went upstairs to see Margaret and Bill, and Mel's wife, Patti, went along in case Bill's tux needed any last-minute alterations.

The staff had let Bill rest most of the day, and Kevan had taken Margaret to get her hair done. As it became apparent that they really were going to go through with it, Margaret had begun preparing Bill for the big occasion. And now the more she talked about Terry's wedding blessing, the more excited Bill became.

Margaret and Patti decked Bill out in his tux, and figured out that they could just slip the drive lines under his cummerbund. Bill really looked terrific, and he knew it. Staffers kept dropping in to tell him so, and he'd reply clearly, "Thank you very much." When they asked if he wanted to rest a little more before the blessing, he'd answer, "No! I'm too excited." Margaret got dressed up, and Polly presented her with a corsage. The closer it got to 6:00 P.M., the more antsy Bill became. Larry switched him to the Heimes and settled him in the wheelchair. They had to lock the chair's brakes in position because Bill kept trying to wheel out of the room. He couldn't wait.

Downstairs, the kids walked through a quick rehearsal, and then waited as Margaret, Polly, Larry Hastings, and Peter Heimes brought Bill downstairs. Margaret wanted to push the wheelchair, but Polly insisted on doing it herself, saying that Margaret had been under too much stress. Of course, everybody knew that although the press was excluded from the ceremony, Strode was taking pictures, under the agreement with *Life*, so whoever pushed Bill was sure to be all over the magazine. Staffers sometimes kidded Polly about how many photos of Bill she managed to show up in.

They parted the curtain that separated the makeshift chapel from the rest of the hospital, and Polly wheeled Bill in. The room was lit with the soft glow of dozens of candles, and packed with family and friends. Bill's strapping sons were lined up on either side of the entrance, looking sharp in black tuxedos. Up ahead, his daughters stood smiling in beautiful dresses. And there, in seats on either side, were many of Bill's longtime friends. As his wheelchair went down the aisle, Bill kept grabbing his sons' hands and squeezing them.

"Hi, Dad!" his boys said. "You look great in your tux!" When Bill looked toward the end of the line, he saw Stan grinning and giving him the thumbs-up the way Bill had always done at his football games. For a moment Bill broke down in tears.

As soon as Bill and Margaret were settled into places at the front, the ceremony began. Someone switched on a tape of an organist playing "Here Comes the Bride," and Julie walked down the short aisle. Father Sylvester gave a brief blessing. This was followed by a couple of readings from Patti, both of them short, to avoid tiring Bill. Another reason they had to hurry was that at the last minute, someone realized that the candelabra had been lit right beneath the emergency water sprinklers, and if the candles weren't snuffed out soon, the whole system would douse the wedding party.

Afterward, Bill stood up from his wheelchair and, with very little support, posed for some wedding pictures with his family. It was amazing: As he stood in his tux with the rest of the wedding party, Bill blended right in. You'd never have known he had an artificial heart except for the two drive hoses that peeked out from under his sash.

After the photo session, the group went downstairs to the briefing room, where the Stonemill Band was playing, and tables were laid out with hors d'oeuvres, punch, beer, and two cases of champagne—a wedding gift from Polly. Julie, who'd worked on her wedding arrangements for months, was stunned to see such a beautiful ceremony and reception materialize in less than thirty-six hours. The people at Humana, and especially Polly, had really outdone themselves.

At the reception, hospital staffers blended in with the family. Dr. Jarvik flew in for the occasion, bringing along his ex-wife and their two kids. Bill smiled when he saw him. Dr. DeVries and his wife also showed up, although they didn't stay long. The whole Schroeder family still had a lot of angry feelings toward him, but they greeted him politely. After all, Bill would never have lived to see this day if DeVries hadn't saved his life, and they knew they still had a long way to travel with the doctor.

Bill was the center of attention at the reception, and tried to talk with everyone who came to shake his hand and pose with him for snapshots. This day was definitely his, but that was fine with the bride. She could see that she was marrying into an exceptional family, and that today's celebration honored that family's heart: Bill himself.

Jarvik, unaware of Bill's swallowing problems, tried to help Bill celebrate by giving him champagne from a plastic goblet. Margaret and the kids made a mad dash to stop him.

"Hey, Dr. Jarvik! He can't—!"

"Oh, a little bit won't hurt him," Jarvik said as he put the goblet to Bill's lips. "The stuff's good for you, isn't it, Bill?"

Bill eagerly helped hold the goblet, clearly loving the taste of the champagne. He kept trying to drink it, even though he couldn't swallow it. Finally, Terry got the goblet away from him, but Bill kept reaching for more as Terry explained the problem to Jarvik.

Still, Bill was probably having the best time of all of them. He enjoyed watching everybody as they laughed, danced, talked, and ate. The reception wasn't exactly like one back home, but they were a family together again, even if just for a couple of hours. When the band struck up one of Bill's favorites, the snappy, old-time tune "Will the Circle Be Unbroken?" the family formed a big circle, clapping and singing along. Bill, of course, was part of that circle. Sitting in his wheelchair between Margaret and John Lammers, the nurse, he clapped his hands and tapped his foot to the beat.

John leaned over and whispered, "Doesn't it just make you want to get up and dance, pal?"

Bill nodded and smiled.

"Well," John whispered, sensing another challenge for his patient, "why *don't* you?"

Before anyone realized what Bill was doing, he was on his feet, standing shakily, swinging his arms and bouncing at the knees. He danced that way for less than a minute before he had to sit down again, but still, nobody could believe it. *This* was the guy who was too sick to go to Jasper?

The party went on until late in the evening, and Bill stayed almost the whole time before he got tired and had to go to bed. The rest of the wedding party split up again to change back into regular clothes. By this time, they were all laughing and stumbling over each other.

The kids had to do some fast talking to persuade Margaret to go back to Jasper with them. She hated leaving Bill, but they finally convinced her that he'd probably just rest until she returned. Terry and Julie promised they'd find her a ride back the following night. When the group left the hospital, they spotted some TV crews who had learned of the festivities and were hoping for some shots of the Schroeders. By that time, some of the folks from Jasper didn't care and just partied their way on out the door, waving beer cans and shouting greetings at the stakeout.

The bus ride home was a long one, and it was well past midnight before the Schroeders finally collapsed into their beds. When alarm clocks went off a few hours later, they were exhausted. They couldn't imagine having to do it all over again. But

there was no time to think. They had to be at Mom and Dad's
house by 8:00 A.M. to talk to the *Life* reporter. This was the only
time they could all get together for an interview.

The family gravitated toward the kitchen table the way they
always did whenever they gathered to talk. Margaret and the kids
had been living day to day, discussing each problem as it came
up, trying to anticipate new ones, but they had never met to review everything that had happened. The reporter, Donna E.
Haupt, only asked a question or two before all their pent-up feelings came tumbling out—the good and the bad memories, happy
ones and sad ones, funny and scary. They were still fuming over
Dr. DeVries's decision, and those feelings came out, too. It was
such a relief to talk about the ordeal with someone who wasn't
connected with Humana or a friend they'd feel they were burden-
ing with the same stories. As happened any time a bunch of
Schroeders got together, they were all telling stories on each
other, cutting in and improving on each other's versions, supplying sound effects, and jumping up from their chairs to act out
particularly dramatic moments. Soon the kitchen rang with the
old boisterousness of so many other family gatherings. The *Life*
reporter let her tape recorder run for a couple of hours.

By the time the interview was finished, the morning was
half over, and the wedding was just a couple of hours away. That
meant trouble. A Dubois County wedding is a huge all-day event,
requiring all kinds of preparations. The guys get up early in the
morning to wash their cars together and decorate the vehicles with
paint, streamers, and flowers, which the girls make from colored
plastic trash bags or tissues. The cars, vans, and pickup trucks
form a larger wedding procession after the ceremony, as newlyweds and guests travel around town, stopping at a couple of
bars, and sometimes visiting elderly or ailing relatives who
couldn't make it to the church. They all end up at a reception hall
where they eat a big dinner. Then there's dancing until the wee
hours, to a live band that usually starts with polkas and country-
western, then switches to rock-and-roll as the older folks get
weary and drop out.

Now the Schroeders were way behind schedule. The wedding photographer had arrived to take pictures, and nobody was
ready. A mad rush followed with the kids pounding on the
bathroom door, yelling for each other to hurry up, and asking, "Is
this on straight?" and "How do I look?" Their wedding finery was

already wrinkled and sweaty from the night before, and several had lost cufflinks or other accessories in the scramble to get back on the bus and come home. But somehow they all got themselves decent-looking and drove off for St. Joe's.

Everyone was so rushed they didn't worry about the press camped outside the church. An ABC News crew was set up in the balcony to film the ceremony, on the condition that they provided videotapes to a media pool as well as to the Schroeders.

Of course, it was a beautiful wedding with about four hundred guests in the majestic old Catholic church. Margaret left a space beside her in the pew where Bill would have sat. During the ceremony's traditional "passing of the peace," the bride and groom stepped down from the altar to greet Julie's dad with a handshake and give her mom a rose and a kiss. Then they moved across the aisle to greet Margaret the same way. Terry hugged his mother for an extra-long time.

After the wedding, the parade of cars and vans made the usual round of bars, toting cases of beer and the remaining champagne from Polly. After everyone arrived at the reception hall, they sat down to a huge dinner, then danced for hours and drained several kegs of beer. Dr. Jarvik tagged along. He danced up a storm, grabbing Cheryl's bridesmaid's hat and modeling it. Everyone kept thinking that if Bill could have been there, he'd have been right in the middle of it all.

Late that night the newlyweds said their good-byes and drove off on their honeymoon—with Margaret beside them in the front seat. Terry and Julie were headed for the Poconos, but they'd assured Margaret that Louisville would be right on the way—sort of. The three returned to Audubon and looked in on Bill, who was sleeping soundly. Then Margaret yawned discreetly and said she probably should sleep on the couch in Bill's room, just in case he needed her. So Terry and Julie went up to her room and spent their wedding night on the sixth floor of the hospital.

CHAPTER SIXTEEN

The next couple of days, Bill slept a lot, but his sleep was restless because he was frequently coughing to clear secretions in his throat. He continued to have occasional fevers, and still required nutritional supplements. But by Monday he felt up to having Strode photograph him for the cover of *Life* magazine—and well enough to insist that his surgeon be in the photo with him. DeVries was happy to oblige. Strode posed the doctor and patient side by side. Bill wore a jogging suit and a T-shirt that read I ♥ WALKING. DeVries wore a green scrubsuit, and a surgical mask hung casually around his neck. Bill was happy to be with his pals again, and kept trying to say things to them. While Strode focused his camera, DeVries draped his big arm around Bill's shoulders.

"Okay," Strode said. "Can you give us a smile, Bill?"

Just before the shutter snapped, Bill whispered, "Say 'shit'!" DeVries couldn't help laughing. Bill grinned, too. That shot was sure to turn out well.

Meanwhile, another *Life* reporter, Jeff Wheelwright, visited Louisville to interview David Jones, Humana's chairman and chief executive officer. Wheelwright asked some tough, skeptical questions about Humana's motivation for backing the artificial heart program, and about all the free publicity from the extensive media coverage. Humana concluded that *Life* was doing a hatchet job on the hospital company and the artificial heart program. A few days later Donna Haupt called the Schroeders. She told them that she had begun to get a runaround and couldn't obtain interviews with doctors or hospital staffers. If Humana wouldn't cooperate, she'd just have to say so in the article, which could make the company look as if they were trying to hide something.

George Atkins told the Schroeders that employees were indeed reluctant to help with an article that might hurt the program

267

for which they were working so hard. After all, Humana was under no obligation to accommodate the magazine's contract with the Schroeders. The family tried to explain that they weren't after a totally positive or negative article. It didn't take a genius to realize that they had all endured some emotionally wrenching times after Bill's implant, and that they'd probably face more in the future. But the artificial heart had also given the Schroeders some precious, irreplaceable moments with Bill—and, they hoped, many more to come. However, what had begun as a simple, true-life story about a family had turned into a test of wills, with the family caught in the middle. Eventually, a compromise was reached in which *Life* submitted written questions in advance.

The resulting article was touted as the inside story of a medical experiment, but it didn't really say anything new. It seemed to the Schroeders that the story had been written before the reporters ever got to Louisville, with a few blank spaces to be filled in with comments from the family. The media picked up on a couple of isolated quotes from Margaret: "Bill thought he'd either die or be better. If he had anticipated the hardship this has been on the family, he might not have done it. . . . Now I see it as more of a research experiment. The longer he lives, the more information they will get. Only for us, it's just so hard sometimes." The family didn't see why these quotes were such a big deal. Any realistic person would have had second thoughts. Bill couldn't have known at the time he signed the consent form— nobody could. Surely no one expected them to feel otherwise.

By late March the medical team was firming up plans to discharge Bill to the apartment. The Schroeders knew that this interim step was necessary; staffers had compared it to pushing birds out of the nest. But now, with the move so near, it began to sink in that Margaret and Bill would still be far away from the family, friends, and community that gave shape to their lives. By now it was becoming clear that no matter how much better Bill got, he'd never be 100 percent again. All of his progress would be relative, with good days measured against bad ones. A good day now was when Bill was talking a bit, in not much pain, and eager to get out of bed.

On bad days, when complications confined Bill to bed, Margaret ached to hear him talk the way he used to, tell her how to handle everything, hear him making his own choices again.

Her thoughts kept drifting back to that December evening, minutes before the stroke, as the two of them were eating supper, talking about nothing in particular. If only she'd known that stroke was coming, she would have asked him so many, many questions. Now that chance was gone forever. In her diary she wrote:

> I feel so lonesome. No one to talk to. No one to share with and love me. Sometimes I feel like I'm in this spider web and it gets tighter and tighter around me.

The weekend after Terry's wedding, some of the kids visited their parents and arranged another van ride, this time around the parking lot at a suburban mall. Bill enjoyed the trip, speaking clearly in short sentences and nodding enthusiastically as the kids pointed out sights along the way. Since he seemed to be doing rather well, they persuaded Margaret to make an overnight visit home. When Terry and Julie brought her back early the next morning, they couldn't believe how much Bill had improved. His condition had always been unpredictable from day to day, sometimes even from hour to hour, but this was amazing. Margaret wrote: "Bill changed so much. He was ready to get up and go. He could talk up a storm—I never heard the like—and *wanted* to walk."

As springtime settled in, Bill grew increasingly restless and eager to take walks down the hall and go for wheelchair rides outside. More tests showed that he was swallowing better, so he began taking pureed foods and liquids, and relied less on the feeding tube. The last weekend in March, the medical team informed the Schroeders that Bill would probably be discharged the following Saturday.

Nurse Kevan Shaheen, the patient coordinator who had supervised much of the remodeling of the apartment, took Margaret to see the place where she and Bill were about to move. It would be a five-minute walk from the hospital, across the parking lot and a four-lane thoroughfare, to the boxy, four-dwelling complex. The apartment's living room was tastefully decorated in soothing tones of gray, peach, and cream, and had a foldout couch, easy chairs and tables, and a TV. Elegant, brass-framed prints of Louisville landmarks hung on the walls. The living room opened onto a kitchen with an oven, range, sink, refrigerator. The back door led to a large wooden deck with a ramp sloping to the asphalt driveway.

The living room was roughly the size of Bill's hospital room. A short hall led to a back bedroom, which could be closed off with a sliding wooden door. Inside, a queen-sized hospital bed, draped with a beautiful handmade quilt from Appalachia, took up most of the floor space. Opposite that room was a recessed area just big enough for a single bed and a dresser. That area adjoined a bathroom adapted for a wheelchair user. Throughout the apartment there were wall outlets to supply the Utah with compressed air.

The only other obvious difference in the apartment was a Med-Call system, the type often used in homes of elderly and handicapped persons. Alarms about the size of a doorchime were located on a bedroom wall, in the bathroom and living room. An emergency button on the box alerted a central switchboard where an operator would ask whether help was needed. Margaret would also have a remote alarm to wear around her neck or carry in her pocket. A special white phone in the hall was a direct line to the heart institute.

The apartment was lovely but, not surprisingly, Margaret had mixed feelings about moving there. Initially, at least, nurses would staff the apartment around the clock, while teaching Margaret to take over the nursing duties. She was eager to learn to administer Bill's medicines and watch over the machinery so that she could care for him herself if they moved back home. But at the same time, the prospect of such responsibility was frightening. Although she and the rest of the family were looking forward to bringing Bill a step closer to home, there were still many practical questions about what they had to do along the way.

The family couldn't help wondering whether Bill was being pushed out of the hospital prematurely, perhaps to make room for another artificial heart patient. After all, DeVries himself had insisted just three weeks earlier that Bill was too sick to make a 180-mile round trip. Why was he sure that Bill was now ready to leave the hospital for good?

The family were also disturbed by a change in the nursing plan. Humana had discovered that although the apartment was just across the street, residential zoning restrictions prevented the hospital nurses from caring for patients there. So Audubon contracted with Humana Care Partners, the company's home-healthcare agency, whose nurses worked for patients who didn't need hospitalization. This change was hard for the family to accept: They'd heard lots of talk about the importance of "consistency of nursing care" for patients—but now a whole new set of home-care nurses would have to be trained to look after Bill.

Throughout that week, Bill's condition was unpredictable as ever. He seemed tired all day, and ran fevers at night. As more people began to hurry in and out of his room for last-minute preparations, he seemed anxious about the activity. Margaret tried to reassure him, hoping that he couldn't sense her own fears and apprehension. Now, if Bill had any trouble in the hospital, help was just seconds away. But in the apartment it would be several long minutes before help arrived.

On Friday, the PR department asked the Schroeders about letting the news media tour the apartment and photograph the interior. Margaret didn't like the idea. Why should the whole world be allowed into their new home when Bill hadn't even seen it yet? Besides, it was just a regular apartment—providing her first real privacy with Bill in more than four months—so why did reporters have to nose around in there?

The press insisted to PR officials that footage of the apartment would be an important addition to the debate over artificial heart patients' "quality of life." Finally, another compromise was reached that allowed a TV crew to photograph the apartment and pool the film.

Saturday, April 6, 133 days after Bill received his artificial heart: He was running a slight temperature that morning, but his fever was still so unpredictable that it might well be gone in time for the move that afternoon. All the gifts from well-wishers were packed in boxes. The walls of his room looked strangely bare without family pictures and get-well cards. Throughout the morning, staffers came to congratulate him and give Margaret a hug.

The family met with the medical team to set the day's agenda. They agreed to send Margaret, along with Moni and Mel, with DeVries while he briefed the press. Meanwhile, some of the other kids and grandchildren who had come down for the day would go ahead to the apartment to await their arrival. The briefing room was packed with reporters. DeVries gave a medical update on Bill's condition, and then let reporters question the Schroeders.

How did they feel?

Margaret stepped to the microphone and smiled. "Today is really important to me, because we're going home in a sense. We were in the air force for almost fifteen years, and 'home' was wherever we were at. So we're going home."

The press conference went smoothly, and afterward everyone hurried back upstairs to get Bill ready to go.

Finally, after several delays, Larry Hastings switched Bill to the Heimes and hefted it onto his shoulder. This was it. Margaret wheeled Bill down the hall, and all along the way, patients and staff hurried up to shake Bill's hand or pat him on the back. Just past the lobby's glass doors reporters and onlookers were crowded into roped-off areas on either side of the short walkway. At the end, the Schroeder boys stood waiting beside the van. She took a deep breath, murmured some words of reassurance to Bill, and Larry led the way outside.

The crowd began to applaud, and Bill waved stiffly in response. Reporters yelled questions about how it felt to be leaving. Bill moved his lips, struggling to speak, but no one could hear him. As the boys positioned Bill's wheelchair on the van's lift, reporters shouted more questions, and Bill answered with a raised fist, as if to say, "All right!"

Terry had his camera, and stepped back to take snapshots of his dad's proud moment. "Hey!" a network TV reporter shouted. "Get out of the way. Hey! Get that guy out of there!"

Terry whirled around and glared. "Shut up! I'm his *son*, all right? Geez!" He wasn't about to move until he finished getting his pictures. As the lift slowly raised Bill's wheelchair level with the van's floor, reporters turned their questions to Margaret. What would she serve for Bill's first meal in the apartment?

For heaven's sake! With all she had to worry about, she hadn't given any thought to what they'd *eat* there. She managed to say something about fixing Bill some German food, then added, with a smile, "Hopefully he'll feel like helping me. He's a better cook than I am!"

With Bill safely aboard, Margaret climbed in beside him. Mel hopped into the driver's seat and flipped every accessory switch he could find in order to give his dad a proper send-off, with sirens wailing and lights flashing. Louisville police stopped traffic and escorted the van across the street. A camera pool stationed on the hospital roof filmed the procession.

As they neared their new home, Margaret pointed out to Bill all the people who had come out to greet him. Neighbors stood in their front yards waving, and some local kids held a large, hand-lettered sign which read: WELCOME, MR. AND MRS. BILL SCHROEDER. More reporters were waiting in a roped-off area beside the ramp.

While the boys helped get Bill's wheelchair out of the van, some neighbor children gave Margaret a hand-picked bouquet of flowers. The rest of the family waited on the deck of the apartment as the grandkids jumped up and down, shouting, "Welcome home, Grandpa!" As Bill was wheeled up the ramp, the media pressed in close, asking how he liked his new home. Bill managed to answer, "Fine." Just before he was wheeled inside, Bill obliged the cameras with another wave.

The family then gave Bill a quick tour of the apartment. Lots of reporters were still hanging around outside waiting to catch a glimpse of Bill's first venture out of the apartment. No telling how long they'd camp there, so the family quickly decided that maybe if they gave the press a little more, they'd leave Bill and Margaret alone for a while. Bill was still doing well and, after all, it was a proud day. Besides, the Schroeders had really been touched by all the strangers who turned out to wish them well. So they wheeled Bill to the front door. As soon as the door opened, cameras and microphones on long poles appeared from nowhere. People cheered and shouted congratulations. Bill returned their waves and blew kisses.

After a couple of minutes, the boys brought Bill back inside and helped him into a firm chair with an adjustable footrest like a recliner. Sitting beside the TV, with his feet propped up and the Heimes pumping away on a nearby kitchen chair, Bill looked the way he had back home in Jasper, relaxing in his old La-Z-Boy. The apartment soon filled with the familiar sounds of the Mill Street house as family, spouses, spouses-to-be, and grandkids celebrated this historic move. In fact, it became so crowded that many went outside to sit on the front and back steps. Because the move had been widely publicized in the local media, drivers honked and waved as they went past. Hospital workers also stopped in to wish the Schroeders good luck and have a drink or sip some champagne, which Polly brought as a housewarming gift. They took turns sitting beside Bill, asking if they could bring him anything and how he liked his new home.

Each time, Bill replied, "Fine." It seemed incredible to them: He just looked so *natural* sitting there.

A couple of hours later, as the gathering began to thin out, Bill was tired and ready to rest. With one of his sons on either side, Bill slowly walked back to his bedroom. The family realized the hallway was barely wide enough for the three to walk through at the same time. When they reached the bedroom, they realized something else: The small room's layout would make it even trickier than in the hospital to help Bill in and out of bed. There was barely enough room to fit the Utah beside the bed. Next to the Utah sat the shoebox-sized monitor, which made shrill grinding noises whenever anyone made a printout. On the other side of the bed stood the feeding machine, a boxlike device on an IV pole, which regulated the nutritional supplements in the feeding tube and beeped loudly when the liquid ran low. Those machines had been scattered around the hospital room; now they were all squeezed alongside the bed.

The family helped Bill into bed, positioned the Utah alongside it, and set the Heimes on a chair near the foot of the bed. Technician Larry Hastings started up the Utah, then turned his back to Bill and crouched between the two drive systems. "Okay, Bill. Going to switch you back to the Utah now."

Larry pulled the drive tubes out of the whooshing Heimes and turned to plug them into the Utah. But as he tried to swivel between the machines, the drive lines got caught on the bedpost. Everyone lunged for the tubes. Larry quickly turned around and unsnagged them, then lifted them over the bedrail, and hurriedly plugged them into the Utah. It was unnerving to see Bill disconnected for that long, but his heart missed only a few beats, and he seemed okay.

The family were relieved that the move had gone so smoothly. Bill had made history again. Now if he and Margaret could build up their confidence about living away from the hospital, to become comfortable with all the machinery and work out the logistics of everyday life with an artificial heart, the next step would be to move back home.

By evening only Margaret, Bill, and a nurse remained at the apartment, along with Terry and Julie, who planned to stay overnight on the foldout couch. Suddenly Bill's condition changed again: His fever shot way up and he vomited. Until the early hours of the morning, Margaret and the nurse went through the familiar routine of changing the bed linens, and soothing his fevered skin with wet towels and rubbing alcohol. If this first night was any indication, their stay in the apartment was going to be long and stressful.

CHAPTER SEVENTEEN

Sunday, Apr. 7. Easter Sunday was a long, quiet, sad day for us. Had Communion here at the house. Bill slept most of the day. The kids all were at home.

Monday, Apr. 8. Was up at 4 A.M. helping with Bill. Such long days. Then taking him into the living room three times a day. Bill had fever off and on all day long. The generator malfunctioned and the alarm went off. A burned wire.

A number of problems with the apartment became obvious right away. First, as the medical team had promised, the apartment was much quieter than the hospital. However, the Schroeders were surprised to discover that without a constant hum of activity—staffers going in and out of the room, interruptions by the intercom, conversations out in the hall, the TV nearby—the noises from the artificial heart and drive system were more noticeable. Anyone who stood even a few feet beyond the end of the bed could clearly hear the Jarvik-7's ticking, and the small, boxy bedroom somehow seemed to amplify the whooshing of the Utah.

The relatively small size and layout of the rooms meant that when Margaret helped Bill move around, he had to take a couple of steps at a time, then let her reposition the big machine, or turn it around a corner, or maneuver it through some other tight space. The first floor of the Mill Street house was about the same size, so they realized they'd face the same problem if Bill went back home, which almost certainly meant that they would have to widen the doorways and perhaps knock out a wall or two.

The building's basement was packed with heavy machinery supplying the Utah's electricity and pressurized air—massive air compressors, control boxes, a maze of intake and outake pipes, and spare air tanks, all of which would take up at least half of the Schroeders' own basement. Next to the backyard deck, a generator about the size of six refrigerators was installed to take over in the event of a power failure. The whole system was linked to alarms to alert the heart institute of emergencies.

Humana had done an impressive job outfitting the apartment, but the machinery's very size and complexity caused new worries for the family. Would all *that* have to be done to the Mill Street house? Would the Schroeders have to add a special room to their home to accommodate everything? Who would pay for the installation? Here, maintenance and repairs would be taken care of by the heart institute and the company that installed the system, but who would be responsible in Jasper?

Then there was the problem of getting used to new nurses. The plan called for at least one registered nurse to be in the building at all times, visiting the apartment a few times each shift to chart Bill's progress and teach Margaret how to take vital signs, check the Utah's readouts, and administer medications. Initially, the nurses would be in the apartment around the clock, but as time went on, they would retire upstairs to a vacant apartment to give the Schroeders privacy, and let Margaret get used to looking after Bill, which she was eager to do.

That was the theory. In practice, Margaret not only had to learn to care for Bill with minimal assistance, but also keep house, buy groceries, do laundry, cook meals, and find some time for them just to enjoy being together. Margaret felt it would make more sense to have nursing aides who would help with some household duties, too, since she insisted on caring for Bill herself. But the medical team maintained the nurses should perform the duties for which they were trained.

Margaret also felt it wasn't fair that she couldn't choose which nurses were assigned to Bill. After all, if she and a nurse didn't get along, she couldn't just leave and go to her room—her room was right there. As in the hospital, some of the home-care nurses seemed more dedicated than others, and for various reasons, they were a somewhat transient group. It was upsetting for Bill to have so many strangers coming in to do things to him and his machine.

It became clear that at the apartment, there would be more work to be done and fewer people to do it. Because the hospital no longer supplied the couple's meals, Margaret began getting up at 6:30 each morning to start breakfast by the time the nurses looked in at the 7:00 A.M. shift change. Since breakfast was always Bill's best meal, she'd make enough to feed three, in hopes that he'd eat well. When the nurse came in, they'd get Bill cleaned up for the day. Occasionally, they'd try to give him a shower, but the bathroom was as small as the one in the hospital, so it was hard to manage without extra help. Margaret also tried to make sure that Bill always wore regular clothes instead of a hospital gown. It was tricky to get Bill up and dressed and have a hot breakfast ready for him at the same time.

The apartment might have been ideal for a patient and spouse both capable of maneuvering for themselves. But the stroke had changed everything; this was hardly what Bill and Margaret had envisioned in that first discussion with Dr. DeVries. It wasn't like the old days when Bill used to bound out of bed, wrapping his bathrobe around him as he padded into the kitchen to start breakfast, then sat back with the morning paper. Now just getting him on his feet and helping push the Utah from the bedroom to the kitchen took at least five minutes.

As time went on, the rest of his daily routine continued much the same as in the hospital. Dr. Mudd, the psychiatrist, often dropped by to have coffee with Margaret in the mornings and talk things over. The security guards who were stationed outside the door around the clock continued to check in several times per day, as did the heart technicians, who had lived upstairs during the first week. Lab technicians came regularly from the hospital to draw blood and take other tests. Bill was taken to the hospital three times a week for physical therapy, riding in the van or, if the weather was good, in the wheelchair. When Bill was hospitalized, staffers always used to drop by his room to say "Hi" as they began or ended their shifts. But now far fewer came to see him. Visits from DeVries and his associates also tapered off. Although the couple welcomed a little more privacy, Bill, who loved being around people, seemed disappointed that all the visits had ceased so abruptly.

Again, all the Schroeders could do was acknowledge that things hadn't turned out as they'd hoped. Unless Bill and Margaret proved they could make the apartment situation work, they'd never move back to Jasper. The most encouraging sign was that Bill was still trying hard. Whenever he felt okay, he resisted

279

help, and wanted to brush his hair or his teeth himself—but, even so, someone always had to hand items to him.

The apartment did offer a few advantages: Margaret was glad she could help give Bill his medicines, regulate the feeding machine, and read the computer's graphs that monitored heart activity. "Never thought I could learn to do all this stuff," she wrote. "I sleep some and keep one eye open to watch things."

The apartment was also more convenient for the kids. They could visit their parents in a more homelike atmosphere as they watched TV together or played cards. They could step into the kitchen and let Margaret rest while they fixed her a sandwich and made sure she ate it. During one visit, they fried up some fresh catfish they'd caught, so Bill could enjoy a taste he had missed for months now. On warm spring mornings, the kids would help haul the Utah out on the back porch so Bill could get some fresh air. They also slept over in the apartment on the foldout couch, although nurses still came through the living room several times throughout the night, carrying flashlights to check on Bill and make printouts from the noisy monitor beside his bed. The kids couldn't imagine how their parents endured such interruptions night after night.

When Mel and Terry visited the apartment the first weekend after the move, they found their mother worn out. So they told her to rest while they took Bill for a van ride. No place in particular, they told her. Of course, it never was as easy as just wheeling him out to the van and taking off. Arrangements and scheduling had to be made through the heart institute. The technician who usually went along on the van rides was Brent Mays. The Schroeders were grateful for this because he was providing his services during his off time.

That afternoon, they had no destination in mind. Bill just seemed happy to be out on the road again, sporting sunglasses and his beret from Dr. Jarvik. They wound up driving along the Ohio River. Brent suggested that they surprise Dr. Lansing, who lived nearby in a mansion overlooking the river. Lansing was indeed startled when he looked out his front door and saw Bill Schroeder in his wheelchair beside the large, horseshoe-shaped driveway. The doctor greeted them warmly, jokingly offered Bill a beer, and took him on a tour of the grounds. After about a half hour, the group said their good-byes and took off again.

On the way back, they decided to make another house call:

this time on DeVries. Bill stayed in the van while Mel went to the door and asked one of DeVries's kids to tell his dad that Bill Schroeder wanted to see him. Soon the doctor and some of his family came out of the house, all of them a little incredulous. By now Bill was tired, but he perked up at the sight of his surgeon. The group only stayed about ten minutes because they knew Margaret might be getting worried. Sure enough, as they pulled up to the ramp behind the apartment, she was standing on the deck, asking why it took more than two hours to go for a little van ride around Louisville and didn't they know it was time for Bill's medicines?

But all in all it had been a great afternoon. Bill had obviously enjoyed the ride, and the success fueled everyone's hopes that in a few more weeks, he might work up to a ninety-mile trip to Jasper.

CHAPTER EIGHTEEN

Meanwhile, artificial heart research was proceeding quietly in a few other medical centers. The week after Bill left the hospital, there was a dramatic burst of activity in the field, as if his move across the street had somehow broken through a barrier.

In Sweden, Dr. Bjarne K. H. Semb implanted a Jarvik-7 in a fifty-three-year-old man named Leif Stenberg. Doctors in Stockholm had prepared for the implantation with advice from the University of Utah and Symbion, and Dr. Jarvik himself flew there for the operation.

Back in Louisville, at Jewish Hospital—the institution that Dr. Lansing had left for Audubon—a sixteen-year-old boy with a human heart transplant was recuperating after being kept alive for a few days with a makeshift artificial heart fashioned from two "ventricular assist devices," or VADs. The experimental pumps, were being used increasingly to assist the lower chamber, or ventricle, of an ailing heart until the muscle had recovered enough to pump on its own. Using two VADs in tandem as a temporary artificial heart had been done only a couple of times before.

At Audubon, just one week after Bill was discharged, DeVries implanted yet another artificial heart, this time in a sixty-two-year-old Illinois man named Jack Burcham. However, just when such operations had begun to seem almost routine, this one became an ordeal. After DeVries removed Burcham's diseased heart—listening to Willie Nelson and the sound track from *The Big Chill*—he was shocked to find that the inner contour of the chest cavity left a space that was too small for the Jarvik heart. DeVries had to shave part of the breastbone, and because the Jarvik's chambers were joined only by Velcro, he was able to twist the heart to make it fit. However, the unexpected difficulty jolted the medical team, and again dramatized the trial-and-error nature of the whole program. Burcham not only required massive transfusions during the prolonged operation, but was returned to surgery the next day to stop the bleeding from the suture lines connecting the remnant of his heart and the Jarvik-7—a problem similar to the one that had sent Bill back for a second surgery.

In mid-April nurse Sandy Chandler arranged for Bill to visit a country club which had a small private lake where he might be able to go fishing. So on a windy Saturday afternoon, Margaret and some of the family loaded up the van with fishing tackle, and took Bill to the lake. Margaret pushed his wheelchair up along the shore as Mel and Terry baited a hook and cast the line for him. The fish weren't biting, but it didn't seem to matter; Bill was enjoying just taking in the scenery and feeling the breeze coming off the water. Terry threw out another line, hooked a fish, and brought the pole to his dad, just as Bill had done when teaching Terry to fish. Bill took the pole, felt a firm tug, and eagerly began reeling in his catch. He managed to bring out a small bass. It was by no means a trophy, but Bill looked delighted as he proudly lifted it for a snapshot.

The group stayed for another hour, desperately hoping that Bill could catch one of his own. But he got only a couple of nibbles, so the boys each hooked another bass and let their dad reel them in. Bill was tired by that time, so they took him back to the apartment. It hadn't been the same as fishing at the forty acres, or tossing bread in the pond to watch catfish swim up and snap for it, but Bill had loved every minute of that trip.

A few days later, Margaret had lunch with some members of Jack Burcham's family. Burcham was not doing well. Before he received the Jarvik-7, Burcham's kidneys had been deteriorating. He had continued to weaken from the stress of two surgeries, so DeVries put him on kidney dialysis.

Two nights later, Polly phoned Margaret with some sad news: Burcham had died, only ten days after his implant. With little warning, blood had begun to seep into his chest, gradually squeezing shut the left atrium, one of the two upper chambers of the natural heart that were connected to the Jarvik. Doctors told the media that the bleeding had probably been caused by the anticlotting drugs, coupled with the fact that he was on dialysis.

Mel, who happened to be staying overnight at the apartment, was watching TV with his dad the next morning when the story of Burcham's death was broadcast. Since no one had told Bill that Burcham had died, Mel was careful not to say anything, but he watched his father closely for a reaction. As Bill watched the report, a look of concern spread over his face. Then he shook his head, frowning, as if to say, "Oh, no."

By the next afternoon, when DeVries faced the reporters, many critics were calling for an end to the artificial heart program. The surgeon stood his ground, arguing that such setbacks were part of the experimental process. DeVries admitted that the artificial heart had probably cut short Burcham's life by days or weeks, but he emphasized that the experience had produced valuable scientific information that would help future patients. "There's no question that we can take care of patients now better, after four patients, than we could after one, after two, or three," he said, and added that he planned to implant another artificial heart as soon as he found a suitable patient.

It was a difficult time for everybody involved in the project. The FDA was scrutinizing DeVries's work more closely, forcing him to provide much more documentation of his results. He also faced growing criticism from the medical community and from ethicists. He often countered with the story of his mentor at the University of Utah, Dr. Willem Kolff, who invented the kidney-dialysis machine. Kolff had lost sixteen patients on the device before it started prolonging lives. Similarly, DeVries argued, many more artificial hearts must be tested in humans, and much more scientific information collected, before anyone could decide whether the invention was worthwhile. Maybe, he acknowledged, the artificial heart would indeed prove impractical or too expensive, but if the experiments were stopped, no one would ever find out. Even if the device itself didn't work, the data produced might lead to spinoff medical discoveries that would prove even more valuable.

As DeVries began to spend more time traveling to defend his work and advise new artificial heart programs, the Schroeders saw less and less of him. They wondered whether DeVries sometimes found it difficult to visit Bill now. After all, he was a surgeon used to operating-room heroics—not following someone through a difficult, long-term convalescence. Obviously, DeVries was proud that Bill had survived this long. However, his patient had exchanged one set of medical problems for another. The fact that Bill was suffering stroke complications had to be a constant reminder that, at least in part, the doctor had failed.

Toward the end of April, some of the kids took their dad for a ride to Bill Strode's house, about a half hour out into the country. They toured around a little among the rolling fields and looked at a lake, but Bill soon became tired and ready to go back. That Sunday night, after the kids had gone home, Margaret noticed something different about Bill. "I feel so lost and alone here," she wrote. "Bill is in serious trouble, I believe. He is very weak and tired."

Back home, Jasper's Strassenfest committee had just voted to honor the Schroeders at this August celebration of the town's German heritage. After all, during his TV interview, Bill had grandly invited the whole world to his "little town of Jasper" for Strassenfest. Even if Bill hadn't moved back to Jasper by then, everyone had high hopes that he could at least make a trip to ride in the town parade. Three committee members arranged with Margaret to visit Bill and present him with a certificate honoring the Schroeders as official host family for the fest.

But the day they were to come, Bill was doing poorly.

Wednesday, May 1. Bill got up late. He ate breakfast. He sat here and acted strange. He couldn't talk.

John [Lammers, the nurse] came and talked to me. He helped me get Bill up. Bill couldn't talk to me. He went back to sleep. When he woke up, he had a fever and couldn't use his one side. . . . Stan and Terri were here and Stan thought Bill wouldn't talk to him. I knew something was wrong.

I called up Kevan and she called Dr. Yared. [DeVries's associate] Dr. DeVries is out of town. . . . Cheryl, Terry, and Julie, came down, too. The doctors think that Bill had another stroke or seizure.

It was too late to call the Strassenfest committee to reschedule, and they arrived at the apartment decked out in full Bavarian costume with a photographer from the Jasper *Herald*. Margaret apologized and explained that Bill was too sick to see visitors. That kind of news was sure to travel all over town within hours, but they couldn't worry about it now.

No one was sure what was wrong this time. Margaret thought perhaps Bill should be readmitted to the hospital, but the doctors concluded that the best thing to do was to sit tight. If the problem was another "seizurelike episode," they knew that it would soon pass—even though no definitive explanation had ever been found for them. The doctors told Margaret that in their judgment, the results of several neurological tests so far didn't warrant a readmission to the hospital. They would keep a close eye on him, and give him more blood and wait to see if he perked up.

On Thursday, May 2, the family was still playing wait-and-see. Now they had an additional problem: Mel and Margaret had agreed to a live remote appearance on ABC's *Good Morning America*, to help promote the *Life* magazine article. Margaret hesitated to leave Bill, and Mel wondered how to explain his mother's absence. If the media suspected that Bill was too sick for her to leave him even for a few minutes, camera crews might stake out the apartment.

By the time the driver from ABC arrived to pick them up, Bill seemed stable, so Mel was able to persuade Margaret to go, provided that they come back immediately after the interview. They followed out of the apartment to find a plush, six-door limousine waiting for them. As they zipped along, bystanders peered through the tinted glass, trying to see who was inside. After all, many celebrities were in town for the Kentucky Derby, which would be run that weekend. The driver took them to the downtown convention center's underground garage, and stopped next to what looked like an abandoned trailer. The driver then directed Margaret and Mel inside the trailer. Junk was piled everywhere as if it had been dumped months earlier and left there. The TV crew greeted them and tacked a dark blue blanket on one wall and set two folding chairs in front. That was it. Mel and Margaret had to laugh. You get into a fancy limo and it drops you off at an abandoned trailer.

As they took their seats, the crew hid microphones in their clothing and gave them earpieces to hear interviewers' questions. This was going to be a new experience—twice as bad as facing a roomful of reporters—because they would have to sit there with the camera staring at them and act as if it was perfectly normal talking into thin air.

Once the interview got under way, it went quickly. Margaret and Mel hoped that their eyes and voices didn't betray their new worries about Bill, but there wasn't even a monitor—much less an interviewer's face—to look at. Margaret was asked to elaborate on her comments in *Life*, but there wasn't much more she could add. Mel described his dad's van rides.

The interview switched to another remote with Dr. Christiaan Barnard, the surgeon who performed the first successful human heart transplant. Barnard emphasized that human heart transplants were far superior to artificial hearts. The Schroeders didn't get a chance to respond. Had they been able to, they would have explained that when Bill was dying, he was ineligible for a transplant because of his diabetes and his age. Ironically, a few heart surgeons had recently expanded their criteria to include patients over fifty and even diabetics—another example of how heart surgery was advancing so quickly. Maybe if Bill's symptoms had developed just six months later, he could have received a human heart instead of an artificial one. But even if he wanted a human heart now, he would be disqualified because of his stroke and other complications. Such what-ifs were painful to consider. Those doors had also closed behind them forever.

CHAPTER NINETEEN

By Saturday, May 4, Bill was even more weak and lethargic. He hadn't spoken a word in four days, and fluid building up in his lungs made it increasingly hard for him to breathe. DeVries and Fox examined Bill at the apartment that morning, but still hesitated to transfer him back to the hospital unnecessarily. These kinds of symptoms had recurred from time to time, and again it might only be that he needed another transfusion.

DeVries gave Bill some blood through an IV in the jugular vein. Because Bill was receiving anticoagulants, the tiny wound continued to ooze blood for more than an hour after the transfusion was finished. Finally, DeVries had to close the wound with two stitches. The episode left Margaret exhausted with worry and fear.

The next day was no better. Bill had developed a cough, his chest congestion increased, and, for the first time in weeks, the nurses had to suction him. Now he found it harder to breathe, and the Utah's alarms were going off everytime he coughed. For much of the afternoon, Kevan hurried back and forth between the apartment and the hospital, checking on Bill and bringing more supplies. Margaret was so worried about him she was afraid to leave his side, even for a minute.

Rod, who had spent the night, also hesitated to leave, but he had to get to work the next day, and there wasn't much else he could do there. So Margaret faced another long, quiet Sunday evening. Bill was asleep almost all the time, and when he was awake his eyes had a distant look. He seemed more lethargic than ever, and she could see that his right arm and leg looked unusually weak.

On Monday Bill slept almost all morning. At least that meant he wouldn't cough and set the machine off or require being suctioned so often. DeVries examined him that morning; late that afternoon, Larry Hastings came to the apartment with the Heimes, saying that doctors had given orders for X rays and a CAT scan. An ambulance was waiting outside the apartment to take Bill over to the hospital.

An oxygen mask was put over Bill's face to help him breathe, while paramedics strapped him onto a stretcher. As Margaret followed the stretcher out the back door and onto the deck, she saw a TV camera crew bearing down on her husband. She couldn't believe it. How in the world had they found out? Bill looked so pale and helpless under that oxygen mask, so weary from struggling for breath, his eyes just staring. For a moment, all she could think of was footage of traffic accidents on the evening news, with TV crews competing for closeups.

After the long, exhausting weekend, Margaret felt some relief to be back in the hospital, where the doctors and staff could help shoulder the burden. Bill was wheeled directly to the X-ray department to film the action of the heart. In an adjacent room, Margaret watched a monitor as a technician pointed out the ghostly outline of the heart's synthetic parts, moving steadily, back and forth, against a background of blue. For a moment, she was completely fascinated by its valves, which looked like white circles as they floated silently, purposefully. It was such a wonder that those metal parts were really inside of her husband's chest, helping to keep him alive.

The heart seemed to be working correctly, which was a relief, since the alarms on the Utah had been sounding. Next Bill was placed in a CAT scanner, a huge, doughnut-shaped device that would take cross-section X rays of his body, slice by thin slice, like cutting a loaf of bread. While Margaret watched through a small window, Dr. DeVries and Dr. Fox studied a monitor as the machine scanned deeper and deeper into Bill's brain.

DeVries hurried out of the room and took Margaret aside. "Margaret, the news is bad," he said. "Bill's having a brain hemorrhage. He's bleeding inside his brain."

Margaret was too stunned to respond.

They weren't sure why or how long it had been bleeding, DeVries said. Maybe tiny blood vessels weakened by his diabetes had broken, or perhaps another clot had lodged in the brain and broken a vessel. In any case, they would have to discontinue the blood-thinners right away.

Margaret just looked at the doctor. She couldn't say a word.

DeVries told her that stopping the blood-thinners meant that Bill might develop more clots, which could cause another stroke, but at that moment the hemorrhage was an immediate threat to his life. If the bleeding continued even after the blood-thinners were stopped, her husband might need brain surgery.

Brain surgery! Never in a million years had she expected to hear something like that. Somehow she gave the response that had become automatic: "Well, do what you have to do for him."

As Bill was rushed to coronary intensive care, Margaret followed as far as the conference room, where DeVries joined her and tried to explain what had happened in more detail:

The hemorrhage was actually another type of stroke—and, what's more, the blood could further injure the brain if it wasn't reabsorbed into the tissues naturally or drained by surgery. Just as with the other stroke, it would be days or weeks before the doctors could assess the amount of brain damage. The bottom line was that they'd have to wait and see.

Margaret tried to take in all this information. Another type of stroke? Bleeding into his brain?

DeVries reminded her that Bill's first stroke had been embolic, meaning it was caused by clots, or emboli, that lodged in the brain. This new stroke was hemorrhagic. They might never know the cause of the bleeding, but the tiny pool of blood in the brain was causing similar effects—drowsiness, paralysis of his right side, inability to talk.

Nurses came to comfort Margaret and DeVries left to check on Bill. Everything seemed to happen now in slow motion; all their words were coming at her so slowly. This couldn't be happening. Just a month ago, many of these nurses had hugged her in an emotional good-bye, wishing her and Bill good luck on the next step of their journey. Now, as they embraced, some had tears in their eyes again.

Margaret was too stunned to cry, or maybe too scared. All she thought about was that she couldn't let herself fall apart now. Not when she had to give Bill whatever he needed. And the kids—her kids were going to be so upset about their dad. She couldn't fall apart while her family needed her . . . and all these people around her who had become like family. She couldn't lose control when she had to be strong for all of them.

After a while, Margaret glanced up and saw a familiar figure in the doorway. Dr. Salb knew he didn't have to say anything; he just came in and hugged her. Margaret could hold back no longer, and finally wept in the doctor's arms for several minutes. Then the two sat and talked for a long time. Salb assured her that if he knew Bill Schroeder at all, that man wasn't about to give up yet. But deep down, they both wondered how Bill could stand any more.

Margaret called home with the news and cautioned the kids not to rush down because there was nothing to do but wait. Terry and Julie soon arrived anyway, having planned to visit Audubon after work that evening. Bill was asleep when they went in to see him. Since Jasper was on Central time and Louisville was on Eastern time, visiting hours were nearly over when Terry and Julie reached the hospital. When the nurse informed them that it was time to leave, Terry was furious. He hadn't driven all that way just to spend a few minutes with his dad, even if it only meant sitting by his bed. Terry argued with the nurse, and angrily called DeVries at home to complain. DeVries gave orders to let Terry visit an extra half hour.

The next morning, the staff met with Margaret to inform her that unlike Bill's previous hospital stay, the Schroeders' visiting hours would now be restricted in accordance with regular policy. Bill needed his rest, they said, and the family's comings and goings would interfere with nursing care. But the Schroeders had been at Audubon so long that the hospital felt like a second home, and it was hard for them to accept the restrictions, especially after the medical team had regularly bent rules for them in the past.

CHAPTER TWENTY

The big wait began. Bill was sleeping almost around the clock now. Margaret was allowed to go into his intensive-care room for only a few minutes at a time throughout the day. She wasn't sure whether he recognized her. She sat by his bed, holding his hand, just wishing she could give him some of her own life to help him through this. Bill had been trying so hard in the apartment; now he lay helpless again. This was probably the toughest part of all. It was as if Bill kept on climbing along a slippery trail, only to have something knock him back down again as soon as he neared the top. It just wasn't fair, she kept thinking.

The Schroeder kids had already taken off so much time from work that they couldn't afford to take much more. But Moni came in for a few days, and the rest visited that week in the evenings. They'd sit close to their dad, take his hand, gently tell him who they were, urge him to hang in there and keep fighting. They'd ask him if he knew them, and encourage him to squeeze their hands, but Bill didn't respond at all. The few times that he did open his eyes and look at them, they'd strain to see a hint of recognition.

Whenever they left his room, they'd ask themselves and each other if maybe Dad had tried to respond but just couldn't. Or maybe he didn't understand what they were asking, or all the medications had him too doped up. They would all read for themselves what—if anything—their father was trying to say with his eyes. But the cold truth was that they just didn't know. They wondered if maybe this really was the end. Maybe Dad was finally ready to give up. Nobody could say he hadn't fought long and hard enough.

There wasn't much to do for him then, so they concentrated on getting Margaret out of the hospital, even if for just a couple of hours to eat or go shopping. She looked so tired and

preoccupied, and the family knew that she couldn't hold up forever under this kind of stress. She insisted on taking a beeper
with her and only an hour or two would pass before she'd ask to
go back to Audubon.

Once again, Bill endured test after test—all the usual
blood work, plus an arteriogram, in which his blood was tagged
with radioactive dye so its path could be traced on X-ray film.
The doctors still weren't sure whether he would need brain surgery. A CAT scan later that week suggested that the bleeding had
stopped, but the prognosis would be uncertain for several days.
DeVries held off briefing the media until he could give some more
definite answers.

That Sunday Mel appeared on a live remote for *This Week
with David Brinkley*, along with Dr. Lansing. Mel was asked the
old question about whether, in hindsight, Bill would do it all
again. People still didn't understand that without the artificial
heart, Bill had faced certain death. Mel compared this question to
that of the ballplayer who contends that if he'd known he was
going to be thrown out at second base, he wouldn't have tried to
steal it. The Schroeders felt that future artificial heart candidates
would have to make their own choices based on the experiences
of Bill and others.

The next day in the hospital briefing room, DeVries and
Fox told the press that Bill's prognosis was extremely guarded.
Reporters repeatedly asked DeVries whether he and the family
had discussed turning off Bill's artificial heart. The doctor insisted that they were nowhere near that stage, but the media kept
pressing for details: Who would make the decision, who would
turn the key off, where the key was kept. DeVries tried to deflect
such questions, but the reporters wouldn't let up. Flustered, De-
Vries finally answered: "He's still a living, responding, injured
organism that still has recoverable ability. . . . I think it would
be very unfair to him to start that dialogue at this time, because
we just don't know where he's going."

Nine days after Bill's second stroke, the doctors were convinced that the hemorrhage had completely stopped. This was
good news, but the family couldn't see any outward signs of improvement. Bill was still sleeping almost all the time. When the
nurses had to suction him, he didn't resist—and that just wasn't
like Bill at all.

DeVries joined the kids in urging Margaret to get away for

a few days. She was exhausted from trying to care for him in the apartment, and this new stress was bound to catch up with her sooner or later. Bill was stable, DeVries assured her, and improvements in his condition would be easier for her to see after she'd been away for a while.

Margaret knew she felt run down, and that she should probably have a checkup with Dr. Salb, since it had been about six months since her last one. And there was an additional incentive to go home: Stan and Terri's baby was due any day now. Margaret was eager to bring back to Bill a firsthand description of the new grandson or granddaughter, so she agreed to let some of the kids drive her back to Jasper.

Back home, Terri was admitted to the hospital that afternoon, so Margaret stayed in Jasper an extra day, hoping to see the baby. In the meantime, Dr. Salb adjusted her medications because her blood pressure was low. She waited around all day for the baby to be born, but it turned out to be a false alarm, so a couple of the kids drove her back to Louisville that night.

CHAPTER TWENTY-ONE

The next morning, Stan called Margaret at the apartment, and she immediately hurried over to see Bill. She rushed into his room and without even bothering to remove her jacket or set down her purse, she squeezed past the Utah, grabbed Bill's hand, and planted a big kiss on his cheek.

"Hi, sweetie! Guess what?"

Bill opened his eyes.

"You're a grandpa again! Terri and Stan had that little one, honey! It's a baby boy, and they named him after you! Lukas *William*. What do you think of that?"

Bill seemed to be listening intently, but she couldn't be positive that he understood. Later that day, she walked down to the hospital gift shop to buy some "It's A Boy!" cigars, and gave them to everyone who came into Bill's room, telling each of them about little Lukas William, and making sure that Bill heard every word.

The next morning, Bill appeared more alert. For the first time since his second stroke, Margaret felt sure that he recognized her. Terry visited that evening, and Bill seemed to know him, too. There was something different in Bill's eyes, a look of understanding that hadn't been there before. Terry brought a snapshot of little Lukas, and Margaret taped it to the Utah so Bill could see it whenever she reminded him of his grandson.

Margaret had to see that baby, so Terry took her to Jasper that night. As she held Lukas for the first time, Margaret tried to remember every little detail to tell Bill. Lukas definitely looked like a Schroeder, with his grandfather's dark eyes and definitive eyebrows. She was thrilled to see the baby, and felt a little more at ease during this visit than she had on others because Bill was sleeping so much that there wasn't much she could do for him. She even let herself relax enough that night to play Bingo with

297

Terry and Julie at a local community center where she and Bill had been regulars, always arriving early to stake out a table and staying until the last number was called. Throughout the evening, friends, acquaintances, and strangers came over to ask Margaret about Bill. Margaret quickly learned to fall back on the family's standard answer: "He's doing as well as we can expect."

When she called Audubon early the next morning, she was shocked to learn that Bill had already been moved out of intensive care and back to his old room. She couldn't imagine why they would move him out so soon. She had wanted to be there to help Bill through that transition, but she felt powerless to do anything, because she couldn't get back to the hospital until that night.

As usual, friends and family called the house throughout her visit to check on her, so she didn't think twice when the phone rang around lunchtime.

"Margaret, this is Gary Rhine at the hospital. Apparently Bill had another seizure, and the doctors need your approval to run a CAT scan." Gary told her that Bill was resting comfortably, and the scan should give them more information.

She told him to go ahead and do what had to be done, and to tell Bill she'd be there as soon as she could. Dazed, Margaret hung up the phone and paced through the empty house. Maybe they shouldn't have moved Bill so soon. The nurses were watching him twenty-four hours a day, but she still couldn't stand the thought of his going through all this without some family there. Now, of course, she blamed herself for taking it easy. She *knew* she shouldn't have left him, and it would be hours now before any of the kids could get off work and take her back. She sat down in Bill's old easy chair, buried her face in her hands, and began to cry.

Minutes later, Mel and Cheryl came by for lunch and found their mother weeping. Tearfully she explained the situation, and they both decided to take off work early to drive her back to Louisville. When she got back to the hospital, Bill instantly recognized Margaret and his two kids, and was so glad to see them that he started crying. Apparently the seizure had had no lasting effects.

But the episode had further strained relations between the Schroeders and the hospital staff. With all the complications that had occurred, the family were frustrated and angry that Bill had been moved so soon after the hemorrhage. The staff, in turn, complained that the family's visits were making Bill too agitated. Another meeting with the medical team was held, at which the Schroeders complained that if Bill was going to be on the regular cardiovascular floor instead of in intensive care, their visiting hours had to be more flexible. The Schroeders knew they were guilty of pushing the limits, of having large numbers of people in Bill's room, of staying past regular hours—and they were well aware that they weren't exactly the quietest family around. But they agreed to play by the rules. Margaret settled into a routine of staying overnight at the apartment and coming to Bill's room around 9:00 A.M. to spend the day at his side until about 9:00 P.M.

During her spare time between visits, she began to see more of Murray Haydon's wife, Juanita, and the other wives of patients there for human heart transplants. Juanita had moved from her Louisville home into the apartment across the hall from Margaret's, and they checked in with each other at the beginning of each day, often walking over to the hospital together. At night a security guard would walk them back and check inside each apartment to make sure they were safe. There developed a small circle of implant and transplant wives that grew and diminished as ailing husbands were admitted and discharged. Many transplant recipients and their families stayed in touch, returning often to the hospital for checkups and to see the friends they'd made during their stay. Hardly a day passed that they didn't gather for lunch, a cup of coffee, or just a small chat in the hallway. On days when Bill was doing better, Margaret would listen to the other wives and console them, and if she or Bill had had a bad day, the others were there for her, too.

Amazingly, by late May Bill began to show a few signs of improvement. No one could believe it: Even after the massive stroke in December, and the second one caused by a brain hemorrhage, plus all the other complications, Bill wasn't about to give up. He was determined to climb back into the ring and keep punching. He could move all his extremities now, and could squeeze family members' hands when they asked him to. It had been almost three weeks since he'd spoken, but the family sensed that Bill understood what they told him because of the attentive expression

299

in his eyes and the fact that he even grinned occasionally when they kidded him.

One smile came when they teased Bill about a remedy a nurse had devised for him to correct a condition called "drop foot." As the muscles around Bill's ankles grew weak from disuse, his feet began to droop to the side. One of the nurses suggested that he wear oversize high-top basketball shoes to support his ankles. Margaret bought him some right away, following the nurse's advice to choose size 12s, so they'd slip on and off easily. The Schroeders knew that if Bill could talk, he'd be the first to crack a joke about how funny he looked lying there in a hospital gown with an artificial heart, wearing big white shoes that made him look like Mickey Mouse. When they teased him about this, Bill grinned a little. He'd begun to smile again, and right then that was enough to hang on to.

On Memorial Day Terry brought Margaret home for a cookout with the kids. They spent the afternoon relaxing at a friend's cabin on Beaver Lake, just around the bend from the cinder-block cabin that Bill and the boys had built one summer. That evening, Mel drove Margaret back to the hospital.

They were astonished to find that Bill looked so much better that he even seemed to want to get out of bed. Margaret and the nurse pushed the chair up beside the bed, and Mel lifted his dad and gently swung him onto the seat, making sure that Bill didn't try to stand. Even that small accomplishment was a giant step, and Bill enjoyed sitting up after a month lying in bed. He stayed in the chair for about thirty minutes and seemed to tolerate it well. It was even more encouraging to see that Bill was determined to get out of bed instead of giving up.

Margaret spread the good news the next morning, and staffers began getting Bill out of bed on a regular basis. Actually, a person confined to bed for a long time shouldn't just get up all of a sudden because the blood flow to the brain is temporarily reduced, causing dizziness and headaches, and the weakened legs tend to buckle. The proper method is to strap him to a horizontal tilt table, then move one end up slowly, over several sessions, increasing the angle and duration until the person is able to stand on his own. They tried putting Bill on the tilt table during the next few days, and soon he was able to stand with the board's support. When she saw Bill standing for the first time in weeks, Margaret realized just how thin he had become. He was

300

down to 160 pounds, which he probably hadn't weighed since high school. His weight on admission to Audubon had been unusually high due to fluid buildup, but it was still striking to realize that since November, Bill had lost some eighty-seven pounds.

By early June Bill began to bounce back so dramatically that even the doctors were at a loss to explain it. But the Schroeders were sure of one thing: His amazing recovery took off immediately after Bill achieved another cherished goal—seeing that new grandson.

Stan and Terri had decided that the only place to christen little Lukas William was in Bill's hospital room. On June 2 they came to Audubon along with several family members, including Terri's parents, grandparents, and a brother and sister; Mel, Patti, and their girls; Terry and Julie; and Rod and his girl friend, Lori. They were joined by Polly, Kevan, Dr. Lansing and his wife, and, although the Schroeders hadn't seen much of Dr. De-Vries lately, he and his wife also came.

Everyone gathered around Bill's bed as Terri held Lukas, and Father Rusty, who had continued to look in on Margaret and Bill almost daily, performed the sacrament. Bill lay propped up, watching as the priest said a prayer and began the Catholic baptism. Rod was named the baby's godfather, and Terri's sister was named godmother.

After the ceremony, Margaret wanted Bill to hold the baby, so she had Bill crook his arm on his pillow. Bill was tired now, so he kept his eyes closed as Stan gingerly set little Lukas beside him.

"Dad," Stan said. "Here's your grandson. We named him Lukas William, after you. He looks like you, too, doesn't he, Dad?"

Bill kept his eyes closed. "Now look, honey," Margaret said, "they've come all this way. You'd better look there and see what you've got!"

Bill opened his eyes and stared at the tiny person next to him. Stan watched closely for his father's reaction, but wasn't sure whether Bill knew who this was or not. Lukas began to cry and Bill looked at Margaret as if to say, "What in the world is *this?*"

Margaret picked Lukas up and soothed him. Afterward, Bill's eyes followed that baby all around the room. Margaret was convinced that Bill had caught on to what was happening, and since she had always understood him better than anybody, the others gave him the benefit of the doubt. After the christening, the families went over to the apartment, where members of the hospital staff joined them. This occasion was not only important for the family, but for the medical team as well, confirming that what it was doing was worthwhile.

Three days later, Bill was placed on the tilt table for a fifteen-minute session. As Margaret watched, the nurse asked Bill how he was doing and, as usual, searched his eyes for an answer.

"Okay," Bill said distinctly.

Margaret and the nurse hardly dared to look at each other. Finally, the nurse asked, "Did he say what I think he said?"

Margaret hurried over to hug and kiss her wonderful husband. It had been more than a month since she had heard his voice. If he could say "Okay" today, who knew what he could say tomorrow, next week, next month? As a matter of fact, the whole day turned out to go *extremely* well for him. Word flew along the hospital corridors and, as usual, staffers from all over came to see for themselves—doctors, nurses, administrators, technicians, security, PR officials, dietary, the cleaning crew, and anyone else who'd met Bill during his first stay at Audubon. Bill greeted each of them with a wave, and when Gary Rhine, the social worker, told him good-bye on his way out the door, Bill responded with a very clear "good-bye!"

The rest of that week, Bill's room was full of laughter and smiles. He began to talk in short, understandable sentences. He could maneuver in and out of bed with more ease, and was much more aware of his family and his surroundings. Maybe that grandson had been just the right medicine after all. Dr. Fox repeatedly examined Bill, shaking his head in amazement. Margaret pressed the neurologist to explain why Bill was suddenly doing so well, but Fox would shrug, point toward the ceiling, and say, "Don't ask me—ask Him up there. I've never seen anything like it before!"

Bill began to sit up in the chair a few times a day. Whenever he was returned to his bed, the nurses would first spread out a sheet on top of the regular sheets and use it to scoot Bill to the center of the mattress. One morning, as a couple of staffers helped Bill back into bed, a male nurse who had difficulty getting enough of the sheet to grasp, muttered, "I'm having a hard time getting any," then added jokingly, "Oh, well, that's the story of my life." Bill burst out laughing, which in turn set the staff laughing. *That* was the Bill Schroeder they all knew and loved.

Ever since Bill had moved to a regular room, the home-care nurses had cared for him twenty-four hours a day. One of them, Mrs. Fish, was a stickler for cleanliness, and never felt that her shift was complete unless she had given Bill several sponge baths. Bill never complained, but he wasn't crazy about the scrub-downs either. That week, Mrs. Fish told Margaret that she planned to increase her weekly workload from three shifts to five. Bill overheard them, and exclaimed: "Ohhhh, *mercy!*"

Whenever Margaret walked into the room, Bill's eyes would sparkle and he'd reach for her and kiss her. He was swallowing better, eating solid foods again, and rarely required suctioning. The whole medical team was excited.

A few days later, when Stan and Terri brought Lukas to visit, Bill was strong enough to cradle the baby on a pillow in his lap. They put Bill in the wheelchair, gave Lukas to him, and the group traveled the hospital corridors as Bill made sure everyone admired his grandson. Bill seemed to love the grandkids' visits most of all. The younger grandchildren would climb into his lap, just as they used to when he babysat for them, and the older ones would tell him all the things they were doing now that school was out.

But increasingly the kids' visits gave him mixed feelings, because they meant that Margaret might ride home with one of them for a few hours. Margaret informed Bill whenever she was about to go home, and carefully assured him that she'd be back soon, but sometimes he became very upset, unable to understand why he couldn't go along. When she returned to his room—usually the next day—sometimes he'd turn his head away as if he were angry. But after a few minutes, he'd turn back, grab her hand and hold it close to him, and say tearfully, "I *missed* you."

By mid-June there was more good news about Bill's condition: CAT scans revealed that the blood clot from the hemorrhage had almost completely dissolved. The everyday pace picked up again, Bill had to start all over with the physical therapy, occupational and speech therapy routines. That would never be easy, but Bill seemed to manage even better than he had after the first stroke. The Schroeders were also more accustomed to the therapists and their methods now, and hospital staffers, in turn, understood better how to interact with the family. The argument about Terry's wedding was now in the past, and, with Bill doing much better, everyone was looking toward the future. Maybe he would get well enough to make a trip back home after all. And what better time than the first weekend in August, during Jasper's Strassenfest? Of course, the family knew not to count on anything, but Strassenfest gave them all, including Bill, a goal to strive for.

During this time, the media and the general public were largely unaware of how much Bill had improved. Ever since De-Vries announced the cutback on information about his patients, most news about Bill and Murray Haydon came from brief, weekly updates on a telephone recording line set up by the hospital. Haydon had remained in intensive care ever since his second operation, intermittently using a respirator because of breathing complications. In early June Haydon suffered a minor, transient stroke that briefly left him partially paralyzed. Many news organizations, especially those that focused on the more sensational aspects, seemed to lose interest—maybe because there were no longer colorful quotes or dramatic events to report but only day-to-day, tedious problems.

In June Margaret agreed to do a couple of interviews. At the hospital she taped a segment for a show called *Beyond 2000*, an Australian version of *60 Minutes*. Margaret also accepted an invitation to appear live on Oprah Winfrey's morning talk show in Chicago—but there was a very special reason for her decision. The program would include all four wives of the men in whom DeVries had implanted artificial hearts: Margaret, Juanita Haydon, Jinx Burcham, and Una Loy Clark. Mrs. Clark had continued to send Margaret warm, newsy letters of encouragement, assuring her that she didn't expect any letters back because she knew from her own experience that all of Margaret's energies would be focused on Bill. Mrs. Clark, a devout Mormon, had endured two years of a special sort of loneliness as the wife, and then widow, of the only man in the world with a permanent artificial heart. Margaret had experienced a similar loneliness, and jumped at this opportunity to meet her.

In late June Margaret flew to Chicago with Juanita Haydon and Donna Hazle from PR. They were whisked by limo to a hotel where Mrs. Burcham and Mrs. Clark had already checked in.

When they stopped by Mrs. Clark's room, Margaret immediately recognized the prim, grandmotherly woman with thin-rimmed spectacles. Mrs. Clark recognized her, too, and there was no need for words. The two simply embraced, and when they pulled away, each was in tears.

All the women talked and cried and laughed together until late that evening. The next morning on the live show, they answered questions from Oprah Winfrey, the studio audience, and viewers who phoned in. Margaret told the audience that she didn't mind the media for the most part. "I think that a part of our lives belongs to you people out there, because you're behind us one hundred percent." She bristled at a question whether Bill had become just an experimental subject. "He's not a guinea pig, in no means," she said. "He's still my husband."

When Margaret returned to Louisville, she learned that Bill was doing so well that he'd just returned from a van ride with Mel, Patti, and the girls. They'd taken off with Brent Mays that afternoon, not sure where they would be going. Mel drove downtown, and when they neared a bridge spanning the Ohio River, he decided to keep on driving across, right into Indiana, returning Bill for the first time to his home state.

Afterward, Bill seemed not only worn out, but a little lonely and depressed until Margaret came in, bubbling with excitement from her trip and, most of all, from meeting Mrs. Clark. Bill was so glad to see her that after the rest of the family left, he kept patting the mattress and motioning for her to climb into bed with him.

"Bill," Margaret said, "I can't get in *bed* with you! Not here!"

Bill looked perturbed. "Why NOT?" he asked again and again.

He was so insistent that Margaret finally asked herself the same question. She couldn't think of a good answer, so she moved his IV lines aside, climbed in next to him on the side farthest from the whooshing Utah, and hugged him close. Bill was soon fast alseep, so she got up and went to the apartment for the night. After that, she was no longer embarrassed about crawling into bed with Bill in the hospital. It just seemed like the natural thing to do.

A few days later, Dr. DeVries started Bill again on regular doses of heparin, a blood-thinner. Bill had gone a long time without blood-thinning drugs—ever since the brain hemorrhage—but DeVries knew that if they hesitated much longer to start the anticoagulants, Bill would almost certainly have another stroke. Again, the doctors would continue to experiment with Bill's drug regimen as they struggled to find the delicate balance between too much anticoagulation and too little. When they gave him too much, he developed nosebleeds, seemed especially tired, and bled longer than normal after blood was drawn from him. The doctors would believe they had it regulated, then Bill would develop bruises and prolonged nosebleeds, and they'd have to cut back on the anticoagulants.

Because the heparin had to be given intravenously on a regular basis, DeVries began using a subclavian catheter, a thin, flexible tube that was inserted through a four-inch needle into a vein beneath the collarbone. This procedure was painful and frightening; the doctor had to wear a surgical mask and gloves, and push the needle carefully through the skin, into the artery, then insert the catheter and stitch it into place. Medication could be administered and blood could be drawn through the tube, thus avoiding having to stick Bill daily. But to prevent infection, the subclavian had to be changed every three weeks.

Bill continued to get out of bed each day. He still had occasional fevers, though not as bad as the ones in February. The doctors still didn't know their cause, but all along tests had been showing that Bill's blood was being infected intermittently, possibly as a result of all the needles used for IVs. Doctors tried using a variety of antibiotics to battle the infections. Bill was also given tests that showed he had a slight liver infection.

But overall Bill apparently was doing well. He'd begun walking again, and seemed to welcome getting out of his room and being among people again. Many other patients on the cardiovascular floor also looked forward to his walks and would line the hallways to watch his efforts.

One of those patients made a special effort to speak with Margaret in the cafeteria just before his discharge from the hospital. He asked her to give Bill a message from him and several other patients: "Every day I was in here," the man said, "I knew about what time Bill would be going for his walk, so I'd get up and stand by the doorway to watch. As he walked past me, I would just think to myself, 'What a courageous man. What a gift of courage for all mankind!' I just wanted you to know I have the greatest admiration for you both." Margaret was so surprised, she didn't catch his name. But if anyone had set out to boost Margaret's spirits and make her feel that people hadn't stopped caring about Bill, no one could have done a better job than that man.

CHAPTER TWENTY-TWO

Bill steadily regained his strength. With each day that passed, the family let themselves hope a little bit more that Bill might really be well enough to attend Strassenfest. By now he was riding in the van about once a week, and his stamina had increased so dramatically that he could tolerate forty-five-minute excursions. So on July 6, Mel, Patti, the girls, and Margaret decided to see if he could go farther. This time they would take a trip to Brent Mays's Indiana farm, about a forty-five-minute drive each way.

The family and Brent loaded Bill in the van, then climbed in along with a nurse. As they left the parking lot, the whole group was figuring: *Let's see, a ninety-minute round trip . . . you could probably make it to Jasper in an hour and forty-five . . . so if Dad can make this trip, he should be able to handle a trip home . . .*

Brent lived on a large, rolling farm with his wife, Michelle, who was a coronary-care nurse who also happened to be Dr. Lansing's daughter. When the van pulled into the driveway, Michelle was outside watering down one of their horses. Bill had loved horses since his boyhood summers on his grandparents' farm a few miles outside of Jasper. The family got him out of the van, and, as the grandchildren petted the horse, Bill rubbed the animal's nose. It was a windy day, but the sun was shining brightly and all the rich greenness of summer must have brought back memories of the forty acres. But the long, winding drive had made Bill tired, so they loaded him back into the van, and returned to the hospital. By then Bill was exhausted, and slept the rest of the day. However, they had been out on the road for ninety minutes—Bill's longest ride yet.

The next day Brent was reprimanded by his superiors for not taking more precautions for such a lengthy ride. The heart institute laid down the law: From now on the Louisville police were to be informed any time Bill was to ride farther than five miles from the hospital. That seemed a little much to the family; for one thing, every news organization monitored police scanners, and the Schroeders could visualize the caravan of reporters and photographers that would follow them whenever they got out on the road. Some hospital staff also worried that if Bill was seen near a public place he would be mobbed. Actually, every person who had ever come up to meet Bill—during his wheelchair rides through the hospital or crossing the street outside the apartment—was polite and friendly. So the family agreed that they'd learned their lesson: From now on, if asked, they'd just tell the heart institute they weren't going farther than five miles away.

The kids began taking Bill for rides every weekend, and he became increasingly eager to get out of the hospital. Weekend rides were no problem, but weekdays, Bill was on a tight schedule of rehabilitation and testing, and he had to be at the hospital to take his medicine at prescribed times. The family were always searching for someplace special to take him. Jim Smith, one of the security guards who looked in on Bill, mentioned that he had a relative who worked for the Louisville Redbirds baseball team, a minor-league club that had been drawing record crowds that summer. Maybe they could take Bill to a game. Dr. DeVries was all for the trip, provided that Bill really wanted to go and that somehow they could keep him out of the bleachers and away from the crowd. When the family asked Bill if he wanted to go to a ball game, he answered with a definite "Surrrre!"—and that was all the encouragement they needed.

Everyone knew the outing would be tricky. It would be the first occasion Bill would be near a crowd for any length of time. They'd have to take him in the van and let him watch the game from his wheelchair. Jim Smith found out that the Redbirds would be willing to set up a portable fence at the end of the third-base line, so that Bill could sit in his wheelchair on playing-field level. The wall around the base of the bleachers would keep away the overly curious. It just might work.

The Redbirds were to play a doubleheader against the Oklahoma City 89ers on July 19. All four Schroeder boys took off from work that day and went to Louisville. When they arrived, Bill was ready to go. Margaret and the nurse had helped him dress in one of his Jarvik-7 T-shirts, sweat pants, and a Redbirds cap. He was waiting just as eagerly as he used to on the front porch when they planned to take him fishing. The Schroeders had insisted that this trip be kept hush-hush: just a night out with Dad and the boys, as close to normal as possible. None of them wanted to have to pass through a corridor of reporters and photographers on the way to or from the game. The PR staff reluctantly agreed not to announce the trip, although they did arrange a police escort.

Bill was talking up a storm as the four boys, Brent, and nurse John Lammers wheeled him into the van and piled in themselves. A police car led the way, followed by a car containing Jim Smith and and the captain of security Tom Biondolillo; then came the van and another police car in back. The drive took just a few minutes, and when the procession reached the stadium gate, a waiting security vehicle pulled in front to lead the way.

The game was just getting started. After the first inning, they got Bill out of the van and pushed him through a gate that led to the playing field. The portable fence enclosed an area bounded by the wall at the base of the bleachers and the left-field wall. The rows of seats just above the area had also been roped off because the assigned space wasn't large enough to accommodate them all. At first, the group didn't attract much attention.

The Schroeder boys took turns sitting beside Bill and pointing out the sights. Being on ground level at the end of the left-field foul line made it hard to see all the action, but Bill looked happy just to be in the ball park, to hear the crack of the bat and the roar of the crowd.

An early-evening ball game in the middle of summer! How could he not love it? Bill used to coach his kids' teams, looking like a small mountain as he crouched along the third-base line, hands on his knees, yelling instructions. From time to time, he'd also umpired. When Terry pitched for Jasper High, Bill had faithfully attended every game, and when Terry played at his junior college in Illinois, Bill had even traveled to out-of-town games. Whenever Terry received a game ball for hitting a homer, Bill would inscribe it with the date, the inning, the score, and the count, and toss it gruffly to his son as soon as he came home for supper.

When Rod went off to find a rest room, he overheard a radio broadcast of the game, just as the announcer mentioned that Bill Schroeder was attending. So this wasn't going to be different after all. Rod came back and told his brothers that the word was out. Sure enough, as the game progressed, news crews showed up and started photographing Bill through the gate and from the bleachers. The boys took turns being interviewed in the stands to keep the media away from their dad.

The Redbirds' owner, A. Ray Smith, came down to the field to say hello. Bill shook hands and said clearly, "Thank you for having me here." They had a brief chat, and Smith gave Bill a sackful of Redbirds souvenirs, including another cap, a baseball, a beachball and towel, and a warm-up jacket. Smith invited the boys upstairs to the clubhouse. Never ones to pass up a free drink, the boys took turns watching an inning or two from the plush accommodations.

Between innings, the third-base ump came up to shake Bill's hand and wish him the best. Some of the players also jogged over to say "Hi," including one of Terry's former team-mates who now played for the Redbirds. Terry reminded his father that they'd played together at Southern Illinois. It was hard to tell whether Bill recognized him, but he smiled broadly as he shook the player's hand and looked at him carefully in an effort to recall. Throughout the game, park and team officials came over to meet Bill, which of course he really enjoyed. Spectators kept a respectful distance, although someone seated nearby yelled, "Hang in there, Bill! We're all proud of you!" Bill answered with a wave and a grin.

The Redbirds won, 3 to 2. There was still one more game to go, but the boys had agreed that nine innings would be enough for Dad. Now that word of Bill's visit was all over the radio and the TV crews had called even more attention to him, some of-ficials asked if the stadium announcer could formally recognize Bill's presence. The boys agreed to wheel Bill briefly into the outfield to face the crowd, and maybe he'd give them a wave.

The announcer then asked for everyone's attention, and the noise of the crowd died down as the four boys wheeled their father out onto the grassy field.

"Ladies and gentlemen," the loudspeaker droned, "we'd like to inform you that our attendance tonight is 15,957—plus one very special guest. May I draw your attention to left field, where we are honored to have with us a very brave person: none other than artificial heart patient *Bill Schroeder*."

The boys had expected polite applause, maybe even some

cheers. Instead, the entire crowd immediately rose to its feet and gave him a long, deafening ovation.

It caught them all off guard. Terry leaned over and whispered, "Look at everyone, Dad! They're all standing!" All these people, standing up for Bill and cheering him on—it was unbelievable. The boys had to swallow hard. Even Bill seemed surprised, but after a moment, he began blowing kisses to the crowd, as if he'd hit a grand slam in the bottom of the ninth.

Brent was frantically motioning from the sidelines, saying over and over, "Let's get OUT of here!" He was afraid that things might get out of hand. So the boys wheeled their father off the field and loaded him back into the van. By the time they returned to the hospital, Bill was exhausted but happy, and proudly showed off each of his souvenirs to Margaret.

CHAPTER TWENTY-THREE

BILL's surprising recovery peaked and leveled off. There were days when he simply didn't feel well and resisted getting out of bed. Sometimes he would get depressed and begin crying for no apparent reason. The fevers still came and went unpredictably. Blood infections were an ongoing problem. And he continued to endure test after test. But overall, at this point, the days when Bill felt relatively good outnumbered those when he felt bad.

In late July Dr. Salb dropped by for a visit. Some of the kids were there, too, and Margaret suggested that they all wheel Bill over to the apartment, which he hadn't seen since his first stay there. The trip took about ten minutes, and the apartment's air conditioner provided welcome relief from the muggy summer heat. Margaret fixed everyone a cool drink, then sat down to talk with Dr. Salb. Bill didn't seem pleased to be there, and wasn't saying much. About twenty minutes had passed when, out of the blue, Bill announced, "Let's get the hell *out* of here." No one knew whether something in the apartment had triggered that statement or whether Bill was simply tired. But he made it clear that he didn't want to be there, so they didn't stay much longer.

A few days later, Bill was eager for another van ride, so some of the family took him to a nearby park, where he sat with Margaret and watched their granddaughters show off on the playground equipment. Again, bystanders kept their distance, wondering aloud if that could really be Bill Schroeder, or politely asking the security guard if they could meet him. The fact that Bill did well on another public outing was especially encouraging, because now Strassenfest was just days away.

Back in Jasper, the kids were preparing for Bill's homecoming on the day of the Strassenfest parade. They knew there was no guarantee that Bill could make it. The decision wouldn't

315

be made until the day before, but everyone was getting ready on the assumption that he would be able to come. Stan, Terry, and Rod built a wheelchair ramp for the house. Cheryl rearranged furniture so Bill could maneuver indoors, and planted flowers in the front yard.

Since the Schroeders were to be honored as official host family, Margaret thought it would be nice for them to wear something to make them stand out. The family still wore their Jarvik-7 T-shirts from time to time, so she decided to have a new set made. She knew that Bill would want them to be black and gold, in honor of the Jasper Wildcats, and she ordered enough that everyone, from Bill to Lukas, would have one. The shirts had SCHROEDER FAMILY printed on the back. Friends and relatives also expressed an interest, so she ordered fifty more; those had BILL'S BACKERS on the back. They sold out within hours. And when hospital staffers, doctors, and other Jasper residents heard about the shirts, hundreds more had to be ordered.

Bill's trip home seemed increasingly likely, in part because Dr. DeVries would be in Jasper that weekend, having accepted an invitation to be the parade's grand marshal. DeVries had visited Jasper before, as keynote speaker before a packed house at the Dubois County Heart Association's fund-raising dinner in February. The friendly, famous surgeon had been a big hit with the locals, and they were happy to roll out the red carpet for him again.

Now logistical preparations began in earnest. The staff and family decided that if Bill did indeed make the trip, they'd take him home on Saturday morning, just hours before the parade. A series of police and security escorts was arranged. PR would set up a media center in a vacant bank building across from the courthouse, and present DeVries at a press conference the morning of Bill's visit. Exactly when Bill returned to the hospital would depend on his condition, but if all went well, he'd ride in the van at the head of the parade.

By Friday, August 4, Bill was continuing to maintain strength, and his condition seemed stable. Of course, he became very excited at any mention of going home to Jasper. DeVries gladly gave the okay for Bill to go, just before the doctor, his wife, and five of his children went ahead to Jasper to get an early start on the weekend's activities.

Jasper's Strassenfest (German for "street fair") is four days of good old-fashioned small-town summertime fun. Streets down-town are blocked off, and wooden booths, strung with lights, go up overnight. There are homemade quilts and wood carvings for sale, along with all kinds of foods, like bratwurst and sauerkraut, sugary flat cakes called elephant ears, ice cream, fresh-squeezed lemonade—and of course, in the beer garden, all the German brew you can drink. Bavarian bands in full costume play on the main stage in front of the courthouse, and amusement-park rides are set up for the kids. There are horseshoe and volleyball tourna-ments, and all kinds of crazy contests, such as bed races, keg tosses, and motorized-barstool relays. All the proceeds go to local charitable organizations and community improvement projects. Each year the festivities are capped by the parade, which snakes its way downtown and around the courthouse square.

On Friday afternoon Dr. DeVries and his family faced off against the Schroeders in a friendly game of volleyball, which ended with the Schroeders victorious, 21 to 16. The doctor also good-naturedly took a turn sitting in the cage of a dunking booth. Terry couldn't resist this opportunity, and plunked down his money right away. What a chance to use the old pitching arm! DeVries had to know he was in for it. Terry wound up and hurled the ball as hard as he could—not at the target, but right at De-Vries. The ball hit the cage and bounced off, but the doctor was so startled he nearly fell off his seat. Terry laughed and made a couple of unsuccessful shots at the bull's-eye before letting some little kids play out the rest of his turn.

The next morning at Audubon, it seemed as if Bill & Com-pany would never get away from the hospital. He was supposed to be in the van and on his way to Jasper by 9:00 A.M. Margaret knew it would take a long time to get him ready, so she was at his room by six that morning. Bill was now receiving a constant flow of heparin through a new, smaller pump that could be worn under his shirt rather than be attached to an IV pole. But the nurse on duty was having a hard time regulating the dosage and struggled with it for a couple of hours, making several phone calls to the medical team's blood specialist.

Terry and Julie arrived at the hospital about 8:30 A.M. Terry was going to drive the van, which would take Bill and Mar-garet, a nurse, technician Brent Mays, and Lawrence Barker, a former coronary-care nurse who had been trained as a heart-drive technician. The procession of vehicles would include the Kentucky State Police, followed by a car with security guards, then the van, and an ambulance bringing up the rear.

Finally, everything was set—and Bill and Margaret were on the road together again, side by side, and this time they were finally headed for home. Bill sat in the van's backseat beside Margaret and leaned his head on her shoulder. When they crossed the Ohio River, the Indiana State Police took over the escort. All along the way, television crews pulled up alongside the van and pointed their cameras inside as everyone waved.

Up at the Mill Street house, a flatbed eighteen-wheeler was parked by the side of the house. A wall of television cameras extended from one end of the trailer to the other, all aimed at the front sidewalk leading to the Schroeders' front porch. That morning the kids had been busy painting signs to greet their dad. Across the wrought-iron porch fence was draped a homemade banner that read WELCOME HOME DAD. They'd tied balloons and yellow ribbons all along the front of the house. Rod had borrowed a large portable flashing sign spelling out the family's congratulations, and arranged for a friend to videotape Bill's visit. Some neighbors who lived on a grassy slope across the street had arranged slats of wood on the steep bank to read WELCOME HOME BILL.

Every Jasper cop was on duty that day. They roped off a small area in front of the house and blocked traffic, which probably wasn't necessary since about two hundred people were milling around in the street. Reporters walked around interviewing neighbors and trying to find the closest spot possible to the front sidewalk. Helicopters hovered high above the house. Some of the Schroeder kids were selling T-shirts and black and gold trucker's caps that said GET THE WILL OF BILL. Strode, along with a new photographer, was taking pictures for Humana. DeVries, in a suit and wearing a carnation, and his wife, Karen, who wore a corsage, arrived and took places on the front porch as they checked and rechecked the camera they'd brought to take pictures of the historic occasion.

Every few minutes, police radios crackled with reports on the van's progress. "They've turned off the interstate." "They've made it through Ferdinand." Everyone was getting really excited now. Police were asking the family and the PR people last-minute questions. With each new report, all the Schroeder kids felt more restless.

The long ride on the highway was tiring and uncomfortable for both Margaret and Bill. But when they got off at the Ferdinand exit, Bill perked up and eagerly watched the scenery going past. Margaret and Terry pointed out all the familiar sights: Fleig's Café in Ferdinand, where they used to go for fried chicken on Friday nights; Highway 162, flanked by acres and acres of corn-fields now summer-high; the Bretzville turnoff, which would have taken them to the forty acres. Bill looked all around and nodded enthusiastically.

The closer they got to Jasper, the more they saw hand-lettered signs in yards and store windows. Yellow ribbons were tied everywhere—on traffic signs, telephone poles, and mail-boxes. All along the way, drivers were waving and honking their horns. On the outskirts of Jasper, the van passed Holy Family church, where Bill and Margaret were married. The marquee at Dippel's Food Center read WELCOME HOME, BIONIC BILL. They passed the Schnitzelbank German restaurant, crossed the small bridge over the Patoka River, near Druthers' Restaurant. People on porch swings and in lawn chairs waved and cheered. They were almost home.

Back at the house, word came over the police radio that the van was just five minutes away. It was finally happening. None of the kids could keep still now.

From behind the rise at the end of Mill Street, a police siren wailed as the car crested the hill, blue lights flashing. The van was right behind it. Police ran ahead to clear a way through the crowd. The several seconds that it took for the van to cruise down the street seemed like forever. Terry carefully pulled the van as close as possible to the curb, and Mel gave him the thumbs-up.

Brent and Margaret took several minutes to move Bill into the wheelchair. They put the Heimes on his lap and coiled the drive lines on top for him to hold. Mel opened the door, and suddenly the van became filled with the noise of the crowd and cameras snapping away. People were pressing in close as the po-lice and security tried to keep them back.

The new Humana photographer ducked under the rope and crouched in the front yard, taking pictures. The other reporters were furious and began yelling, "Get him out of there!" The pho-tographer turned around and shouted angrily, "Hey, I'm working for HUMANA, buddy!" Some family members and the police finally persuaded him to get out of the way. The last thing they needed now was a commotion.

As Brent and Lawrence wheeled Bill out onto the lift and began to lower it, applause and cheers went up from the crowd. All the Schroeders gathered along the sidewalk, saying, "Hi, Dad! You're home! You're home!"

Bill sat squinting in the sunlight for a moment, just looking up at his house—the house where he was born and raised, where he had brought his six kids and wife to live with his own ailing father. Margaret and the kids were talking to him, pointing out the banner on the front porch. Then the grandkids came up, and he reached out to hold their hands. Stan wheeled him up the ramp, then turned the wheelchair around to face the crowd. Bill waved and everyone cheered again. Margaret bent over and asked him to wave to all the television cameras; so he did.

Stan pushed the wheelchair on through the front door and into the living room. The family had waited so long for this moment. Terry leaned close to his father. "See, Dad? I *told* you I would get you home!"

Bill looked around the room: the green shag carpet, the dark panelboard, the drop ceiling; the corner glass cabinet with Margaret's collection of dishes, cups, and saucers he'd added to over the years, some from his mother, others from his overseas tours of duty and out-of-town union trips. All around the room were the other knickknacks Bill had carefully selected for Margaret at yard sales; on the walls, framed photos of the kids' senior class pictures and weddings; the old couch, draped with the afghan Margaret had crocheted; in the corner, his old La-Z-Boy recliner; his kids all around him, smiling, the grandchildren holding his hands. And Margaret.

"We're *home*," Bill said. "We're home now."

Many relatives had gathered, and were now filing past Bill's wheelchair. For some, it was the first time they'd seen him in nearly a year. The folks from Margaret's side, who'd all settled near the forty acres, were there. Sometimes Bill had to look at them for a few seconds before he remembered every one.

Margaret's younger brother, Riley, came up to him and said, "Hi, Bill," unsure if he'd be recognized. Bill and Riley had been the biggest kidders in the family and always swapped jokes any time everyone got together.

Bill slowly took his brother-in-law's hand in both of his,

and exclaimed, "Riley!" Bill looked at him as if he just couldn't believe it, and began to cry. Some of the relatives weren't ready for that, and they quickly moved out to the kitchen or to the back porch, so Bill wouldn't see their tears. They all remembered Bill Schroeder as the big strapping guy who was the life of every party, the master of ceremonies, who could never sit still, who could cook up a storm in the kitchen, who always phoned them to organize some family gathering or other. And now Bill had brought them together again for the most extraordinary gathering of all.

"We're home," Bill said again, looking around the room. "We're home. I don't ever want—" He didn't finish the sentence.

Strode gathered the Schroeders together for a couple of family portraits. By now Bill was tired, so the boys and the technicians helped settle him in the room that used to be his father's. It was a tight squeeze getting through the doorways of the small house. They switched Bill to the Utah, which was running now on reserve air tanks, and let him nap for about an hour. DeVries left for a press conference in the basement of the Dubois County Bank, where he told the media: "No wonder he wanted to come back—this is a great town."

Since many of the reporters and photographers circling the house hadn't budged, the kids and Margaret stepped out on the front porch for an impromptu press conference, where they got all the usual questions.

As the cameras rolled, the family tried to sum up their feelings. "There was a lot of tears," Mel said. "Everybody was hugging and kissing each other. Dad cried a lot. We all did." He wanted to say more, but couldn't find words to convey that it had been the strangest feeling he'd ever had in his life, something he'd never felt before and might never feel again—butterflies mixed with a kind of warmth inside, and a glow outside.

A lunch of German food soon arrived, catered by the Schnitzelbank restaurant. The Schroeders invited the Humana personnel to join them in snacking on sandwiches, dumplings, and hot potato salad.

Bill woke from his nap, and Margaret wheeled him into the kitchen—their kitchen: the cabinets he'd built and stained a redwood color while recuperating after his first heart attack; the kitchen table on which he'd shown off his cooking, and where he'd won so many card games; on the counter the relish made with corn that he and Margaret had grown at the forty acres and canned together. There were the flour and sugar canisters that Bill had made for Margaret in ceramics class; the picture of "The Last Supper" displayed beside the refrigerator; the back door, which had never stopped opening and slamming during the summers—and the backyard, which always had so many bare spots when the kids were young, where he'd taught them to pitch Wiffle balls and run football plays.

Margaret helped him eat a little of the German food, and he told her it tasted great. All too soon, it was time to go. Everything had happened so fast. Bill had spent barely two hours at home, but now it was time for him to lead the parade. Margaret pinned a corsage to his shirt, and the technicians switched him back to the Heimes and rolled the Utah into the rear of the van.

The family brought Bill back to the van and put him in the front passenger seat, and designated Mel as driver. There was no place for Margaret to sit close to Bill, so she decided just to kneel beside him. A few photographers had lingered for some parting shots of Bill, and of course, the cameras closed in on the van. Bill handled it well and just waved back. They drove to the parade's starting point, about a block away. A police car pulled in front to lead the way, and started off with its siren blaring. The rest of the Schroeder family followed in open convertibles plus Dr. DeVries and his wife in another car.

Two Jasper police officers walking alongside the van which moved slowly. None of the family were prepared for what happened next. More than fifteen thousand people had turned out for the parade, about five thousand more than usual. People were lining both sides of the streets, standing or seated on bleachers and lawn chairs. As the silver-and-blue van approached, the whole throng rose to its feet, like waves in the ocean, cheering and clapping. Bill waved back enthusiastically.

The Schroeders brought candy to toss along the parade route. Mel threw some out the driver's window, and handed some to his parents. Bill tossed the candy out his window, and even though it didn't land very far away, he loved watching the children run after it, and kept reaching for more to throw. Every once in a while, Margaret would spot one of Bill's old friends in the crowd, and Mel slowed the van to a halt so they could come over and say "Hi." Many Jasper residents waved signs congratulating Bill and wishing him well.

The Humana PR folks had arranged a cordoned-off section of bleachers for the media at two strategic corners of the courthouse square, promising a good view of Bill and his van leading the parade. The route took them around the courthouse, and right past the main stage that served as the center of activities for Strassenfest.

By this time Bill was very tired, almost too tired to wave anymore, so when they passed all the cameras, Margaret held his wrist to help him wave at the press. It was too bad that this was what the cameras recorded and replayed on the evening news, because ten or fifteen minutes earlier, Bill had looked so strong.

Photographers jumped out of the crowd and pushed up close to Bill's side of the van, some holding up their cameras without looking and snapping away. It was confusing for Bill. Mel tried to speed up, but there were too many photographers darting back and forth in front of the van. Finally, somebody yelled at Mel to roll up Bill's window, so the reflection would prevent the cameras from getting good shots. That was the end of *that* problem.

Brent remembered that the van was equipped with a public-address system. He switched it on, and Margaret made an impromptu speech of thanks to the good people of Jasper. By now they'd nearly completed the parade route. The family had dreaded this point. After all that had happened that day, who was going to tell Bill it was time to go back to the hospital? Fortunately, he was so tired that he didn't seem bothered when the van turned and headed for the interstate. He looked as though he was doing fine sitting in the front seat, so they decided against moving him to the wheelchair in the back. All along the route, there were still signs and yellow ribbons.

They took a break at a truck stop about halfway to Louisville. A number of news crews, which had followed the van, also stopped to film Bill when Lawrence Barker, the technician, opened the door to let him stretch. By the time they returned to Audubon, Bill wasn't the only one who was exhausted. They put him to bed right away and switched him back to the Utah. Mel drove Terry's car back that evening, and, since they expected Bill would rest most of the next day, Margaret returned with Mel for an overnight stay at home.

What a day! Sure, it had been a lot of trouble, a lot of logistics to work out. But if someone had asked any of the Schroeders that day if all the fears and worries, the stress and the hardships had been worth it, the answer would have been undoubtedly, absolutely *yes*.

CHAPTER TWENTY-FOUR

The next days after Strassenfest were difficult. As often happens with stroke patients, Bill began to have episodes of being irritable and angry. When he was upset, even Margaret had a hard time calming him down. At times he was so uncontrollable that the nurses had to give him Valium.

There was more news that disturbed the whole family. The medical team informed them that Bill would again be discharged to the apartment the following Sunday. A week or two before Strassenfest, Dr. DeVries had indicated that he believed Bill was ready to move back across the street, and new nurses were already being trained to watch over the Utah.

The family wondered if DeVries was under some kind of pressure—to give the program a boost perhaps—or if the doctor feared being criticized for keeping Bill hospitalized but declaring him healthy enough to attend Strassenfest, or if Bill had become too unruly and his presence too disruptive for the day-to-day workings of the cardiovascular unit.

Living at the apartment was beginning to sound more like being in a nursing home, a situation Margaret and Bill had vowed never to let the other endure. As far as the family were concerned, this "transitional" period now seemed like a waste of time. Much of their apprehension concerned the quality of life versus quantity of life. If Bill was well enough to leave the hospital, it seemed to them that he was well enough to come home to Jasper to live out whatever time he had left among family, where he had wanted to be all along. If he wasn't well enough, he should stay in the hospital, where there were nurses he knew and trusted. What would really be achieved if he was living just half a block down the street? Besides, regardless of what Bill had meant, they vividly remembered his last visit to the apartment when he'd said: "Let's get the hell *out* of here!"

325

Of course, the Mill Street house wasn't equipped yet for an artificial heart patient, and outfitting it would take weeks, if not months. A new staff of nurses, therapists, and drive technicians would have to be hired to care for him in Jasper, and a doctor would have to take on the responsibility of visiting Bill regularly. The Schroeders weren't sure whether everything would work out, but they felt they should at least try. A compromise was reached: Bill would return to the apartment, and in the meantime DeVries would look into arrangements for letting him move to Jasper. Maybe they could go ahead and equip the house and let Bill try an overnight stay, then a weekend, and if all went well, he could work up to being there all the time.

The Schroeder family remained wary of moving back into the apartment, but what were they supposed to do? If they wanted to raise a fuss, they could go to the media with their concerns. They also knew there was no way they could keep Bill alive without the help of the doctors and hospital workers; they would have to work together. More and more, Margaret began to feel that the family and the medical team were trapped together in some kind of a spider web.

The weekend after Strassenfest, Bill and Margaret moved back across the street, with less fanfare and media coverage than before. The routine began again. Bill was especially unhappy at once more having to get used to new nurses. All Margaret could do was tell him that if they tried really hard, they might be able to move back home to Jasper sometime soon.

There were some good days, just simple quiet times together, when little things reminded them of what it was like back home. Some mornings, Margaret and Bill would push the Utah onto the back deck to have coffee and watch the birds at a feeder in a nearby yard. They might watch a soap opera together or flip through a scrapbook. When Bill was feeling especially good, he helped her dry the dishes, just as they had after the big holiday meals they'd always cooked together. Margaret was so excited the first time Bill helped with the dishes that she ran for her camera and took a picture of him.

Bill still found ways to be so funny sometimes, teasing Margaret or acting smart with the nurses. When the kids visited him, they'd watch Bill carefully try to pick up an object, concentrating hard as he grasped and painstakingly lifted it almost to where he wanted it—only to drop it at the last second. Then he'd yell, "SHHHHHHHHEEEE-ITTTTT!" with such exasperation that the kids had to turn away so he wouldn't see them giggling. When they turned around, he'd be pointing at them, saying, "Uh-HUH! *Caught* ya!" as if he was irritated but still proud of himself for getting a laugh. It was so great to see his old personality shining through at times like that.

Bill went on some more van rides, including one with Dr. Jarvik, who took him fishing. September 2 was another wonderful day: Bill and Margaret's wedding anniversary. The kids all came down to celebrate. They took their parents to the Red Lobster seafood restaurant along with Brent and Captain Tom from security, where DeVries and his wife met them in a specially reserved room. Bill had a wonderful anniversary. He was so glad to have family all around him, to celebrate thirty-three years of marriage, and to visit with his friends from the hospital. The Heimes was discreetly tucked under the table, and everything seemed very natural, just another anniversary dinner. As on every family occasion, Bill tried extra hard to participate and do things for himself. Margaret was thrilled because he ate well and even managed to pick up one of the restaurant's big cut-glass tumblers to drink without help.

But good days grew fewer and farther between. At times, Bill still became belligerent. Part of that behavior was an effect of the stroke, but then he was also enduring plenty that would make anyone frustrated and angry. He frequently had to get used to new nurses, many of whom were newly trained to work with artificial heart patients, and he got nervous whenever they came near the Utah. From Margaret's diary:

> Wednesday, Sept. 4. Bill woke up in a good mood. He woke me laughing. He thought we were alone. Soon as we talked, there was the nurse's head over the Utah. He gets so disgusted.
>
> Got him up to eat and his stomach starts hurting him. Back to bed, didn't eat much. . . . They are going to give him a G-I series for his stomach.
>
> Bill sleeps a lot. I went to cardiac rehab. . . . I walked to McDonald's and got chicken nuggets to eat for me and the nurse.
>
> Bill is lonesome and wants someone to talk to him. I crawl up on the bed and watch TV with him. You can al-

most forget the heart and machine at times. Then something always happens, like the nurse walks in, pill time, blood pressure, temp, or some silly thing like that.

By late summer the medical team and Margaret felt that somehow Bill had become more aware of being tethered to the machine. He would point two fingers at Margaret and then at himself, noting his two arms and hers, then his two legs and hers. Next, he would point to his Utah and then beside her, where Margaret's Utah would be, and give her a questioning look. It was difficult for him to find the words, but he would go through the series of pointing again and again and ask, "Why?"

She would play the usual Twenty Questions to find out what he meant, asking if he was saying he wanted her to have a Utah. Bill would nod vigorously and say, "Yes!" What could she tell him? All she could do was remind him that he needed that machine, and that if they just kept trying, maybe they could go home again and be with the kids and grandkids.

About this time, DeVries brought a Boston ethicist, George Annas, to meet Bill and left him at the apartment for a couple of hours to observe a typical morning. Bill was sitting up in a chair, trying to eat breakfast, but he was having a difficult time. He was tired and his stomach was hurting him. Annas tried for quite a while to talk with him. "How do you like your machine, Mr. Schroeder?" Annas asked.

"I hate it!" Bill answered. *"I HATE IT! I HATE IT! I HATE IT!"*

Margaret was stunned. "Well, you heard it yourself," she said. "I've never heard him say that before!" Later, when they were alone, she climbed up into bed with Bill, held him close, and asked, "Honey, what do you mean that you hate your machine? Is it the noise you hate? You know that if you didn't have the machine, you'd be gone and the kids and I wouldn't have you anymore. Is it the noise, sweetie?"

Bill nodded and kissed her. But sometimes she wondered.

CHAPTER TWENTY-FIVE

Visiting their parents had become part of the Schroeder kids' regular routine. It got to the point where it would have felt strange *not* to drive to Louisville at least once a week. And with each visit, they saw that their mother looked a little more tired than the time before. As Margaret had said on Oprah Winfrey's show, it was the unpredictability of things that was so wearing.

For example, one Friday night in September, after a day when Bill had been particularly restless, Margaret was getting ready for bed, hoping for an uneventful weekend. Bill was sleeping soundly. About 11:00 P.M., the nurse came in to make her last check on him before shift change. After a moment, she said, "Margaret, I can't get Bill to respond."

"Oh, he's probably just sound asleep," Margaret said. "Come on, Bill." He didn't respond, so she shook him a little. Still no response. She shook him harder, but he wouldn't open his eyes.

Margaret helped the nurse take his vital signs, which showed nothing abnormal. The nurse was certain that something was wrong, especially since Bill wouldn't wake up for Margaret. The nurse called the hospital, which in turn set emergency procedures in motion. Margaret kept trying to wake Bill, but he just lay motionless. "Bill, if you don't wake up for us, they're going to take you across the street to the hospital." Margaret was puzzled—it just didn't make sense. The alarms on the Utah weren't even going off.

An ambulance and a technician arrived. Bill was switched to the Heimes, strapped once more onto a stretcher, and rushed over for a CAT scan. By the time they got there, the news was all over the hospital that Bill was back. Nurses John Lammers, Bill Binggeli, and George Roth, and Captain Tom Biondolillo from

329

security hurried downstairs to see what was wrong. Dr. Fox was also called in. The scan room and observation area were now filled with people. Margaret told them she didn't think anything was wrong with Bill. This wasn't like the other times.

"Well, we'll just find out," they assured her.

After the scan the group waited as Dr. Fox studied Bill's test results. Captain Tom tried to lighten the mood with a joke. Margaret was still watching Bill, and suddenly she thought she saw him smirk.

"Bill?" She couldn't believe it. She nudged John. "Look at him!"

Bill peeked up at them with one eye. John saw it. A few seconds later, Bill did it again, and this time Captain Tom saw it, too.

"Well, I'll be damned!" John said.

"Hiya, Bill!" the captain said.

Bill had always liked the guards. He opened both eyes and slowly held up a stiff hand. "Hi, Cap!"

John was trying not to laugh. "You old turkey! You just wanted to get out and go cattin' around on a Friday night, didn't you?"

Bill folded his hands behind his head and grinned.

Dr. Fox stepped into the hall, and suddenly Bill was unresponsive again. For some reason, Bill had never liked Fox. The family hadn't liked him either at first, probably because he was always the bearer of bad news. They'd been upset by his grim assessment on TV after Bill's first stroke, but had come to appreciate that he was often right. Fox also performed the strangest-looking tests: running a toothed tracing wheel along the soles of Bill's feet, holding a cloth with red dots up to Bill's face and moving it back and forth, pinching him, or reaching behind Bill's head and snapping his fingers. Of course, they were standard neurological tests for responsiveness—but they drove Bill crazy, and whenever Fox left the room, he would give Margaret a look that said, "Who WAS that guy, anyway?"

Now when Fox turned his back for a moment, Bill peeked at him.

John was getting worried. "Bill! If you don't let the doctor know you're all right, he's going to admit you. You'd better tell him, or you're going to have to start seeing my ugly face all the time again."

Fox turned around. Bill was wide awake and grinning from ear to ear. He'd been caught. Fox asked him, "Well, how are you feeling, hotshot?"

Bill just shrugged, as if to say: "So-so, I guess."

Fox ordered a few more tests, just to be sure. However, the tests showed that all was fine. By the time Margaret and Bill got back to the apartment, it was 4:00 A.M. Margaret put Bill to bed and fixed coffee for everyone who'd been up all night with him. They talked for a while. Had he really been playing possum, all the way over to the hospital? Or had he had some kind of spell, maybe a "seizurelike episode," and then come out of it in the scan room? Nobody would ever know for sure. However, Margaret and some of the nurses agreed that he was just showing some of his old spunk, the rascal. At about 5:30 Margaret crawled into bed with him. Bill was still wide awake. He grinned, wrapped his arms around her, and held her with surprising strength. Soon they both fell asleep, but in less than two hours, it would be time for shift change, Bill's morning medication, breakfast, and another day.

The next afternoon, when Mel and his family visited, Bill was tired and cranky. Early that evening, the Utah's alarms sounded, indicating that the power source had been cut and the machine was running on the reserve air tanks. There were some tense moments as the family frantically checked the Utah and the drive lines and called Brent Mays. Bill was worried, too, seeing them so anxious. He clutched his granddaughter Melanie close, saying over and over, "Well, DO something!"

A hospital maintenance worker was alerted and came over to check the equipment in the basement. But the worker had been there only once before, so he wasn't sure what to look for. In exasperation Mel checked the fuse box and discovered that two circuit breakers had blown. He switched them back over, the air compressor kicked on again, and the alarms stopped.

Now it was time for Mel's family to go back home. Just another predictably unpredictable weekend, and another long Sunday evening for Margaret.

In mid-September when Una Loy Clark came to Louisville for some fund-raising events sponsored by the American Heart Association, she and Margaret had a joyful reunion at the apartment. That morning one of DeVries's associates had been there to stitch a new subclavian catheter into place. Bill was still in bed, sore and tired, when Margaret brought in Mrs. Clark to meet him,

331

telling him she was the wife of Barney Clark. Bill's eyes brightened, and he nodded. He definitely knew who she was, and he watched her every move. Mrs. Clark didn't want to wear him out by staying too long, so she greeted him pleasantly, kissed his forehead, and said, "I just want you to know how much I love and appreciate you and what you're doing."

Bill looked into her eyes and said plainly, "We do it for others."

Early the next morning, two hundred or so "graduates" of Audubon's cardiac unit would kick off their annual walkathon for charity by taking a lap around the dirt track at Churchill Downs. Somebody suggested that the group be led by a horse-drawn surrey carrying Bill and Margaret, Mrs. Clark, Mrs. Haydon, and Jack Burcham's widow, Jinx, who was in town for the weekend's events. It might be a nice outing for Bill, Margaret was told. Afterward, a brunch would be held honoring his contributions and those of the other recipients.

So at 5:00 A.M. the following day, Margaret got up to get Bill ready for the buggy ride. Cheryl, Julie, Mel and his family, and Moni and her kids also came down to Louisville for the event. Bill hadn't slept well at all, so he was still weary when they loaded him into the van and headed for the track.

When they got to the Downs, Mel pulled the van up alongside a horse-drawn, fringe-topped surrey with three rows of seats. Dr. Lansing was in the front seat, next to two drivers, one dressed in a cowboy outfit and another wearing a top hat and tails. Mrs. Burcham and Mrs. Clark sat in the rear, and Mrs. Haydon sat on the middle bench. The group didn't know how Bill would be transferred to the buggy, but he managed well, standing from his wheelchair with assistance, then stepping right in. Technician Lawrence Barker got in beside him, set the Heimes on the floor, while Margaret hopped in the back row, where she could sit behind Bill and keep her hand on his shoulder to reassure him.

The sun was just coming up over the racetrack's twin spires, and the morning was surprisingly chilly. Margaret draped a hospital blanket over Bill. A high-school marching band played a couple of songs, then the ride began. Humana had sent out press releases, so plenty of reporters and photographers were there to cover the event, and some jogged alongside the buggy all the way around the track, calling out questions to the Schroeders and Dr. Lansing.

After the surrey had taken a lap, the driver brought it to a halt to wait for the marching band and for the walkers to finish their walk. Reporters started pressing up close to the surrey, trying to interview Bill.

"How are you feeling, Mr. Schroeder? How do you feel?"

At first Bill answered. "Feeling great," he said clearly. Margaret patted his shoulders and tried to reassure him. But now too many people were pressing up close to the surrey and shouting:

"Did you enjoy the ride? Did he enjoy the ride, Mrs. Schroeder?"

When Moni saw that the surrey had stopped, she ran over to see what the matter was. She had to push and shove her way past the reporters to get to her dad and give him some room. Bill was crying now.

Finally, they got back to the van and headed to the hospital for the awards breakfast. Bill had become chilled from the morning ride, and he was exhausted—he never had much energy after being up for two hours—and started complaining loudly while Lansing was making a speech. Mel told one of the coordinators of the event that if they wanted to give Bill an award they'd better do it right away. A presentation was hastily made, after which the family took Bill back to the apartment, where he slept most of the rest of the day.

As usual, Moni and Cheryl tried to convince Margaret to come home for a rest. They were surprised when Margaret agreed that she was pretty tired. Maybe she'd go home on Thursday and have a long weekend at home. Perhaps she could get someone from the hospital to look after the apartment and fix Bill's meals while she was gone.

Moni and Cheryl stayed with Bill so Margaret could go with the other wives to an evening picnic and outdoor concert, part of the weekend's fund raisers. She returned late and talked for a while with her daughters before collapsing into bed as soon as the nurses changed shifts at eleven. The next morning Moni and Cheryl took Margaret grocery shopping before heading back home. That evening, once again it was just Margaret, Bill, and the nurse.

Sunday, Sept. 15. Well, the day is "up-to-here" and very lonely. Am tired and sleepy. Have things to do like wash and do dishes and strip bed, etc. Tomorrow is another week and I can't see how I can face the days to come. It gets harder all the time.

That entry turned out to be more than prophetic. The very next morning, as she was getting ready to make breakfast, Margaret collapsed in the hallway and lost consciousness for several minutes. Sandy Chandler, who was filling in for a home-care nurse that day, shouted to the security guard and helped Margaret onto the couch.

Moments later, Mel called to check in and firm up plans for Margaret's trip home that weekend. Sandy answered and told him that Margaret had fainted, her blood pressure was low, and a neurologist was on his way to examine her. They'd call him as soon as the doctor was through.

Mel hung up, but he couldn't take his eyes off the phone. After twenty minutes, he called back. The neurologist, an associate of Dr. Fox's, got on the phone and repeated the information Sandy had given him, but added that just to be safe, he wanted to admit Margaret for some tests.

That sounded a lot more serious than just a fainting spell. "Do you think it warrants someone coming down right away?" Mel asked.

There was a pause. "Yes, I think that would be best."

Mel hung up and started down the list of his brothers and sisters. Again and again, as Mel explained what he knew, the reaction was *"Who?"* Anytime Mel called the kids at work, they half expected to hear that something had happened to Dad—but now Mom, too? Some of them took the rest of the day off, telling their bosses they didn't know when they'd return.

Mel reached Louisville first, and went to the apartment to check on his father. Even before Mel knocked on the door, he could hear his dad calling out for Margaret. Mel tried to calm him, saying that Margaret was in the hospital, so he'd have to work with the nurse for a while and do what she asked. Bill acted as though he didn't understand, as if he suspected that Mel was telling him a lie so Margaret could leave for a while.

As each family member reached the hospital, he or she was directed to Margaret's room, just down the hall from Bill's old room. Their mother was lying in bed, extremely groggy. She'd wake up a little whenever one of them came into the room. "Is that you?" she'd ask slowly. Her words were slurred and hard to understand. She'd say, "I'm okay. How's your dad? Tell him I'll be back later today. I just need some rest." She kept saying that her head hurt, and that she was having trouble moving one side of her body. The kids assured her they'd take care of Dad.

Out in the hall, Mel stopped John Lammers, and asked hopefully, "Did they give Mom something to sleep, a sedative or something?"

John gave him a somber, knowing look and shook his head. "We didn't give her a thing."

The kids couldn't believe it; this was exactly what Dad had been like. Terry and Stan stayed that night with Bill, who remained confused and irritable. Cheryl took over for the next couple of days, going back and forth between the hospital and the apartment, looking after both parents. On Thursday, the neurologists told Margaret she was going to have to take it easy. The collapse had been a warning. The test results were inconclusive. It could have been a combination of low blood pressure and exhaustion. But it could also have been a transient stroke. At any rate, she was sent back to Jasper with strict orders for six weeks of rest. Patti looked after her at the Mill Street house the next couple of days. Margaret's speech was still a little slurred and her head sometimes throbbed with pain. The kids decided that any thought of their parents moving back home had to be put on the back burner. The priority now would be getting Mom well again.

Things at the apartment would have to be different from now on. A nurse's aide from the agency came in to take care of basic housekeeping chores, prepare meals, and help the nurse. This was the arrangement Margaret had wanted all along so that she could have more time for herself and Bill.

Now that Margaret was not there, Bill became confused and angry. They had been together from the beginning, and he was upset not having her close. Back in Jasper, Margaret felt terrible about being away from him. The family took turns visiting Bill every other night, but their presence only seemed to bring out their father's frustration. He became irritated when he saw them, and sometimes it took most of the visit to calm him down. Then it was time to leave, and he would become agitated again. When it became clear that they had to go home, he would cry and shout, "Then go! *Go!* Just *go!*" The nurses would be left with the difficult job of trying to calm him down. As soon as the family returned and stopped by the Mill Street house, Margaret would be eagerly waiting to ask how Bill was doing. The kids were caught in the middle. All they could do was emphasize the good, say that he missed her, and not mention how upset he'd been.

It tore them up to leave him, and they often wondered whether they should take a leave of absence from work. However, they knew their parents wanted them to carry on with their own lives. Also, since they were by no means wealthy, they had to keep drawing a paycheck. But the idea of Bill staying in the apartment without any family at all made the place seem more than ever like a miniature nursing home.

While Margaret was home, the medical team arranged for Bill to undergo stroke rehabilitation at a center a few miles away. That meant getting him up and ready for a twenty-minute van ride at either end of a grueling session. Often Bill resisted going. The family had to question whose interest was being considered. Bill's condition seemed so precarious, and he had had so many brushes with death before. All the family wanted to do was have more time with him; everybody knew that his artificial heart wouldn't last more than a couple of years. If Bill was a terminal patient, how much sense did it make to try to rehabilitate him? Of course, everyone wanted Bill to be the best he could. It was hard, though, to imagine how he could improve if rehab left him so drained that he'd collapse and sleep for hours, missing lunch and sometimes supper.

After two weeks at home, Margaret felt better. She was still a little unsteady on her feet at times. When she was tired, her speech had a slight slur, and her handwriting was loose and disjointed. But she was beside herself with worries about Bill. She called the apartment every day to find out how he was doing. The answer was always the same: "He's doing fine." She didn't buy it for a minute—Bill had never been fine for two weeks in a row, especially in that apartment.

Margaret had a checkup with the neurologist, who agreed to let her visit Bill one evening, provided it was just for a couple of hours. She went to the apartment full of joyous anticipation, only to find Bill tearful and angry at her. She realized that some things had changed: They were parting Bill's hair on the wrong side, and letting him nap in a chair instead of putting him back to bed. He had definitely lost a lot of weight, and was having trouble moving his left leg. This wasn't the same man she'd seen two weeks ago. In Margaret's eyes Bill was doing terribly, and they weren't caring for him the way she would have—but then, nobody could do that. It was upsetting to see him this way and to hear the nurses insist he was doing fine, and even more frustrating to have to leave him after only a couple of hours, and let the nurses perform the duties she'd been doing.

The family had another meeting with Dr. DeVries and worked out a routine in which Bill would get up and have breakfast by 8:30 A.M., go across town to rehab, return by 12:30, and have a nap. Margaret's visits were limited to a few hours at a time, for her benefit as well as his, according to the doctors. Bill would become upset whenever she had to return to Jasper. Sometimes when she wasn't looking, he would take her purse and hide it under the sheets, knowing that she couldn't leave without it.

As the days went by, Bill's fevers returned. He began to have seizures, which led to more EEGs and tests. Also, he wasn't eating well. One evening, when Margaret arrived, Bill reached out to her and said tearfully, "I tried, honey, I really tried!" She could only hold him close and whisper, "I know, honey, I know. This thing is just bigger than the both of us."

On Saturday evening, November 9, one of the nurses called Margaret at home and indicated that Bill was getting worse. Terry rushed her to Louisville. They arrived around midnight to find that Bill's temperature had gone up, he was increasingly lethargic, and everybody was concerned that sooner or later, he was going to have another stroke.

CHAPTER TWENTY-SIX

November 11, 1985: One year to the day when Bill was first admitted to Audubon for tests, he was readmitted with a third stroke. As the family gathered around his bed once more, Bill just looked at them and cried, as if he knew that it was about to start all over again. Margaret moved back to Louisville so she could be at his bedside.

Dr. DeVries told the press a week later that Bill's consciousness now waxed and waned. Again, reporters wanted to know if the Schroeders planned to turn off the machine. DeVries said the family were nowhere near discussing that question, which was the truth. He described Bill as "a fantastically durable individual" with an unusual ability to regain his strength: "We chose him for those reasons, and he's behaving as usual."

Since Jack Burcham's death in April, DeVries had done no implants but emphasized that what he had learned from Bill and the other recipients only confirmed his resolve to push on with his work. He had always compared the current Jarvik-7 heart to a Model-T Ford, predicting that further testing could ultimately lead to a device as sophisticated as the space shuttle. He readily acknowledged that human heart transplants were far superior to artificial hearts at this stage of development, and that the field of potential artificial heart candidates had narrowed, thanks to advances in transplant technology.

Increasingly, artificial hearts were being used with success in a few medical centers as a temporary "bridge-to-transplant." Some critics praised such temporary use of artificial hearts, while condemning DeVries's determination to keep on testing the Jarvik heart as a permanent device. He argued that any recipient of a temporary heart should be prepared for it to become permanent, because a stroke or other complication could disqualify that patient for a human heart transplant. And, he maintained, permanent hearts could someday solve the problem of a shortage of donor hearts for transplants: If permanent implants were perfected, the devices would be available off the shelf in any number.

A few days after the press conference, reporters started calling the family again—this time for stories on Bill's one-year anniversary with the Jarvik heart. As the kids fielded many questions about the stress of their ordeal, they realized, among other things, that some of them had put as many as fifteen thousand miles on their vehicles just traveling to and from Louisville.

The anniversary of Bill's admission to Audubon brought back so many memories. Cards and letters began pouring in again, just as they had during Bill's first spectacular eighteen days. But it was very different now. Whenever the kids tried to encourage Bill with talk about another trip to Jasper or coming home for good, he would just look at them, or shake his head as if he knew he'd never leave the hospital again. His weight loss over the past year had made his dark brown eyes seem bigger and more expressive. He even had a strand or two of gray in his beautiful fine brown hair.

Meanwhile, the FDA called DeVries to Washington for extensive questioning. He was still the only U.S. surgeon authorized to implant the Jarvik-7 as a permanent device, and he convinced the skeptical FDA panel that his work should continue. But the agency insisted that now he would have to justify his work with detailed, written reports every three months.

The days stretched on and on. One encouraging change was that now there was a consistent team of home health-care nurses staffing Bill's hospital room around-the-clock: Cheryl Ailiff on the day shift, Trish Haaker in the evening, and Bea Bryant at nights. They were all young, dedicated women who got along fine with the Schroeders. They all traded stories about their families with Margaret, and the nurses good-naturedly took kidding from the Schroeder boys. It was a relief to have a regular nursing team, even if it had taken a whole year to get it established.

Around this time, the Schroeders were approached by Martha Barnette, a twenty-eight-year-old reporter who had covered their story for *The Louisville Times* and later for *The Washington Post*. She suggested collaborating on a book about the family's experience. The Schroeders agreed to give it a try, and Martha began a long series of visits with Margaret and Bill at the hospital, and interviews with family members back home in Jasper.

In early December Glenn gave Cheryl an engagement ring; their wedding was a year and a half away. Again, because the family had no guarantees that Bill could get better, Cheryl and Glenn decided that they would share their good news with their parents in a special way.

First, they visited Glenn's parents and toasted with champagne. Then the couple came to Louisville to see her parents. Bill's condition was largely unchanged. He was still unable to talk, but when Cheryl told him that she and Glenn were now engaged, Bill pointed at her ring, took it in his hand and fingered it, then squeezed her hand tightly. Cheryl was sure that he understood and approved, because he had given them his blessing before he came to Audubon.

She and Glenn also brought along a single white candle. The couple lit a match together while her parents did the same with another. Then the four of them lit the candle together.

"This is a special candle, Dad," Cheryl told him. "We're going to put this on the altar during our wedding ceremony. That way we'll all be there together, no matter what."

Again Bill looked at her steadily, blinked attentively, and Cheryl was certain that he understood.

The day before Christmas Eve, Bill surprised Margaret by waking up and saying, "Hi," his first word in six weeks. Over the next few days he was able to say, "Yes," "No," and "Why?" He also used a red pen to scribble some marks on a piece of paper. Margaret knew it was a love note.

The holidays came and went, and as usual the kids came down to be with their parents. But increasingly they would find Bill asleep. If he was awake, they'd talk to him about what was going on back home, and he might respond with a nod or an occasional smile. However, it was getting harder to find something to say that would interest him, and sometimes, no matter what was said, he would just look at them wearily.

From time to time, the fluids building up in Bill's chest cavity had to be removed. One January morning DeVries had just finished using a needle to drain some of the fluid through his back. The TV was on. Margaret was sitting close to Bill, trying as usual to assure him that this procedure, too, was important. De-

Vries happened to glance up at the TV—just as the space shuttle *Challenger* exploded.

"My God, it blew up!" DeVries said incredulously. "It blew up! Margaret, would you look at that? Turn up the television!"

Margaret hurried over to turn up the volume. "What blew up?" she asked. "What happened?"

"The space shuttle!" DeVries answered, pointing at the set. "It exploded! Look at that, Margaret! LOOK at that!" Margaret stood still, watching the trail of smoke branch, then stop rising.

Suddenly, she was kicked from behind. It was Bill. His dark eyes were bright and alert, and he was moaning and craning his neck to see around her. Apologizing, she moved over as the three watched the spacecraft explode again, and again, and again. Bill had avidly followed all the space shots, rousing the kids out of bed in the middle of the night to watch the moon landings. "A few years down the road," he had always preached to them, "who knows what they'll come up with? Who knows?"

Back home, when the Schroeder kids heard about the tragedy, the news seemed eerily familiar. The astronauts and their families were still on Mel's mind the following week when he traveled to Washington to testify before a congressional committee on science and technology.

"As I thought of what they might be experiencing, I could relate somewhat to their situation," he said. "Though everyone feels for these pioneering people, we all remember their courage to put the advancement of mankind before their own lives. You recall the successes you have experienced, you praise the pioneers of technology, and you dream for the future successes for mankind. This holds true for all new technologies. There's a long way to go, with many problems and questions to be answered with the artificial heart program. But with pioneers like my father, William Schroeder, you get closer each day."

Late that winter, Bill was provided with a new bed. Throughout his hospital stays the medical team had tried several different kinds to see which would be most effective at preventing the skin ulcers that develop in bedridden patients. This latest bed was strange-looking: The mattress consisted of about two dozen navy blue inflatable cushions standing up on their sides within the bed frame, like piano keys or swimming-pool rafts stacked sideways. A console at the foot of the bed could be adjusted to inflate some parts of the bed more than others to make Bill comfortable. It did do a good job of protecting Bill's skin, but now Margaret could no longer sit on the bed next to him or crawl under the covers with him. She had to stand by the bed and put her arms between the cushions to hug him close. Sometimes she wondered if the trade-off was worth it; preventing skin sores was important, but then so was the simple need to be held.

Every day, Margaret stayed as close to him as she could, for as long as possible. Her daily walks from the apartment to the hospital and back had worn a path in the grass beside the parking lot. The days grew longer and longer, the routine more familiar. There was lots more time to think. Sometimes Margaret would sit by Bill's bed and daydream about putting him across her back and pushing that old Utah all the way down the hall to the elevator. In her daydream, she and the family would just take him out of there and put him in the van. They'd all be back on the road together, like it had always been—just Bill, Margaret, and the kids. They'd turn that van toward Jasper and go as far as those air tanks would hold out . . . and then she would just hold him real tight.

Through much of January, Bill remained bedridden. On a good day he might be able to sit up in his chair for a while, but he was too weak for wheelchair rides. He was coughing a lot, which interfered with his sleep, and he had to be suctioned several times a day.

In February he could sit up in the cardiac chair to be wheeled into the hall. But soon he became worn out and was put back to bed. For his birthday he was wheeled down to the briefing room for a little party, but was able to stay only about ten minutes.

CHAPTER TWENTY-SEVEN

Although Bill showed little improvement, the Schroeders took some comfort at least in the knowledge that new strides were being made in heart implantation, thanks in part to Bill's struggle. By the spring of 1986, there had been about two dozen implants of temporary artificial hearts, including not only the Jarvik heart, but others developed at Penn State, in Phoenix, Arizona, and in Berlin, West Germany. A twenty-five-year-old Arizona man who had received a human heart transplant in September after being kept alive for several days with a Jarvik heart—and who had suffered a mild transient stroke while on the device—was back at work as a supermarket manager. The Swedish man who had received a Jarvik heart, Leif Stenberg, had been well enough to hold a press conference in July. He'd spent his days in a Stockholm apartment, and returned to the hospital each night. But he suffered a severe stroke in September, gradually lost consciousness, slipped into a coma, and died in late November. Murray Haydon remained in the hospital, since he had respiratory problems and infections.

In early April the family's regular meetings with DeVries began to take on a different tone. The doctor explained that a biopsy of Bill's liver over the past several weeks showed that the infection was getting worse, and nothing could be done to reverse it. He warned them that Bill's condition could only deteriorate.

The doctor showed the family some charts of the enzyme levels in Bill's liver, a measure of how the organ was functioning. Normally, patients whose levels were in the hundreds would be very, very ill. Bill's were slowly climbing above three thousand. Few people ever survived for long with such high enzyme levels, but again, Bill's artificial heart didn't suffer the damage which would be expected in patients with a normal heart. The focus of the Schroeders' discussions with DeVries now shifted from getting

Bill well to assuring the family members that the medical world was gaining unprecedented scientific knowledge from him, that he had confounded all the doctors' predictions, and that he was still making history every day. What DeVries was saying was that they had to start preparing for Bill's death. It was most likely that the liver infection would spread, and he would lapse into a coma and never come out of it. As time went on, the kidneys might fail, in which case the family would face the question of whether to put him on dialysis. Or his lungs might collapse, and they'd have to decide whether to put him on a respirator. Ultimately, if he were to lapse into a coma for a long time, they would have to decide whether to turn off the artificial heart and let him die.

It was difficult to imagine ever turning off the heart that Bill had wanted so badly, or ending the battle he had fought so hard. But the family unanimously agreed on one thing at this point: no more artificial measures.

At this point, the Schroeders also began to reflect on their own roles in the experiment. They recognized that they had entered the artificial heart program with very little understanding of what a medical experiment entailed. They knew that from the beginning they should have asked more questions. They definitely should have asked Bill what he wanted done in certain eventualities, such as being unable to talk or make decisions on his own or refuse certain tests. They should have discussed frankly how much each member of the family would be able to help out during and after Bill's hospitalization.

If they'd had to do it over, they would have insisted that from the beginning that Bill have a small, consistent team of nurses to follow him throughout the experiment. They would have made sure that a lawyer went over the consent form to advise them of their legal rights and responsibilities. They would have quizzed their family doctors on every aspect of the complications listed in it. The consent form had clearly stated that having an artificial heart meant the risk of stroke, but it couldn't list every implication—that, in turn, stroke might mean grueling, exhausting physical therapy, or, ultimately, a suctioning of his mouth and nose every few minutes. The family would also have tape-recorded more of their meetings with the medical team—something that might have made the doctors feel threatened, but that seemed the only way to be sure that everyone understood what was happening. It was too easy to get caught up in things and never really hear what the doctors had said.

They would have insisted that Bill and the family have regularly scheduled, inviolable private time together. And that, in turn, he be informed it was impossible for the family to be with him all the time—that they should probably spend one day a week away from him, from day one and consistently throughout.

The family also began to understand the trade-offs involved in any medical experiment, whether clinical trials of a new pain-killing drug or a new surgical device. Had they been asked to advise potential candidates for an artificial heart or any other experiment, they would have said:

You have to gamble on the possibility that the experiment might help you, but you also have to recognize that you will be part of a much larger project that may not save your life—that might even kill you—but could save the lives of thousands in the future. You have to accept the fact that, in a way, you will be donating your body to science while you are still alive. And you have to understand that your doctor will constantly struggle to walk a fine line between treating you and gathering data. You must understand and expect that mistakes will be made.

The Schroeders had thought all along that it was the artificial heart which was being tested. Now they realized that the experiment extended beyond the heart, the patient, the apartment—to the family itself. So many situations had come up that had never been faced before, and everyone, medical team and family alike, had had to make things up as they went along. And all of them had changed.

The whole family found themselves more serious than before, less certain that anything in life could ever come easily. The kids found that, in drawing closer to each other, they had lost touch with many of their friends. Their lives had become so unpredictable that they couldn't be counted on to join their old pals for outings or parties, and much of their leisure time was taken up by regular trips to Louisville anyway. They found it hard to start a project at home, even something as simple as painting a fence or planning a gathering, because they never knew if it would be interrupted. Many friends hesitated to bother them, uncertain whether to ask how their parents were doing. Sometimes the ordeal was the only thing the Schroeders wanted to talk about; sometimes they wished they didn't have to talk about it at all. They often felt set apart from everyone else, as if they had moved away for a long time and no longer fit into their old circles.

The Schroeders also were struck by how much DeVries

himself had changed. At the time of Bill's operation, the surgeon had looked like a skinny young man barely out of college. Within a year much of his sandy hair had turned silver, and his boyish, freckled face was deeply lined.

On some level Bill himself seemed to understand that he was still accomplishing something just by being alive, helping provide information that the doctors had never dreamed of obtaining. His medical chart now occupied more than eight feet of shelf space. When DeVries came to visit and tell him how much they were learning, Bill would listen and nod.

In fact, he often seemed more alert than ever during this period. He'd play possum sometimes, but if someone exclaimed at something seen out the window, he'd snap awake and look, too. If the doctors turned their backs to discuss his medical condition, Margaret could see Bill was craning his neck to look around them and listen. The doctors told her that it was possible that he was more alert and perceptive now because the damage from the strokes was continuing to resolve itself. Every once in a while, though, it took him a minute to recognize people.

There was a lot of time to think during those long days at Bill's bedside. Sometimes Margaret would get up to check the Utah console or look at the computer readouts, or just gaze in amazement at the machine that had become a part of her husband, that went wherever he went, and had never ceased its mechanical, life-giving rhythm. She would think back to her roots, in the hilly farm country outside Jasper, remembering how her grandmother used to come into the cabin with her apron full of sassafras roots for tea to thin her blood in the summertime, or hang leeks and herbs from the ceiling to dry for medicines. If Margaret could observe so much change in her own lifetime, she wondered, what was going to happen by the time the grandkids were grown?

Sometimes when DeVries talked to Margaret now, she wouldn't say a word to him. She was sure the doctor must think she was being angry or moody. That wasn't the case at all—it was that he'd gestured with his hands, and she couldn't take her eyes off them. *Those hands took out Bill's heart and put in an artificial one and made him live again. Those hands gave me back my husband.* Whatever their conflicts during the past, whatever the hardships and disappointments, and whatever was down the road, this fact remained: Those giant-sized hands had given Bill and the family some more time, moments that no one could ever take away. Just as nothing could change her gratitude toward Dr. De-Vries, she also knew that she could never find the words to thank him enough. And sometimes she just couldn't say anything at all to him.

Margaret and Bill continued to share little happy moments. Anyone who ever wondered whether the family had considered turning off the artificial heart had only to see the change in Bill's face whenever Margaret walked into the room, how his eyes would become bright and alert, how he'd lift his head for her kiss.

> Monday, Apr. 21. Came to hospital and Bill is sitting up in a chair. He is so glad to see me. He is so rambunctious. He sits up for two and a half hours. He stood on his legs and got back into bed. I had a big wrestle with him to stay in the bed. He wanted to get out and go home.
>
> Dear, sweet Bill. He just realized who I am. He hugged me and kissed me and patted me. I knew he knew me and wanted me beside him.

Bill kept fighting to stay alive, but the complications worsened. His mouth and nose were sore from being suctioned several times a day. The fevers came and went. His abdomen hurt from the liver infection. He continued receiving antibiotics and new experimental drugs to battle ongoing blood infections. The subclavian catheter required changing every few weeks. He had bruises up and down his arms from additional blood work and injections. He often had headaches. Now it was a good day if Margaret could get him to smile or look out the window and watch airplanes on their approach to nearby Standiford Field.

Family discussions with DeVries now centered on trying to bring Bill home one last time, for one night, if not for a weekend. They talked about maybe taking him up to the forty acres to see one final springtime. The kids were so much like their dad—they hated not to be able to *do* something special for him, and coming home was now the only thing they could think of that he would want. They tried to arrange a weekend when they could secure the personnel and equipment to make the journey. The heart institute staff thought they could probably schedule a trip for sometime in May.

But complications were slowly taking over. One Sunday,

when Margaret went back to Jasper for a visit, the family talked late into the night about bringing Bill home. He was so weak now that the long trip might wear him out and cause him physical discomfort. He might sleep the whole time he was home. Although they wanted so badly to bring him home, they finally had to ask themselves for whose benefit would it be? Would it be for Bill? Or for them? It was hard do admid, bet dhe family agreed that such a trip would hurt him more than it would help. So they decided to drop the idea. This decision meant that the family had also finally admitted something else:

Bill was running out of goals.

CHAPTER TWENTY-EIGHT

In late April Margaret took her wedding and engagement rings to a jeweler to have them enlarged because her fingers had remained swollen from arthritis. Bill hadn't worn his own wedding ring for a long time, and during those long hours sitting by his bed, she thought of having his ring melted down to wear on a necklace. She decided it should be in the shape of a heart—Bill's heart, a Jarvik-7. It might sound strange to anyone who hadn't gone through what both of them had endured. But would it really be any different from the way other people represent their own love with a heart? Margaret wanted to show Bill that she loved him just as he was, and she wanted to have a symbol of his heart with her always.

The jeweler did a beautiful job. The tiny Jarvik heart looked like a little silver flower until you looked at it up close. Jarvik himself visited Louisville that month, and told Margaret he loved her idea and thought it would be great to mass-produce the little hearts to give future Jarvik recipients.

Meanwhile, Murray Haydon's own complications had worsened, and he died in mid-June. Haydon had managed to take a van ride to his wife's apartment and a brief trip home a few miles away. But he had remained in intensive care throughout most of his time with the artificial heart. Margaret had grown close to Juanita, and Murray's death hit the Schroeder family hard.

DeVries had told the Schroeders that Bill might die anytime now. And when the family went to pay their respects to the Haydons, it finally sank in that they could no longer postpone their own eventualities. So back home, they set about making arrangements, hoping that nobody would spot them going into the funeral home and alert the media. There were also legal matters to attend to. Before his surgery Bill had stubbornly refused to make out a will; doing so would have meant admitting that the

351

artificial heart might not work. Margaret also followed DeVries's advice to make herself Bill's legal guardian, in case there were ever any question about the family's right to turn off the artificial heart.

As usual, Margaret and the family had to consider the public-relations aspects of Bill's impending death. She informed the PR staff that she didn't want DeVries simply to read a statement from the family at the medical briefing he would have to give. She wanted to bring the family out with her before the media, to show support for the doctor's program, and perhaps answer reporters' questions. The PR officials were a little taken aback. They could remember how shy Margaret had been when she brought Bill to the hospital. But they told her if she really wanted to do that when the time came, they'd see what they could do.

At the same time, as it became clear that Bill was dying, more and more staffers came to visit him and Margaret, offering encouragement and telling Bill that they appreciated his courage and perseverance.

By late June Bill's throat was so swollen and raw from suctioning that it was impossible to keep the feeding tube in it. DeVries told Margaret Bill would have to be fed through a gastrostomy tube, or G-tube, directly into his stomach. He was put under general anesthesia for the operation. But there were problems with the G-tube: The stomach wall was bleeding slowly and it, too, had to be suctioned through the gastrostomy.

Bill began to have spells of choking on the secretions in his throat; he'd gasp for air, turn red, and stop breathing altogether. The nurses would put a rubber bag over his nose and mouth to squeeze air into his lungs (a procedure called "bagging") until he could breathe on his own again. They had to suction him often, sometimes every few minutes. He wore an oxygen mask over his face all of the time now to help his breathing. He had a couple of seizures, not like the earlier episodes where he just stared, but real seizures in which his body shook violently. He coughed frequently to clear the secretions, and sometimes he would be so exhausted that he'd moan loudly. At night Margaret would dream that Bill was slipping down a steep, muddy riverbank, and that she was gripping his hand for dear life.

In late July DeVries advised Margaret that she should consider a tracheostomy, or trach, for Bill. This would mean cutting a hole directly into his windpipe and fitting it with a plastic lid a little larger than the diameter of a pencil, which would open and close as he inhaled and exhaled through the hole. It would not be a pleasant sight. But his mouth and nose were raw from the suctioning, and with a trach they could suction directly from the throat. It might also make his breathing a little easier. But it would also mean the stress of yet another surgery under general anesthesia, and initially Bill might have a hard time getting used to breathing through a hole in his throat. Margaret asked everyone she knew on the medical staff for advice. No one could give her a definitive answer; it was hard to say what was right, they all told her. They took her to meet a couple of patients who'd had trachs. She felt a little woozy the first time she saw one, but decided she could get used to it if she had to, and hoped Bill could, too. The staffers told her she'd just have to make the decision, and not look back. For several days, Margaret sat by Bill's bed and tried to explain the options to him. She'd ask what he wanted to do, but he would just look at her steadily and shrug: He didn't know.

Of all the decisions she'd faced so far, this one had to be the hardest. There was no clear right or wrong. The doctors seemed to think that it would make him a little more comfortable. The biggest drawback would be that it would prevent his ever really talking again—and hearing Bill say something was about the only thing the family had left to hope for.

Margaret didn't want the kids to feel responsible for the decision, so instead of polling them the way she usually did, she spoke only to Mel and Moni. On July 28 Margaret signed a form authorizing the tracheostomy for the following day, and told Mel and Moni they didn't have to come down.

Again, Bill was given a general anesthetic, and again, there was another long wait during the operation. The trach did seem to help his breathing, and he no longer needed the oxygen mask. It also made his sleep less fitful, and he slept most of the next day. But afterward there was a different look in his eyes.

Wednesday, July 30. Bill is staring right past me. It is so scary. . . . There is always something for Bill to cope with. He never has a whole good day anymore.

That week DeVries told a reporter that Bill was "as strong a person physiologically as I've ever encountered in medicine.

He's shown incredible recuperative powers. He amazes me every day."

Friday, Aug. 1. Bill is sleeping as usual. He looks real good. I hope he is getting used to the trach. I think it's really going to help him, but it takes some getting used to. I can't get over how I can see his face. No tubes at all . . .

Saturday, Aug. 2. Bill is sleeping so much. . . . I think Bill is depressed. I think he just doesn't care right now. I hope I can get him to smile again.

Up in Jasper, it was Strassenfest weekend. It was hard to believe it had been a whole year since Bill was there. Sunday was a long, quiet day—no visitors, just Bill and Margaret. Bill wasn't coughing or needing to be suctioned so much. But he looked so weak and tired and miserable. Margaret could see that he was in constant pain. At one point, he reached for her hand. She could never express how much that tiny gesture delighted her. Bill felt the wedding and engagement rings on her finger, and looked at her.

Sunday, Aug. 3. . . . I told him the rings are from him and I love them. I said, "I have your ring on me, too— do you remember that I told you I had this heart made from your ring?" He reached up and felt it. I said, "Do you like it?" He shook his head "Yes."

I was so tickled, for this is the first time since the [trach] operation he has tried to communicate with me. I know he hasn't given up yet.

On Monday, August 4, Bill ran another fever. He was sleeping almost all the time now. Margaret had seen him look weary before, but she would never have imagined that he could look so exhausted, so defeated. All those machines, all those plastic pieces . . .

Late that afternoon, Bill opened his eyes, just barely. The look Margaret saw in them was unbearably sad. She knew that every part of his body was so tired from hurting. What could he possibly be hanging on for now?

She sat watching him for a long time, thinking about this wonderful man, all the happy years he had given her, the six kids they'd raised together. Finally, she leaned close to him, smoothed his hair, and kissed him softly. "Sweetie, you know what?" she whispered. "You can close your eyes if you want to, and just sleep for a long time. It's all right with me, Bill. I'll be right here with you, okay? I know you're tired. You just go ahead and sleep." She was telling him the best way she knew how.

Bill was sleeping deeply when Margaret left his room that evening. By shift change the next morning, Bill was having a hard time breathing. Around 7:30, nurse Cheryl Ailiff tried to awaken him, but his eyes wouldn't open. She could see that something was different. About a half hour later, DeVries came on rounds and made some quick checks for responsiveness.

Bill was comatose. The surgeon instructed Cheryl to call Margaret and Dr. Fox immediately.

A few minutes later, Bill stopped breathing. Cheryl started bagging him. Soon Margaret arrived, and she held Bill's hand and talked to him until Cheryl stopped the bagging and Bill was breathing on his own again.

When DeVries looked up from the other side of the bed, Margaret knew what he was going to say. "It's time we talked, Margaret," DeVries told her. "And I think you'd better call the kids right away."

CHAPTER TWENTY-NINE

Mel was away from his desk when he was paged for a phone call at work. He picked up the phone at the receptionist's desk in the front office, but he didn't recognize the woman's voice on the other end of the line: "Mel, I'm afraid this is that phone call you haven't been waiting for."

He turned the sentence over and over in his mind, finally realizing that he was hearing his mother's voice. Then the words exploded inside him like a bomb.

As the receptionist looked on, Mel began shaking. "What happened?" he asked. Just the night before, Mom had called him to say that Dad wasn't doing very well, but by now that was nothing unusual.

Now she told him there wasn't really time to explain except that it looked like his father's time was at hand. He could be put on a respirator, but the family had already decided against doing that.

Mel tried to assure his mother that the family would stand by that decision. "Okay, Mom," he said, struggling to sound calm. "Okay. Don't worry. I'll call all the kids and we'll come right down."

Margaret told him to be careful and not to drive too fast. Mel ran upstairs to his office, called Cheryl, and told her that Dad was doing worse.

"How bad is he?" Cheryl asked. Mel repeated what Margaret had said, adding that he was leaving for Louisville right away. His quavering voice told her more than his words. Cheryl said that she'd call Stan and Moni while he called Terry and Rod.

Rod was working his regular shift at the wood factory. Mel called the receptionist there, identified himself, saying that he needed to speak with Rod immediately. Someone went to tell Rod he had an emergency call. Everyone there knew that he was Bill

Schroeder's son, and quickly realized what had happened. Rod made his way between the long rows of machinery, trying to stay calm inside, hurrying but not walking too fast, aware that all of his co-workers were watching.

As Mel waited for him to come to the phone, his reeling mind began to focus. What if they didn't make it to Louisville in time? What if Mom had to go through this alone? Or what if only some of the kids made it before Dad died? It just wasn't fair, it wasn't fair. Dad had fought so hard. After twenty-one months, and all the ups and downs, it shouldn't be a shock, but it *was* a shock—it was a terrible one. All this time to prepare, and he had never expected to feel like this. Why somebody like Dad, who had fought so hard for so long, and wanted so desperately to live? Maybe it was just another false alarm. But somehow this time felt different.

When Rod came to the phone, Mel tried hard to keep control as he informed his youngest brother, but there was no way to make it hurt any less. Rod said he'd meet Mel at the Mill Street house.

Mel then called Terry at work. Terry was supposed to take over a delivery route that afternoon for a co-worker who was on vacation.

Mel told him to do what he thought he should, and said all the other kids would leave for Louisville shortly. Terry called his mom and asked how badly Dad was doing. Margaret knew that her kids had gone through plenty of scares before, so she didn't pressure him to come down, but just told him to do what he had to. Maybe Bill could pull through again somehow. Terry told her he'd finish the delivery route as fast as possible, he'd check in between stops, then drive to Louisville immediately afterward.

At the house, Stan and Rod were getting showered and packing clothes. Mel soon arrived, but he grew too anxious waiting, and said he'd meet them at the hospital. Then he ran to his truck and sped out of Jasper.

Along the highway, which had become so familiar, Mel rolled down the window and let the hot wind fill his ears so he wouldn't hear himself crying. Now was the time for that. Later, he'd have to be strong for his mom—they'd all have to. She was there all alone. Had it already happened? Had Dad already died? Was it happening right now? He screamed and cried and pounded the dashboard.

When Mel reached the hospital, he ran to the second-floor offices of the heart institute, unsure where his parents would be. Polly Brown quickly led him to Bill's room. They walked in and saw what looked like a reunion of all the people who'd ever been associated with Bill and Margaret: Dr. DeVries, Kevan Shaheen, nurses Cheryl Ailiff, Trish Haaker, Bea Bryant, John Lammers, Laura Wood, and technician Lawrence Barker. Margaret quickly reached out for Mel, and they hugged for a long time, weeping silently. After a while, when DeVries started talking, he sounded as if he were stumped by some impossible puzzle.

"He stopped breathing," DeVries said, shaking his head, "but now he seems to be breathing on his own again. I don't know. I really thought this was it." He almost seemed to be apologizing to Margaret for telling her to call the kids.

It was a comfort to see that Bill was still breathing. Mel went to his father's side, took his hand, told him that he loved him. There was no need to be afraid; all the kids would be there soon, Mel said. Everyone but Cheryl Ailiff left the room to give them some time alone together. Margaret and Mel stood over the bed, not knowing for sure whether Bill could hear them. Something made them sense that he was still there—but they knew he couldn't hang on much longer.

Cheryl busily started new medicines through IVs, took Bill's blood pressure, and occasionally shone a small flashlight into his eyes to check for responsiveness. Mel stood with his arm around his mother. Margaret just kept looking at Bill.

Cheryl and Glenn arrived within thirty minutes, and the whole sequence of hugging, comforting, and explaining started again. Stan, Terri, Rod, and Lori were next to arrive. It was the first time any of the kids besides Mel had seen the trach, and they felt a little woozy at first. Margaret couldn't reach Moni at home until about 1:00 P.M. Moni said she'd, make preparations to leave, but first she would have to try to reach her husband, Bob, at work.

Bill was lying almost completely still, barely breathing. The kids tried to get their mother to sit down to eat something. The family took turns walking down to the small conference room where they'd assembled so many times before—for the gallbladder surgery, the implant, the return to surgery, after the strokes. The hospital provided them with sandwiches, soft drinks, and coffee.

Then Polly came in and asked her usual questions: "What do you need right now? What can I get you?"

Mel tried to smile. "Right now, Polly, I could use a stiff drink."

Polly left the room. Within minutes, she returned with two cold bottles of champagne. Good old Polly. The Schroeders decided to save it for later.

Shortly before three that afternoon, Dr. DeVries came in and said the blood-gases tests showed the oxygen content was declining. He estimated that Bill would live another two hours at the most. The family members had gathered their composure, but hearing the doctor's words hit home, and there were more tears.

Now the Schroeders turned their attention to Terry and Moni. There was no way either of them could make it to the hospital in two hours. Cheryl phoned Moni again. Moni asked just how bad it was this time. Cheryl assured her sister that this was it, that she should prepare for the worst. That was all she needed to hear, and said she'd come right away. They also tried to reach Terry, but he was still hurrying to finish his delivery route.

By now, word had leaked to the media. Too many people had access to the hallway near Bill's room, and too many of the kids' co-workers in Jasper had seen them leave in a hurry. Dozens of people could have passed along the news. From now on, the PR staff would have to be involved. Donna Hazle couldn't just tell all the reporters that nothing was going on. Since Bill had only an hour or two left, Donna set about scheduling a press conference for 8:00 A.M. the following morning. Donna wrote a brief update for the telephone recording line and had the family approve it.

Margaret and the kids returned to Bill's side, where they stayed for the next two hours. They took turns bending close to his ear, telling him that they loved him, how proud they were of him, and that it was all right. During that time, the strangest feelings came and went. Sometimes they felt as if they all had an empty space somewhere inside of their bodies, like a physical part of them had actually been removed. None of them lost control of their emotions at the same time—it was as if they were taking turns to be sure that at least one among them could be strong and take charge. Sometimes they felt dry, empty, and numb, and sometimes as if they would never stop crying. At other times they felt drunk, as if everything inside was spinning.

Cheryl, the nurse, was fighting tears as she tried to concentrate on her duties, taking blood-pressure readings, and checking blood gases. After each test, the family wanted to know the results and how Bill was doing. So far, she said, he was holding his own, not getting worse, but not getting better, either.

Those two hours ticked by, while they all reached for, held, touched each other. As he had always been, Bill was at the center of his family. The kids also tried to watch out for their mother's condition. She'd been there twenty-one months and they knew she wouldn't leave his side for any reason now. They made sure she sat down at regular intervals and propped up her feet, and they kept checking the clock to make sure she took her medicines on time.

At the end of two hours, DeVries returned, figuring that Bill would be near the end. The doctor was amazed to find that his patient's vital signs were actually improving. Bill's pupils, which had remained fixed when a light was shone in them, were now dilating. DeVries said he'd never seen anything like it.

It became apparent that there could be only one reason that Bill was hanging on: He was waiting for Terry and Moni to get there. It would be his last fight for life.

By 6:00 P.M. Bill had improved even more. DeVries shook his head and apologized. "I don't know. Maybe he's pulling out of it. He looks better to me." He shrugged. The family was somewhat relieved. Terry and Moni might make it after all now. That was important; they'd gone into this as a family, and if it had to end now, they wanted to be together as a family again.

Soon Terry called to find out how his dad was doing. Stan answered that Bill was waiting for him. A little after 8:00 P.M., Moni arrived, only to find that Bill was fairly stable and breathing on his own. She shook her head in amazement. "Every time I get here, he's doing better!" Terry and Julie arrived at 8:30. Now they were all there.

Someone ordered carry-out fried chicken and the family had supper. By late evening, Bill was still doing relatively well, so Lori, Glenn, and Terri decided to return home. Stan and Rod also decided to go home for the night and come back the next morning with fresh clothes for everybody. It seemed like a good idea; Bill was stable, Stan and Terri had to look in on the baby, and besides, Rod was uneasy cooped up in the hospital. It might be days before the end.

The rest of the family walked over to the apartment. They watched the eleven o'clock news as somber announcers reported that Bill Schroeder had taken "a serious turn for the worse" and that all his children had been summoned to the hospital. The kids shared some fond memories of their father, occasionally trying to make jokes to lighten the mood. Margaret couldn't stop moving around the apartment—doing laundry, washing dishes, cleaning. Everyone was tired, but no one felt like sleeping. It was after 1:00 A.M. before they all went to sleep. A few times during the night, the kids heard their mom phoning the hospital to check on Bill's condition. He was still holding his own.

By 7:00 A.M. everyone was up and moving around. Terry and Mel got ready first and drove over to the hospital, passing a camera crew along the way. When the boys pulled into the underground parking lot and hurried toward an entrance, a newsman called out, "How's Dad doing?" but Terry and Mel kept walking.

Wednesday morning found Bill the same as he'd been the night before. Stan and Rod were on their way back from Jasper with clothes for everyone, but the kids were already contemplating going home at the end of the day. The family gathered in the hospital room as doctors came and went. Dr. Hoskins, the internist, examined Bill and looked at his chart. He told the family he suspected Bill had had another stroke. His kidneys were still functioning, but just barely. They'd have to wait and see, but if the kidneys continued to deteriorate, that could be the end. The family had already discussed that eventuality and concluded: no dialysis, no respirator, no more machines. Fox, the neurologist, ran his tracing wheel along the soles of Bill's feet, noting minimal facial response. Fox told them that Bill's condition might be due to a respiratory problem, rather than a stroke. But since he wasn't sure, he ordered an EEG and a CAT scan.

The family was talking quietly in the room when suddenly Bill got an expression on his face as if he'd tasted something awful. He turned a violet blue. Cheryl Ailiff, who'd been talking on the phone, quickly hung up and grabbed the bag to assist his breathing as Margaret and the kids gathered around the bed. Cheryl told them to hit the call button on the intercom and ask for help. Seconds later, the room was filled with nurses. STAT calls went out to Dr. DeVries and the respiratory department.

The nurses again tried to revive him. The Schroeders watched anxiously, helpless again. The phone wouldn't stop ringing. Cheryl Ailiff gave the bag to another nurse so she could answer it and make her report. Soon Bill was breathing on his own again. Staffers were now hurrying in and out of the room. A few minutes later, DeVries came in. He observed Bill's breathing, then looked at his chart, and talked with Cheryl Ailiff. He mentioned doing a "bronch" on Bill, but added that he wasn't sure he should.

As the doctor started to leave, Mel asked him what was going on: Hoskins says a stroke, Fox says a breathing problem. DeVries replied that no one knew for sure, and it was only a guess at that point. The tests should provide answers.

The family took turns staying with Bill by twos and threes. Terry, Stan, and especially Rod restlessly walked the hospital corridors, checking in on their father, then going down the hall to the conference room, which again was supplied with sandwiches and snacks. Mel was running back and forth between Bill's room, the conference room, and Donna Hazle's office to work out the final public-relations arrangements.

An EEG technician ran a brain-wave test on Bill, inserting just under his scalp the now-familiar series of needles attached to electrodes. Terry looked at the wavy lines on the readout. The lines didn't mean much to him, so he asked the technician if things looked okay.

"We'll wait until the doctor reads it," she replied.

It didn't sound good. Technician Lawrence Barker came in and switched Bill to the Heimes. As Mel helped Lawrence and several others lift Bill onto a stretcher for the CAT scan, they all gently explained to him what they were doing. Bill didn't respond at all.

Margaret and Mel accompanied Bill downstairs, along with Captain Tom from security, Lawrence Barker, Cheryl Ailiff, heart technician Melissa Williams, and an orderly. Along the way, people were pulling Margaret aside to wish her luck. By that time, there weren't many people she didn't know, and all of them, from the cleaning crews to the doctors, let her know their thoughts were with her.

As Bill was put through the scanner, the group watched the black-and-white images on the monitor, remembering that dark spots indicated areas of stroke damage. They could see several such spots. As a doctor studied the results, they asked him how the scan looked. He told them that he would have to compare it with previous scans, but it appeared that some new areas were affected.

They took Bill back upstairs. The family looked at Cheryl Ailiff, who was usually talkative and always thoroughly explained test results to them. Now she wasn't saying a word, and trying hard not to cry.

Mel whispered to her, "It doesn't look good, does it?"

Her silence said it all.

When she and Mel were alone for a moment, he asked her what to expect. He didn't really want to know, but felt he had to.

Cheryl understood. First, she told him, the fingernails and feet would begin to turn blue. The body would start getting cold, then slowly turn a light gray. She had looked after Bill for almost a year now, learning to read his large brown eyes, which could stare holes through her if he was angry, and make her smile when something struck him funny. She, like the family, was preparing herself to let go.

It was just a matter of time now. The family were trying to console each other, saying that he was tired, and it was finally time for him to rest. He'd done his work. Damn, had he done his work!

Then it was lunchtime. Bill seemed fairly stable, so the kids convinced Margaret to leave for a quick lunch in the conference room. They talked about how it felt like they were all in some kind of dream. And this seemed the most unreal part of all: Dad had always come up with an answer for everything. Even with an artificial heart, he had always found a way to bounce back. Even the doctors had stopped making predictions. Dad had stared down certain death so many times, and death had always blinked. Maybe he could do it again.

Gary Rhine, the social worker, sat with the family for a while, and asked them how they felt about the past twenty-one months, what the biggest problem had been.

Immediately, everyone answered, "The nursing arrangements." Especially at the apartment, they explained. Trish, Cheryl, and Bea were some of the best nurses Bill ever had—but it had been a whole year before they'd come on the case.

About 1:00 P.M. Dr. DeVries and Dr. Fox came in. The test results suggested that Bill had suffered another stroke, which had damaged the part of his brain responsible for respiratory function. His breaths were growing shallower, and he was taking fewer and fewer of them—only about eight per minute. His lungs were increasingly congested and he was almost too weak to cough. Since the family had already decided unanimously not to prolong Bill's death with artificial measures, DeVries told them that Bill wouldn't be "bagged" anymore. He did say that it might help Bill to have a bronchoscopy, a common procedure for intensive-care patients in respiratory distress. This would involve sticking a long, flexible tube through the tracheostomy and into the lungs to suction them directly. The scope would be over quickly and would involve very little pain. On the one hand, De-Vries told them, suctioning the lungs should make Bill more comfortable, decrease his need to cough, and might stimulate his lungs enough to help his breathing pick up again. But on the other hand, DeVries said, the scope might not help, and Bill's respiratory function would continue to decline until he died.

It was hard for the family to know what to decide at this point. Did Bill really need to go through one more procedure now? Both DeVries and Fox told the Schroeders that they thought the bronchoscopy would make Bill more comfortable, and that would also give them important clues about whether the cause of his respiratory distress was solely neurological—a result of the stroke—or whether it was due to preexisting lung complications. What could the family really say? The doctors said they believed the scope would help Bill, so the Schroeders agreed to it.

The whole family sensed that the end was near. It felt so strange—even now a part of themselves still prayed Dad could somehow come out of this one, too. The family went back down to have a moment with Bill just before the bronchoscopy. Each of them took a turn holding Bill's hand, telling him that they loved him and it was going to be all right.

"This won't take long," DeVries said. "I really don't know if his breathing will pick up again or not." The surgeon suggested that the family leave momentarily because it might be unpleasant to watch, and said he'd let them know as soon as the procedure was over. Moni and Cheryl decided to stay, along with John Lammers, and the rest of the family stepped out into the hall.

DeVries peered through the bronchoscope, then suctioned the lungs. John Lammers stepped out to get the family. Bill's breaths were increasingly feeble now. As the Schroeders filed back in, DeVries told them that it might take a few minutes for Bill's breathing to improve, if it was going to at all. They all gathered around the bed, and DeVries stepped back to give them room. Margaret held Bill's hand close to her. She hadn't told the kids what she had said to him the day before. Now she was crying softly. "Honey," she said, "I've done all I can for you. The rest is up to you now. I love you." She knew he was so tired. It was all right.

The family watched and waited, straining to hear the sounds of breathing over the steady whoosh of the Utah and the ticking of the artificial heart. It was hard to tell whether Bill was breathing at all. They felt a pressure building up inside them, a pressure that squeezed tears from their eyes. The kids tried to encourage their father.

Two minutes passed, then three.

"Come on, Dad."

"You can do it."

Five minutes.

"Hang in there, Dad. It's okay. We're right with you."

Eight minutes.

Bill had tried his hardest, and fought so long. If anyone deserved to rest, he did. But it was just so hard to see him admit defeat. Finally.

Ten minutes.

"Dad, I love you."

It happened just as the nurse had said it would.

For once, there were no cameras, no reporters. Just a few of the hospital workers who had become like family and shared their sorrow. The family hugged each other tightly and told Bill, "It's all over, Dad. We're proud of you."

Margaret couldn't say a word.

DeVries moved closer to the bed and leaned over to check for signs of breathing. He found none.

"I'll send for Dr. Fox," he said. The neurologist would have to make an official determination that brain death had occurred.

A few minutes later, Fox arrived. He didn't say anything, but moved toward Bill and began routine tests to declare a person brain-dead. He shone a flashlight into Bill's eyes, checking for dilation of the pupils. Nothing. He rolled the tracing wheel along the bottom of each foot one last time. No response. He instructed the nurse to bring a pan of ice-cold water as he prepared a large syringelike tube. He filled the tube with water, lifted Bill's eyelids to watch for a reflex as he squirted water into his ear.

First the left ear, then the right. Nothing. It was official now. There was only one thing left to do: turn off Bill's heart.

The family were still hugging each other, comforting themselves and each other with how peaceful Bill looked. DeVries reminded them about something they had discussed earlier: He wanted to run one last test to measure blood flow through the body so they could compare the reading after 620 days with those taken immediately after surgery. The results would indicate the amount of wear and tear on the artificial heart after all this time in a human body. It was a very important test, he'd told them, one that could give them data they'd never had before, since no human being or laboratory animal had lived nearly so long with an artificial heart.

The family had forgotten the discussion about the test and the fact that they'd agreed to it. But once more, they complied. The test would take about half an hour, DeVries said, and he promised he would send for them when it was time to turn off the machine.

So the family struggled to regain their composure and headed out the door to the conference room. At the door the hospital priest greeted them and said he'd be available if they wanted him. Next, Dr. Dageforde, the cardiologist who had admitted Bill to Audubon, offered his condolences. As the Schroeders made their way down the hall, about two dozen nurses were waiting for them, standing along the corridor in a kind of receiving line. Nearly every one of them had taken care of Bill at one time or another, and many of them needed to share their own grief. They all knew Margaret better than any of the family, so the kids waited as she went along the line and embraced each one. Now other people appeared, many in tears, and one by one, they gave Margaret a long, tight hug—doctors, security guards, hospital officials, cleaning crews, respiratory therapists.

The Schroeders finally reached the conference room and sat down, numb. It was still so hard to believe that after twenty-one months with the artificial heart, Bill was really gone. It seemed as if he had just been taken downstairs for some test and any minute they'd be wheeling him back.

There wasn't much time to reflect, though, because almost immediately PR officials came in to discuss the press conference they had planned for eight that evening. It didn't seem strange at all to be working out public-relations questions at such a time; in fact, the family had always been grateful for the way the PR staff had managed to walk the fine line between protecting the family's privacy and providing information to the media.

A hospital administrator, Charlie Mayer, soon came by to work out details of the memorial service for the benefit of the hospital staff who couldn't attend the funeral in Jasper. The family still hadn't heard from DeVries. Every once in a while someone would break the silence by saying some comforting thoughts about how Dad had done what he wanted to do and they'd all supported him, and how maybe this was all for the best.

Moni spoke up: "Well, they say that every time there's a death, a new baby is born someplace. So maybe the next baby boy in this hospital should be named William." Everyone smiled a little.

The door opened and Bea, Bill's nurse on the night shift, came in. She and Margaret embraced for a long time. Then Bea tried to cheer her up by saying that she'd received some happy news that day along with the sad.

"Remember my sister in New Jersey who was pregnant?"

"Uh-huh." Margaret wiped her eyes and nodded. She knew those nurses' families as well as her own. "Did she have her baby?"

"She had *twins!*" Bea said excitedly. "Can you believe it? A girl *and* a boy! She didn't even know she was carrying two babies. The doctors had heard only one heartbeat!"

The whole family looked at Moni. She was just as stunned as they were.

"Well," Margaret couldn't help asking, "what did they name the boy?"

"Andrew William."

The test went on for an hour and a half. Finally, Dr. DeVries came in to say they were ready. One last time, Margaret and all of the kids filed out of the conference room. Everyone along the hallway knew exactly where the family were going, and what they were about to do. As Margaret made her way down the hall, looking straight ahead, many staffers who watched her were thinking back to almost two years before. This was not the same woman they'd had to hold up, literally, after her husband was wheeled into the operating suite or outside his intensive-care room after that devastating first stroke. This woman was not only standing on her own, but walking resolutely, surrounded by her children, determined to finish what they had all begun together.

When the family returned to Bill's room, the technicians were already beginning to move out some of the equipment. They and a few nurses closest to the family quietly lined up along the window. The family gathered once more around Bill's bed.

DeVries said he thought it would be best for all concerned if he turned off the key to the Utah himself. The family had already discussed this and told DeVries they felt it was important for them all to join him. He nodded.

DeVries took the shiny, silver-colored key from its place inside the Utah's cabinet and leaned over to insert it in the lock on the front of the console. As DeVries held it there, Margaret placed her hand on top of his, followed by each of the children. In a single, unified act, they turned the key counterclockwise to the OFF position.

The artificial heart, which had clicked inside of Bill's chest more than sixty-eight million times, stopped.

In the resounding silence, Bill's children moved toward the bed and, one by one, kissed his forehead and whispered to him. Margaret stood beside him, holding his hand. She had begun to cry hard.

Bill had finished his work. The family knew that he was finally at peace. But it was still so hard to turn away and leave him.

Margaret and the kids walked over to the apartment to wait for the press conference to start. It was already four in the afternoon. Mel began writing a brief speech. Meanwhile, the medical team performed an autopsy, removing the heart for further study.

Everything was still happening so fast. The kids all had a drink to relax and to toast Bill's courage. As with every Schroeder gathering, soon all were sharing stories. Polly came by, kicked off her shoes, and sat on the floor with Margaret and the kids as all the good memories of Bill began coming back, the happy and funny occasions: his jokes, the times he played possum, the day a few weeks after he'd had the first stroke when Polly pestered him to blow her a kiss and he flipped her a bird instead. Some of the kids got restless and drove to K mart to buy some clothes—mostly just to get out and move around. Mel stayed and worked on the family's statement, then he and Polly returned to the hospital to have it typed and photocopied for the press.

Back at the apartment, some of the kids sat outside on the porch in the late-afternoon sun, talking about how strange they felt. They went over the statement to the media which Mel had written, adding suggestions. Soon it was time to go to Donna Hazle's office to prepare for the press conference. The family was escorted into the hall outside the briefing room. A quick peek through the door revealed about one hundred reporters and staffers in the audience and a wall of television cameras. Again, the Schroeders wiped their palms nervously as they had during their first press conference. This time, however, their worry was that they might fall apart in front of the media. The room was hushed as the family members filed in and took their places around the podium. Margaret stood close to Mel as he took the statement from his shirt pocket and unfolded it. His voice wavered only a little, right at the beginning:

"We have been through many rough times in the past twenty-one months, but the past two days have been the hardest. We are all saddened by the loss of our father, a truly great person.

"Six hundred twenty days ago, we came to Humana and to Dr. DeVries to take a desperate chance to give new life to a father we all loved so very much. We leave today taking the sweet memories of this brave and pioneering man: his positive attitude at any situation, his forever good humor, a smile and wave for everyone, his determination and will power. All of these attributes helped brighten our lives and the lives of the people around him. We remember all the holiday celebrations, special family times, van rides, the ball game, fishing trips, the return visit home and many other joys of life he shared with us.

"We came seeking no glory or praise. We leave with newly cherished friends. There is an unending list of persons we would like to thank. For those people who took that extra minute to write a line, say a silent prayer, or stop by just to say 'Hi,' along with the many devoted professionals who spent long hours treating and caring for Bill, we extend our thanks. Friendship isn't just something you make or buy, rather it is something you earn. So many people have earned our everlasting friendship.

"We came with the thought of benefiting people in the future. We leave with the knowledge of twenty-one recipients of bridge-to-transplants throughout the world. The future will speak for itself on the contributions Bill Schroeder and the other permanent heart implant patients have made to mankind. These people are truly remarkable individuals. This should not be considered the end of the artificial heart program, but a continuation of the beginning.

"Finally, we started this experiment as a supportive family, sharing our lives with everyone here and with the world. Today we leave you as that same united family, with all our respect and admiration for a pioneer, a father, and a husband that we will never, ever forget."

The family said thanks and quickly left the room. They went directly to the doctors' lounge, where Bill had attended Terry's stag party. About one hundred staffers had gathered there for the brief memorial ceremony conducted by a priest. Margaret gave another short statement, telling the hospital workers that the family felt as though they were among friends. She finished by saying: "I'd tell you how Bill felt about everyone here, but I'll let him speak for himself."

Someone rolled a videotape. There was Bill, rosy-cheeked and grinning from ear to ear, saying: "They've been awful nice to me. Just one super, super-duper crew . . ." Many staffers wiped away tears—they'd all forgotten what Bill's voice sounded like. Afterward many of them said their good-byes to the family, and several asked for maps to Jasper so they could attend the funeral.

The family returned to the apartment. Now it was time to uncork the champagne. The eleven o'clock news came on and, of course, once again the Schroeders were all over the screen. It brought back memories of those first days after the implant. It was so hard to believe it had been twenty-one months ago. It was even harder to believe that it was really over. The family drove back to Jasper that night. Just as in the beginning, nobody slept well.

For the next two days, the family were at the Becher-Kluesner Funeral Home in Jasper for the viewing. Naturally, no matter how much preparing is done for a funeral, there are always a hundred more things to take care of. So many of those who came to pay their respects apparently thought that the family must be relieved to have the ordeal finally over, that Bill's death really was a blessing. It was very hard to explain that even as physical complications had whittled away his dreams, he had still been so full of life for so long. How could they explain that as they learned to keep their hopes flexible, they had been surprised themselves to find joy in the littlest moments they shared with Bill, in his tiniest gestures? How could they explain that until the end he had reached out for Margaret's kiss as soon as she came into his room—and sometimes this alone was enough to keep them both going? Maybe precisely because he had fought so long and so hard, it was scarcely a relief to lose him.

Donna Hazle informed the Schroeders that there was already a long list of reporters wanting interviews as soon as the family was ready for them. In the past, whenever another implant was performed, the press had called the Schroeders for their opinions. The family wondered whether this would be the last of all the questions or just the beginning. It had just become a part of their lives for so long, they weren't sure what was normal anymore.

Dr. Jarvik showed up at the funeral home. He spent a lot of time with the family, even stood with them for a while in the receiving line. He was so young-looking that many visitors asked whether he was one of the Schroeder kids. Jarvik would put his arm around Margaret and grin, saying, "Sure, I'm her youngest kid."

The family was just about to leave the funeral home for the night, when Dr. DeVries called to say he was on his way with his wife and nine-year-old son. The Schroeders stayed, and when the DeVrieses got there, they all had a brief prayer service before Bill's open casket. Several weeks earlier, DeVries had agreed to Margaret's request that he give the eulogy at Bill's funeral. Doctors usually don't even attend patients' funerals because of an unwritten rule about maintaining professional distance. But DeVries had thought it over and decided that if he was going to worry about criticism from some colleagues, he should have started a long time ago. He wasn't exactly sure what to do; he had attended only two other funerals in his life, not for relatives, but for Barney Clark and Murray Haydon. But that evening DeVries told Margaret that he would honor his commitment.

The next morning, there was a steady drizzle under solid gray skies. The family again met at the funeral home for a brief service. One by one, they stepped up to the casket, slipped a photo into Bill's coat pocket, told him they were going to miss him, and said their last good-byes. When it was Margaret's turn, Terry and Mel moved to either side of her so they could walk with her, but she said she wanted to go by herself. The rest of the family stepped back to give her some moments alone with him. She began to sob. They could hear her saying something to him, but couldn't make out what it was.

The coffin was closed and draped with an American flag. The pallbearers gathered—Mel, Stan, Terry, Rod, Moni's husband, Bob, and Cheryl's fiancé, Glenn. It was raining steadily as they lifted the casket into the hearse. The family scattered to their cars and drove to the church. The parking lot was packed, and the family had to pass a line of cameras on the way into the church.

Bill's uncle, Father Othmar Schroeder, led the procession, followed by honorary pallbearers chosen to represent significant portions of Bill's life: technicians Brent Mays and Lawrence Barker, nurses John Lammers and Bill Binggeli, Jasper mayor Jerome Alles, Bill's high-school classmate John Bohnert, John Brown from the union, and Drs. DeVries and Jarvik. Trish, Cheryl, and Bea, the three nurses who had cared for Bill in his final months, were behind them, carrying offerings for the mass. Next came the pallbearers with the casket, followed by Cheryl, Margaret, and Moni.

It was a traditional Catholic funeral mass, with one exception: At the "passing of the peace," Margaret and the kids formed a circle around the casket, and held hands in prayer. It just seemed like the right thing to do.

DeVries's voice was somber but controlled as he gave the eulogy. He praised Bill as a man who loved life, comparing him to a man who plants the seed of a walnut tree, knowing that he may not live to sit beneath its shade. "He has left the world a better place because of his short sojourn," the physician said, adding, "and I shall always love him." After the final prayer, the pallbearers wheeled the casket out of the church. The rain had stopped. The procession drove to the cemetery just two blocks away. The family hardly noticed the line of television cameras facing the tent-covered burial site.

The pastor of St. Joe's conducted a brief ceremony. An American Legion member said a brief prayer and presented the folded flag to Margaret. A Legion squad fired a ceremonial salute. A bugler played "Taps."

Friends and relatives stepped up to sprinkle holy water on the casket. Then it was the family's turn. Each pallbearer took off his rose boutonnière and laid it at the end of the coffin. Each of Bill's grandchildren placed a single flower beside them.

The family stepped out from under the tent and blinked in the bright sunlight. Without looking at each other, they all shared a smile. It was as if, having left this world, Bill had already put in his first feisty request to the real Man at the Top, asking if somebody couldn't do something about getting decent weather *at least* for his burial.

The family spent quite a while hugging relatives and hospital workers. After most of the crowd had thinned out, Margaret turned and looked down to see a sandy-haired, freckled little boy holding up a daisy. It was DeVries's nine-year-old son, William. Another young William, and a daisy—for remembrance.

Bill was finally home. Step by step, Margaret and the kids had brought him back to the town he loved. Now the Schroeders really could be a family again. And as they turned to leave the graveside, without even looking, they were already reaching for each other's hands.

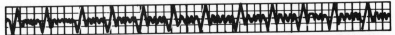

EPILOGUE
March 31, 1987

In Jasper's Fairview Cemetery sits a heart-shaped tombstone with a likeness of a Jarvik-7 etched into its shiny black granite. A few blocks away, construction has begun on Bill Schroeder Field, a complex of baseball diamonds and park facilities.

In recent months, Margaret Schroeder has been traveling around the state as Honorary Campaign Chairwoman for the Indiana Affiliate of the American Heart Association, giving speeches and press interviews at fund raisers for the organization, which hopes to promote healthier living. In addition, Margaret was recently commissioned as a lay minister for her church group at St. Joseph's. She has also learned to drive again.

Moni, her husband Bob, and their two children still live in Sparta, Illinois.

Mel and Patti and their daughters still live on their farm. Mel has spent much of the past year writing extensive recollections for this book, as well as helping his mother with her heart association work, and giving occasional interviews.

Stan and his wife, Terri, have opened a tanning and beauty salon in Jasper. Lukas William is walking and talking up a storm.

Terry and Julie are expecting their first baby in July.

Cheryl and Glenn have bought a house, and plan to marry at St. Joseph's in June.

Rod and Lori became engaged over the Christmas holidays. They will marry in August, after Lori finishes nursing school.

As of March 31, 1987, forty-nine Jarvik hearts have been implanted in dying patients worldwide as temporary bridges-to-transplant.

Epilogue

In January, Dr. DeVries came close to performing his fifth artificial heart implant, even going so far as to have the patient sign the consent form. Shortly before the operation was to take place, however, a human heart donor was found for the patient. DeVries is still seeking another recipient.

Index